Barbara O'Neill Natural Herbal Remedies Complete Collection

1000+ Life-Changing Holistic Remedies, Forgotten Secrets, and Detox Strategies for Self-Healing Beyond Pharmaceutical Dependency

CLARA WHITTAKER

Table of Contents

BOOK 14
HERBAL FIRST AID

BOOK 15
EMOTIONAL AND MENTAL WELL-BEING

BOOK 16
HERBAL SUPPORT FOR FERTILITY AND REPRODUCTIVE HEALTH

BOOK 17
ENHANCING HAIR HEALTH WITH HERBAL CARE

BOOK 18
EYE HEALTH AND VISION SUPPORT

BOOK 19
DETOX STRATEGIES FOR TRUE WELLNESS

BOOK 20 ANTI-INFLAMMATORY HERBAL SOLUTIONS

BOOK 21 HERBAL SUPPORT FOR WEIGHT MANAGEMENT

BOOK 22 STRENGTHENING BONE HEALTH

BOOK 23 HERBAL ALLIES FOR DIABETES SUPPORT

BOOK 24 BOOSTING COGNITIVE FUNCTION NATURALLY

BOOK 25 ORAL HEALTH AND HERBAL DENTISTRY

BOOK 26 ENHANCING IMMUNITY FOR CHRONIC CONDITIONS

BOOK 27 HERBAL SUPPORT FOR LIVER HEALTH

BOOK 28 KIDNEY AND URINARY TRACT HEALTH

BOOK 29 HERBAL REMEDIES FOR ALLERGIES

BOOK 30 INTEGRATING HERBAL WELLNESS INTO DAILY LIFE

CONCLUSION EMBRACING A HEALTHIER, BALANCED FUTURE

INTRODUCTION

A Gateway to Holistic Wellness

UNDERSTANDING THE POWER OF NATURAL HEALING

Understanding the Power of Natural Healing

Natural healing has been practiced for thousands of years, tracing back to ancient civilizations that used plants, minerals, and natural elements to restore balance and health. In today's world, this approach is seeing a resurgence as people seek alternatives to conventional medicine, desiring holistic and preventive strategies that align with their body's natural rhythms. Understanding the power of natural healing begins with appreciating its core principles, the benefits it offers, and its integration into modern wellness.

The Foundations of Natural Healing

At its heart, natural healing emphasizes the body's inherent ability to heal itself when supported with the right tools and environment. It diverges from conventional medicine's often symptom-focused approach, shifting attention toward root causes and long-term wellness. This holistic perspective considers physical, mental, emotional, and even spiritual dimensions, aiming to balance all these aspects for overall health. The following principles are central to understanding this approach:

- **The Body's Innate Intelligence**: Natural healing is based on the belief that the body possesses an inherent intelligence capable of restoring balance when given proper support. Herbs, nutrition, and lifestyle adjustments are viewed as tools to aid the body in its self-healing processes, rather than quick fixes that mask symptoms.
- **Holistic Approach**: This system recognizes the interconnectedness of the body's systems. For example, digestive health impacts immunity, stress levels influence hormonal balance, and mental well-being affects physical vitality. Natural healing practices consider these relationships, aiming to create harmony across all aspects of health.

The Benefits of Embracing Natural Remedies

For many, natural healing provides a more sustainable and preventive form of healthcare. Unlike conventional approaches that may rely heavily on pharmaceuticals with potential side effects, natural remedies often use herbs and holistic practices to address health concerns with minimal risks. Some key benefits include:

- **Minimal Side Effects**: Most herbal remedies are gentle and can be integrated into daily routines without the adverse side effects commonly associated with synthetic drugs. For instance, using chamomile to soothe digestive discomfort or lavender to alleviate anxiety offers safe and effective alternatives.

- **Personal Empowerment:** Engaging with natural healing empowers individuals to take charge of their health. By learning about different herbs, their properties, and their uses, people gain the confidence to manage their well-being proactively, developing a deeper connection with their bodies.
- **Adaptability:** Natural remedies can be personalized based on individual needs. An individual suffering from chronic inflammation, for example, might explore anti-inflammatory herbs like turmeric or ginger and combine them with dietary changes to manage symptoms more effectively. This flexibility allows people to tailor solutions that best fit their lifestyle and specific health challenges.

The Science Behind Natural Healing

Natural healing isn't just rooted in ancient traditions; it is increasingly supported by modern scientific research. Studies have demonstrated the efficacy of many herbs and natural practices, giving credence to methods that have been used for centuries. For example:

- **Anti-Inflammatory Properties of Herbs:** Research has shown that turmeric, containing the active compound curcumin, possesses potent anti-inflammatory and antioxidant properties. This supports its traditional use in managing arthritis and inflammatory conditions.
- **Adaptogens for Stress Management:** Adaptogenic herbs like ashwagandha and holy basil (tulsi) have been studied for their effects on stress and hormonal balance. These herbs help the body adapt to physical and emotional stress, making them ideal for individuals looking to manage modern life's pressures without pharmaceuticals.

Integrating Natural Healing into Modern Life

While the principles of natural healing remain rooted in ancient wisdom, integrating these practices into modern life requires a balanced and informed approach. For someone like Emma, our buyer persona, this means finding ways to blend natural remedies seamlessly into a busy schedule. Modern herbalism has adapted to accommodate these needs, offering convenient forms such as:

- **Tinctures and Capsules:** For those on the go, tinctures and capsules offer an easy way to incorporate herbs like echinacea or milk thistle into daily routines. These concentrated forms provide potent benefits without the need for extensive preparation time.
- **Herbal Teas and Infusions:** Drinking herbal teas, such as lemon balm for relaxation or nettle for mineral support, not only provides therapeutic benefits but also becomes a moment of mindfulness, encouraging a more balanced lifestyle.
- **Dietary Integration:** Superfoods and herbs like spirulina or moringa can be easily added to smoothies or meals, enhancing nutritional intake while supporting overall health. This approach makes herbalism practical, accessible, and easy to integrate into daily life.

In understanding the power of natural healing, it's crucial to see it not just as a collection of remedies but as a lifestyle. It encourages a deeper connection to nature, fosters mindfulness, and empowers individuals to live in harmony with their environment. This holistic approach, combining traditional wisdom with modern science, offers a comprehensive path to wellness that transcends conventional treatments.

BOOK 1

Foundations of Herbal Medicine

The Philosophy of Holistic Healing

EXPLORING THE ESSENCE OF HOLISTIC HEALING

Holistic healing is more than just a practice; it is a philosophy that embraces the body, mind, and spirit as interconnected elements that work together to maintain balance and health. Unlike conventional medical approaches that often isolate symptoms and treat them independently, holistic healing recognizes that true wellness comes from addressing the whole person. This philosophy is rooted in ancient traditions yet remains profoundly relevant today as more individuals seek natural and sustainable ways to manage their health.

Understanding the Interconnectedness of the Body

At the core of holistic healing is the belief that the body's systems are not separate but deeply interconnected. When one area of the body experiences imbalance or dysfunction, it often affects other systems. For example, chronic stress can impact the digestive system, leading to issues like irritable bowel syndrome (IBS) or acid reflux. Similarly, digestive health can influence mood, energy levels, and immunity.

Holistic healing views these interactions as opportunities for comprehensive care. By addressing underlying imbalances, rather than merely treating symptoms, individuals can experience profound and long-lasting improvements in their health. For example, herbalists may recommend adaptogenic herbs like ashwagandha or holy basil to manage stress, supporting not only emotional well-being but also digestion and immunity. This multifaceted approach ensures that the root causes of health issues are addressed rather than just the surface-level symptoms.

Balancing the Physical, Emotional, and Spiritual Aspects

Holistic healing is deeply integrative, recognizing that health is not limited to the physical body alone. It also considers emotional, mental, and spiritual factors as essential components of well-being. Emotional and mental stress, for instance, can manifest as physical ailments, such as headaches, high blood pressure, or fatigue. Therefore, a holistic approach involves nurturing the mind and spirit alongside the body to achieve overall balance.

Incorporating practices such as meditation, mindfulness, and spiritual rituals alongside herbal treatments helps individuals maintain equilibrium in all aspects of their lives. This balance is crucial for holistic healing, as it fosters a harmonious connection between the body and the mind. For example, a person experiencing anxiety might be advised to use calming herbs like lavender or lemon balm, alongside meditation techniques, to calm the nervous system and promote mental clarity. The goal is to create a state of harmony that supports healing from multiple angles, making the results more profound and sustainable.

The Role of Nature in Holistic Healing

Nature is central to the philosophy of holistic healing. Traditional systems, such as Ayurveda and Traditional

Chinese Medicine (TCM), emphasize the healing power of nature and its capacity to restore balance. In these traditions, herbs, plants, and other natural elements are not just tools; they are seen as gifts from the earth, providing essential energy and nutrients that align with the body's own needs.

Herbs like chamomile, peppermint, and ginger are used not only for their physical effects but for their energetic properties as well. Chamomile, for example, is known for its calming effects on both the digestive system and the nervous system, promoting relaxation and digestive health simultaneously. In the holistic philosophy, these plants work synergistically with the body, offering gentle and sustainable support without the harsh side effects often associated with synthetic drugs.

Preventive Care and Empowerment

Holistic healing emphasizes prevention as a key aspect of maintaining health. Rather than waiting for illness to manifest, the philosophy encourages proactive care to support the body's resilience and ability to heal itself. This preventive mindset empowers individuals to take an active role in their health, learning how to use natural remedies and lifestyle practices that enhance their overall well-being.

For someone like Emma Harper, the buyer persona, preventive care is essential. She is a wellness coach who seeks not only to heal herself but to provide her family and clients with effective, natural solutions. The philosophy of holistic healing aligns with her values, emphasizing self-care and empowerment through knowledge. By understanding the properties of different herbs and how they interact with the body, individuals like Emma can feel confident in using these remedies to support their health proactively.

Embracing Individuality in Holistic Healing

Another key component of the philosophy is the recognition that each individual is unique. Holistic healing does not offer one-size-fits-all solutions; instead, it honors the individuality of each person. A treatment plan for one individual might not work for another, even if they present similar symptoms. Therefore, holistic healing requires a personalized approach, taking into consideration an individual's constitution, lifestyle, emotional state, and health history.

This personalized method ensures that the treatment aligns with the person's specific needs, optimizing their path to health. For instance, if two people suffer from insomnia, one might respond well to a valerian root tincture, while another might find relief with passionflower tea, depending on their body's response and tolerance. Holistic practitioners work to identify the most suitable approach for each person, fostering a tailored path to wellness that respects their unique needs and preferences.

In summary, the philosophy of holistic healing is a comprehensive and individualized approach that respects the intricate connections between the body, mind, and spirit. It empowers individuals to take charge of their health through nature's wisdom, preventive care, and a deep understanding of their own bodies, allowing them to achieve balance and long-term well-being.

Traditional vs. Modern Herbal Practices

COMPARING ANCIENT WISDOM AND MODERN HERBAL APPROACHES

Herbal medicine has evolved significantly over centuries, with each culture and era contributing to the wealth of knowledge we have today. The evolution from traditional to modern practices reflects both continuity and adaptation, as ancient wisdom meets contemporary science and technology. Understanding these shifts is essential for anyone interested in herbal medicine, as it reveals how both traditional and modern approaches can complement one another, providing a more comprehensive view of natural health.

Traditional Herbal Practices: Rooted in Cultural Wisdom

Traditional herbal practices are deeply embedded in the history and culture of various civilizations. Ayurveda from India, Traditional Chinese Medicine (TCM), and Native American herbalism are examples of systems that have utilized the healing power of plants for thousands of years. These practices are based on the belief that the body is interconnected with nature and that balance within the body is essential for health.

1. **Holistic View:** Traditional practices often view the body as a whole, emphasizing the interconnectedness of the mind, body, and spirit. For instance, Ayurveda teaches the balance of the three doshas—Vata, Pitta, and Kapha—where herbal remedies are used to restore harmony based on an individual's constitution. Similarly, TCM focuses on balancing the body's energy (Qi) and uses herbs to align and harmonize the body's organs and systems.
2. **Empirical Knowledge:** Traditional herbalists relied on empirical knowledge passed down through generations. Remedies were developed through careful observation and experience rather than clinical trials. For example, the use of echinacea for immune support was practiced by Native Americans long before modern studies validated its effectiveness.
3. **Use of Whole Plants:** Traditional systems often use whole plants, rather than isolated compounds, believing that the synergy of all plant components provides a balanced and comprehensive healing effect. This contrasts with the modern tendency to extract specific compounds for targeted use. The holistic use of plants ensures a more gentle and well-rounded effect, suitable for treating multiple symptoms simultaneously.

Modern Herbal Practices: Integrating Science with Tradition

Modern herbalism has built upon the foundations laid by traditional systems, integrating scientific research to validate and refine practices. This blend of ancient wisdom and contemporary understanding makes herbalism accessible to today's health-conscious individuals, like Emma, our buyer persona, who values scientifically-supported methods alongside traditional approaches.

1. **Scientific Validation:** Modern herbal practices often emphasize clinical research to support the efficacy of herbs. For example, studies on turmeric's anti-inflammatory properties, specifically its

active compound curcumin, provide evidence for its use in managing arthritis and other inflammatory conditions. This scientific backing makes it easier for individuals to trust and adopt herbal practices, knowing they are not only rooted in tradition but also validated by modern research.

2. **Standardization and Precision**: Unlike traditional methods that might vary based on individual herbalists' expertise, modern herbal practices aim for precision and consistency. Standardized extracts, like those of St. John's Wort for depression, allow for controlled dosages, ensuring safety and effectiveness. This approach is particularly important in a contemporary setting where people expect predictable results from their treatments.
3. **Accessibility and Convenience**: Modern herbalism has adapted to fit the fast-paced lifestyle of today's society. Herbal remedies are now available in various forms, such as capsules, tinctures, and teas, making it easy for busy individuals like Emma to incorporate them into their daily routines without extensive preparation. This evolution ensures that herbal medicine remains practical and relevant.

The Synergy of Traditional and Modern Approaches

Both traditional and modern herbal practices have their strengths, and integrating the two can offer a balanced approach to health. Traditional systems provide a holistic understanding of the body and the rich, empirical knowledge of plant-based healing. Meanwhile, modern herbalism contributes precision, safety, and scientific validation, making herbal remedies more accessible and reliable for contemporary users.

1. **Personalized Medicine**: Traditional methods often emphasize personalized treatments tailored to an individual's specific needs and constitution, as seen in Ayurveda's doshas or TCM's Qi imbalances. Modern practices, while standardized, can still integrate this personalized approach by combining traditional diagnostic techniques with modern dosage forms. For instance, a practitioner might recommend a specific herb based on the traditional assessment of an individual's condition but suggest a standardized tincture for convenience and precision.
2. **Safety and Efficacy**: Modern herbal practices have enhanced the safety of herbal remedies by understanding potential interactions and side effects. While traditional herbalists relied on empirical knowledge, today's herbalists can use research to identify contraindications, ensuring safer use of herbs. For example, knowing that St. John's Wort may interact with certain medications is essential information that traditional practices might not have emphasized.
3. **Global Accessibility**: Traditional herbal practices were often localized, with herbal knowledge tied to the native plants of specific regions. Modern herbalism, however, has made it possible for individuals around the world to access a vast array of herbs from different traditions, such as Ayurvedic adaptogens, Chinese tonics, and Western anti-inflammatories. This global exchange of herbal knowledge enriches the practice, offering diverse solutions for a wide range of health concerns.

The integration of traditional wisdom and modern science provides a powerful, well-rounded approach to herbal medicine. Understanding these two perspectives allows individuals to appreciate the depth of traditional practices while benefiting from the precision and convenience that modern herbalism offers.

Essential Remedies for Beginners

Chamomile Calming Tea

INGREDIENTS

- 1 teaspoon dried chamomile flowers
- 1 cup hot water

PREPARATION

1. Steep chamomile flowers in hot water for 5–10 minutes.
2. Strain and drink warm.

Benefits: Chamomile is known for its anti-inflammatory and relaxing properties. It helps soothe the digestive tract and can alleviate stomach cramps and indigestion, while also promoting relaxation and reducing stress.

Peppermint Digestive Aid

INGREDIENTS

- 1 teaspoon dried peppermint leaves
- 1 cup boiling water

PREPARATION

1. Pour boiling water over peppermint leaves.
2. Let it steep for 7–10 minutes.
3. Strain and drink warm or cool.

Benefits: Peppermint aids digestion by relaxing the muscles of the gastrointestinal tract, alleviating gas, bloating, and nausea. It also provides a refreshing and cooling effect, making it ideal for digestive discomfort.

Lavender Sleep Tincture

INGREDIENTS

- 1 tablespoon dried lavender flowers
- 1 cup vodka or other high-proof alcohol

PREPARATION

1. Place lavender flowers in a glass jar and cover with alcohol.
2. Seal the jar and let it sit for 4–6 weeks, shaking occasionally.
3. Strain the mixture into a dark dropper bottle.
4. Use a few drops under the tongue before bedtime.

Benefits: Lavender has calming properties that aid in reducing anxiety and promoting sleep. This tincture helps ease tension and enhances relaxation, making it ideal for those struggling with insomnia or restless sleep.

Ginger Immune-Boosting Infusion

INGREDIENTS

- 1 inch fresh ginger root, sliced
- 1 cup boiling water
- 1 teaspoon honey (optional)

PREPARATION

1. Add ginger slices to boiling water and steep for 10 minutes.
2. Strain the infusion into a cup.
3. Add honey if desired and drink warm.

Benefits: Ginger is known for its anti-inflammatory and immune-boosting properties. It helps fight off infections and soothes the throat, while also promoting circulation and warming the body.

Echinacea Throat Soother

INGREDIENTS

- 1 teaspoon dried echinacea root
- 1 cup boiling water
- 1 teaspoon lemon juice

PREPARATION

1. Add echinacea root to boiling water and steep for 15 minutes.
2. Strain the liquid and add lemon juice.
3. Drink warm to soothe the throat.

Benefits: Echinacea is an immune stimulant that helps reduce the severity of cold symptoms and soothes sore throats. The combination with lemon juice adds vitamin C, enhancing its immune-supporting effects.

Lemon Balm Stress Relief Elixir

INGREDIENTS

- 1 teaspoon dried lemon balm leaves
- 1 cup hot water

PREPARATION

1. Steep lemon balm leaves in hot water for 10 minutes.
2. Strain and drink warm to promote relaxation.

Benefits: Lemon balm has calming and anti-anxiety properties that help relieve stress and promote a sense of calm. It also supports digestive health, making it a versatile herbal remedy.

Garlic Antimicrobial Syrup

INGREDIENTS

- 5 garlic cloves, chopped
- 1 cup honey

PREPARATION

1. Mix chopped garlic with honey in a jar.
2. Let it sit for 2 weeks, stirring occasionally.
3. Strain and store in a dark bottle.
4. Take a teaspoon as needed for immune support.

Benefits: Garlic has potent antimicrobial and immune-boosting properties. This syrup helps fight infections and boosts the body's defenses against common colds and flu.

Dandelion Detox Tea

INGREDIENTS

- 1 teaspoon dried dandelion root
- 1 cup boiling water

PREPARATION

1. Steep dandelion root in boiling water for 10 minutes.
2. Strain and drink warm.

Benefits: Dandelion is a natural detoxifier that supports liver health and promotes the elimination of toxins. It also aids in digestion and helps reduce water retention.

Turmeric Golden Milk

INGREDIENTS

- 1 teaspoon turmeric powder
- 1 cup milk (dairy or plant-based)
- 1/2 teaspoon honey

PREPARATION

1. Heat milk and turmeric in a pot until warm.
2. Stir in honey and mix well.
3. Drink warm before bedtime.

Benefits: Turmeric has anti-inflammatory properties that support joint health and overall wellness. Combined with warm milk, it also promotes relaxation and restful sleep.

Elderberry Cold & Flu Syrup

INGREDIENTS

- 1 cup dried elderberries
- 2 cups water
- 1 cup honey

PREPARATION

1. Simmer elderberries in water for 30 minutes.
2. Strain the liquid and let it cool slightly.
3. Stir in honey and store in a glass bottle.
4. Take a tablespoon daily during cold season.

Benefits: Elderberry is known for its antiviral properties and immune-boosting effects. This syrup helps reduce the duration and severity of colds and flu, providing a natural way to support immune health.

St. John's Wort Mood Lifter

INGREDIENTS

- 1 teaspoon dried St. John's Wort flowers
- 1 cup hot water

PREPARATION

1. Steep St. John's Wort in hot water for 10 minutes.
2. Strain and drink warm.

Benefits: St. John's Wort is commonly used to uplift mood and reduce symptoms of mild depression. It supports emotional balance and helps manage stress effectively.

Calendula Skin Healing Balm

INGREDIENTS

- 1 cup dried calendula petals
- 1 cup olive oil
- 1/4 cup beeswax

PREPARATION

1. Infuse calendula petals in olive oil for 2 weeks.
2. Strain the infused oil and melt with beeswax.
3. Pour into a jar and let it cool.
4. Apply to skin as needed.

Benefits: Calendula has anti-inflammatory and healing properties, making it excellent for soothing skin irritations, minor cuts, and burns. This balm promotes faster skin regeneration and reduces inflammation.

Valerian Root Sleep Aid

INGREDIENTS

- 1 teaspoon dried valerian root
- 1 cup hot water

PREPARATION

1. Steep valerian root in hot water for 15 minutes.
2. Strain and drink before bedtime.

Benefits: Valerian root is a natural sedative that helps promote restful sleep. It calms the nervous system and reduces anxiety, making it an effective remedy for insomnia.

Rosemary Memory Enhancer

INGREDIENTS

- 1 teaspoon dried rosemary leaves
- 1 cup boiling water

PREPARATION

1. Steep rosemary leaves in boiling water for 10 minutes.
2. Strain and drink warm.

Benefits: Rosemary is traditionally used to enhance memory and cognitive function. It improves circulation and has antioxidant properties that protect the brain.

Nettle Mineral-Rich Infusion

INGREDIENTS

- 1 tablespoon dried nettle leaves
- 2 cups boiling water

PREPARATION

1. Steep nettle leaves in boiling water for 15 minutes.
2. Strain and drink warm or cold.

Benefits: Nettle is rich in minerals like iron and calcium, supporting bone health and overall vitality. It also helps alleviate allergies and reduce inflammation.

Holy Basil (Tulsi) Adaptogenic Tea

INGREDIENTS

- 1 teaspoon dried holy basil leaves
- 1 cup boiling water

PREPARATION

1. Steep holy basil leaves in boiling water for 10 minutes.
2. Strain and drink warm.

Benefits: Holy basil is an adaptogen that helps the body manage stress and maintain balance. It supports immune function, reduces anxiety, and enhances overall resilience.

Sage Sore Throat Gargle

INGREDIENTS

- 1 teaspoon dried sage leaves
- 1 cup hot water
- 1/4 teaspoon salt

PREPARATION

1. Steep sage leaves in hot water for 10 minutes.
2. Strain and add salt.
3. Gargle the solution for 30 seconds.

Benefits: Sage has antimicrobial and astringent properties that help soothe sore throats and reduce inflammation. It is an effective natural remedy for throat infections and discomfort.

Marshmallow Root Digestive Soother

INGREDIENTS

- 1 tablespoon dried marshmallow root
- 1 cup cold water

PREPARATION

1. Soak marshmallow root in cold water for 4 hours.
2. Strain and drink the infusion.

Benefits: Marshmallow root creates a mucilage that coats and soothes the digestive tract, reducing irritation and promoting gut health. It is effective for conditions like acid reflux and gastritis.

Aloe Vera Skin Soother Gel

INGREDIENTS

- 1 aloe vera leaf
- 1 tablespoon coconut oil (optional)

PREPARATION

1. Extract the gel from the aloe vera leaf.
2. Mix with coconut oil for added moisturizing effects.
3. Apply directly to irritated skin.

Benefits: Aloe vera gel is known for its cooling and anti-inflammatory properties. It soothes burns, rashes, and skin irritations, promoting faster healing and providing moisture.

Hibiscus Heart Health Tonic

INGREDIENTS

- 1 tablespoon dried hibiscus flowers
- 1 cup boiling water

PREPARATION

1. Steep hibiscus flowers in boiling water for 10 minutes.
2. Strain and drink warm or chilled.

Benefits: Hibiscus has been shown to lower blood pressure and support cardiovascular health. It is rich in antioxidants, which protect the heart and reduce oxidative stress.

Ginseng Energy Booster

INGREDIENTS

- 1 teaspoon dried ginseng root
- 1 cup hot water

PREPARATION

1. Steep ginseng root in hot water for 10 minutes.
2. Strain and drink in the morning.

Benefits: Ginseng is a powerful adaptogen that increases energy levels, supports mental clarity, and enhances physical performance. It helps combat fatigue and improves overall vitality.

Slippery Elm Throat Lozenges

INGREDIENTS

- 1 tablespoon slippery elm powder
- 2 tablespoons honey

PREPARATION

1. Mix slippery elm powder and honey to form a paste.
2. Shape into small lozenges and let them harden.
3. Take one lozenge when needed for throat relief.

Benefits: Slippery elm creates a soothing coating that eases throat irritation and coughing. It's effective for colds, sore throats, and even digestive discomfort.

Thyme Chest Relief Steam

INGREDIENTS

- 1 tablespoon dried thyme leaves
- 2 cups boiling water

PREPARATION

1. Add thyme leaves to boiling water in a bowl.
2. Lean over the bowl, covering your head with a towel, and inhale the steam for 5-10 minutes.

Benefits: Thyme has expectorant and antiseptic properties that help relieve chest congestion and promote easier breathing. It is effective for respiratory issues like colds and bronchitis.

Yarrow Fever-Reducing Tea

INGREDIENTS

- 1 teaspoon dried yarrow leaves
- 1 cup boiling water

PREPARATION

1. Steep yarrow leaves in boiling water for 10 minutes.
2. Strain and drink warm.

Benefits: Yarrow promotes sweating and helps reduce fever naturally. It also supports immune function and can ease symptoms of colds and flu.

Oregano Oil Immune Support Drops

INGREDIENTS

- 1 teaspoon dried oregano leaves
- 1/4 cup olive oil

PREPARATION

1. Infuse oregano leaves in olive oil for 2 weeks.
2. Strain the oil into a dropper bottle.
3. Take a few drops when needed for immune support.

Benefits: Oregano oil has powerful antimicrobial and antiviral properties. It supports the immune system and helps fight infections, particularly respiratory and digestive issues.

Lemon Peel Digestive Bitters

INGREDIENTS

- Peel from 1 lemon
- 1/2 cup vodka

PREPARATION

1. Infuse lemon peel in vodka for 2 weeks.
2. Strain and store in a dark bottle.
3. Take a few drops before meals to stimulate digestion.

Benefits: Lemon peel contains bitter compounds that enhance digestive enzymes, improving digestion and relieving bloating. It also has anti-inflammatory effects that benefit gut health.

Ashwagandha Stress Relief Tonic

INGREDIENTS

- 1 teaspoon ashwagandha powder
- 1 cup warm milk

PREPARATION

1. Mix ashwagandha powder into warm milk until dissolved.
2. Drink before bedtime.

Benefits: Ashwagandha is an adaptogen that supports the body's stress response. It promotes relaxation, reduces anxiety, and enhances sleep quality, making it ideal for overall wellness.

Fennel Seed Digestive Tea

INGREDIENTS

- 1 teaspoon fennel seeds
- 1 cup hot water

PREPARATION

1. Crush fennel seeds and steep in hot water for 10 minutes.
2. Strain and drink warm.

Benefits: Fennel seeds aid in digestion by reducing bloating and gas. They have carminative properties that help relax digestive muscles, promoting better digestion and relief from discomfort.

Burdock Root Detox Infusion

INGREDIENTS

- 1 tablespoon dried burdock root
- 2 cups boiling water

PREPARATION

1. Steep burdock root in boiling water for 15 minutes.
2. Strain and drink warm or cold.

Benefits: Burdock root is a powerful detoxifier that supports liver and kidney function. It helps eliminate toxins from the body and improves skin health.

Comfrey Healing Poultice

INGREDIENTS

- Fresh comfrey leaves
- 1 tablespoon water

PREPARATION

1. Crush comfrey leaves and mix with water to form a paste.
2. Apply to wounds or bruises and cover with a cloth.
3. Leave for 15-20 minutes before removing.

Benefits: Comfrey contains allantoin, which promotes cell regeneration and healing. It is effective for treating bruises, cuts, and other minor skin injuries.

Cinnamon Blood Sugar Balance Drink

INGREDIENTS

- 1 teaspoon ground cinnamon
- 1 cup warm water

PREPARATION

1. Stir cinnamon into warm water until dissolved.
2. Drink in the morning or before meals.

Benefits: Cinnamon helps regulate blood sugar levels by improving insulin sensitivity. It is beneficial for those managing diabetes or metabolic issues.

Horsetail Bone Strength Tea

INGREDIENTS

- 1 teaspoon dried horsetail
- 1 cup boiling water

PREPARATION

1. Steep horsetail in boiling water for 10 minutes.

Strain and drink warm. (#ol#)

Benefits: Horsetail is rich in silica, which supports bone and joint health. It also strengthens nails and hair, providing overall mineral support to the body.

Clove Toothache Relief Oil

INGREDIENTS

- 1 teaspoon clove powder
- 2 tablespoons olive oil

PREPARATION

1. Mix clove powder with olive oil to create a paste.
2. Apply a small amount to the affected tooth.

Benefits: Clove has powerful analgesic and antibacterial properties. It is effective for numbing tooth pain and reducing inflammation.

Licorice Root Respiratory Elixir

INGREDIENTS

- 1 teaspoon dried licorice root
- 1 cup boiling water

PREPARATION

1. Steep licorice root in boiling water for 15 minutes.
2. Strain and drink warm.

Benefits: Licorice root soothes the respiratory tract, alleviating coughs and inflammation. It is effective for respiratory conditions like bronchitis and sore throats.

BOOK 2

Herbal Remedies for Stress and Anxiety

Understanding the Roots of Stress and Anxiety

UNCOVERING THE CAUSES OF STRESS AND ANXIETY

Stress and anxiety are deeply intertwined experiences that affect millions of people worldwide. They manifest when the body perceives a threat—whether physical, emotional, or psychological—and trigger a cascade of responses aimed at survival. While these responses are natural and adaptive, chronic stress or persistent anxiety can negatively impact health. To effectively manage these conditions, it is essential to understand their roots, which often lie in a combination of biological, environmental, and psychological factors.

The Biological Basis of Stress and Anxiety

The body's stress response, also known as the "fight-or-flight" reaction, is an ancient survival mechanism that prepares the body to react to perceived danger. When the brain senses a threat, it activates the hypothalamic-pituitary-adrenal (HPA) axis, which releases stress hormones such as cortisol and adrenaline. These hormones increase heart rate, sharpen focus, and redirect energy to essential bodily functions needed for immediate survival. While this response is beneficial in short bursts, constant activation of the HPA axis can lead to physical and mental health issues.

Persistent stress and anxiety can cause an imbalance in neurotransmitters like serotonin and dopamine, which regulate mood and emotion. For individuals like Emma, who may juggle various responsibilities as a wellness coach and a caregiver, this imbalance can become a chronic state, making it difficult for the body to return to a relaxed state. Moreover, genetic predispositions can make some people more susceptible to these imbalances, increasing the likelihood of anxiety disorders.

Environmental and Lifestyle Triggers

Environmental factors and lifestyle choices play significant roles in the development and persistence of stress and anxiety. Factors such as work pressure, financial concerns, or family responsibilities can overwhelm the mind and body, leading to a state of chronic stress. In modern society, many individuals face constant stimuli from their surroundings—digital devices, social media, and work notifications—all of which can overstimulate the nervous system and prevent relaxation.

Emma, like many professionals and caregivers, might find herself navigating high-pressure situations daily. Her environment may not always provide the opportunity for recovery or downtime, which is essential for maintaining balance. Without moments of rest, the nervous system remains in a heightened state, making it difficult to break the cycle of stress and anxiety.

Lifestyle factors also contribute significantly to stress levels. Poor nutrition, lack of sleep, and insufficient physical activity can exacerbate the body's stress response. Caffeine and sugar, while common go-to stimulants for energy, can also intensify feelings of anxiety when consumed excessively. On the other hand, not getting enough nutrients like magnesium or B vitamins, which are crucial for nervous system health, can leave the body more susceptible to stress.

Psychological Influences and Thought Patterns

Beyond the physical and environmental factors, psychological elements are often at the root of stress and anxiety. Cognitive patterns—such as negative self-talk, perfectionism, and catastrophic thinking—can perpetuate feelings of anxiety, creating a loop where stress becomes self-sustaining. For instance, when individuals interpret daily challenges as threats, the body responds as if in danger, even if the actual risk is minimal.

Emma's situation may involve not only external pressures but also internal expectations. As someone dedicated to helping others achieve wellness, she may place high standards on herself, feeling obligated to meet the expectations of her clients, her family, and herself. This type of perfectionistic thinking can drive stress levels higher, as it creates an environment where anything less than perfection feels like failure. Additionally, unresolved past traumas or negative life experiences can shape an individual's response to stress, making them more prone to anxiety when facing everyday challenges.

The Influence of Social and Relational Factors

Human beings are inherently social, and the quality of one's relationships can either alleviate or exacerbate stress and anxiety. Supportive relationships can buffer the impact of stress, providing emotional support and a sense of belonging. Conversely, conflict, isolation, or unsupportive relationships can amplify anxiety. For people like Emma, who may balance roles as a professional, a partner, and a caregiver, maintaining healthy and supportive relationships is crucial but not always easy. Strained relationships or feelings of isolation can further increase stress, even when the individual is successful in other areas of life.

Social comparison, often intensified by social media, is another significant contributor to stress. Seeing curated images of others' seemingly perfect lives can lead to feelings of inadequacy or self-doubt, intensifying stress and anxiety. For someone involved in wellness coaching, the pressure to appear as an ideal example of health and balance may be particularly high.

The Cumulative Effect of Multiple Stressors

In most cases, stress and anxiety arise not from a single source but from a combination of various factors. Biological predispositions, lifestyle habits, psychological patterns, environmental pressures, and social influences often work together, creating a cumulative effect that overwhelms the individual's ability to cope. When these stressors are ongoing, they can lead to chronic stress and long-term anxiety, affecting physical health, relationships, and overall well-being.

Understanding these interconnected roots is crucial for anyone seeking to manage or support others in managing stress and anxiety. By addressing each layer—biological, psychological, environmental, and social—holistic and effective strategies can be developed. For Emma, this holistic approach means considering all aspects of her life and developing methods to balance and harmonize them, ensuring both her personal well-being and her effectiveness in guiding others.

The Best Herbs for Calming and Relaxation

KEY HERBS FOR SOOTHING THE MIND AND BODY

Herbal remedies have been used for centuries to promote calmness and relaxation, offering natural solutions for stress and anxiety. These herbs work in harmony with the body, gently modulating stress responses and supporting nervous system health without the dependency often associated with pharmaceutical options. Understanding the specific herbs that aid in calming the mind and body allows individuals, like Emma, to incorporate these powerful plants into their routines and enhance overall well-being. Below are some of the most effective herbs for calming and relaxation, each offering unique benefits and applications.

Chamomile: The Gentle Calmer

Chamomile, a staple in herbal medicine, is widely celebrated for its calming and soothing properties. This herb is often used as a tea to help alleviate mild anxiety and promote restful sleep. The active compounds in chamomile, such as apigenin, interact with receptors in the brain, providing a mild sedative effect that encourages relaxation.

Chamomile is particularly beneficial for those who experience digestive discomfort related to stress. By calming the stomach muscles, it not only soothes digestive issues but also alleviates tension in the body, making it a versatile option for managing stress holistically. For Emma, who balances various responsibilities, a nightly cup of chamomile tea can be a simple, effective way to unwind after a busy day, offering both digestive and mental relief.

Lemon Balm: Easing Tension and Lifting Mood

Lemon balm is another gentle but powerful herb known for its ability to reduce stress and uplift mood. Often used in tinctures, teas, or capsules, lemon balm works by calming the nervous system and supporting cognitive function. Its mild sedative properties make it ideal for those experiencing restlessness, nervous tension, or mild anxiety.

The herb's pleasant lemony scent is also known to have aromatherapeutic benefits, enhancing its relaxing effects. Studies suggest that lemon balm can improve mood and cognitive performance, helping individuals stay focused and calm even during stressful situations. For those like Emma, who may encounter daily stressors in both professional and personal settings, lemon balm can be incorporated into morning or afternoon routines to maintain clarity and relaxation throughout the day.

Valerian Root: A Natural Sleep Aid

Valerian root is a well-known herb for promoting deep, restorative sleep. It is often used in cases of insomnia or difficulty relaxing at bedtime, as it acts on the central nervous system to reduce anxiety and facilitate sleep. Valerian's sedative effects are due to compounds like valerenic acid, which increase the levels of gamma-aminobutyric acid (GABA) in the brain, a neurotransmitter that has a calming effect.

Unlike stronger sedatives, valerian root offers a gentle and natural way to support sleep without the grogginess associated with pharmaceuticals. It's particularly effective for those who experience a racing mind or physical tension when trying to rest. Emma, who may struggle with finding time for proper sleep due to her busy schedule, could benefit from a valerian tincture or tea as part of her bedtime routine, ensuring she gets the rest needed to manage her responsibilities effectively.

Ashwagandha: The Adaptogenic Ally

Ashwagandha is an adaptogen, a category of herbs that help the body adapt to stress and restore balance. This herb has been used in Ayurvedic medicine for centuries to promote mental clarity, reduce anxiety, and enhance resilience to stress. Ashwagandha works by regulating cortisol levels, the body's primary stress hormone, helping to stabilize mood and energy levels.

Its adaptogenic properties make it suitable for long-term use, supporting overall well-being rather than just providing temporary relief. For Emma, who seeks sustainable solutions that align with her wellness values, ashwagandha can be an excellent addition to her daily regimen. Whether taken as capsules, powders, or infused in teas, it offers a versatile approach to managing stress while also boosting energy levels.

Passionflower: Tranquility and Mental Clarity

Passionflower is another herb that plays a significant role in calming the mind and body. Traditionally used for its sedative and anxiety-relieving properties, passionflower helps increase GABA levels in the brain, similar to valerian root, thus promoting relaxation. It is especially effective for those dealing with restlessness or nervousness that disrupts concentration and clarity.

This herb is often found in tinctures, teas, and capsules, providing flexibility for different preferences and routines. For someone like Emma, who may need to maintain focus and composure while managing her wellness business and family life, passionflower can be a helpful tool for staying calm and collected during high-pressure situations.

Holy Basil (Tulsi): The Balancer of Stress

Holy basil, also known as tulsi, is another adaptogenic herb revered in Ayurvedic medicine for its profound effects on stress and anxiety. Tulsi helps balance stress hormones, reduces inflammation, and supports immune function, making it a comprehensive herb for overall health. Its adaptogenic nature means that it not only calms the mind but also revitalizes the body, offering both relaxation and energy.

Holy basil tea is a popular preparation, providing a calming ritual that helps the body unwind. For Emma, integrating holy basil into her routine—whether through tea or capsules—can support her in managing daily stressors and maintaining energy levels without feeling overwhelmed.

By understanding and incorporating these herbs, individuals can create personalized, effective strategies for managing stress and enhancing relaxation. Each herb offers a unique set of benefits, allowing for tailored approaches that suit various needs, making herbal medicine both adaptable and empowering.

Remedies for Stress Relief and Mental Clarity

Passionflower Relaxation Tincture

INGREDIENTS

- 1 teaspoon dried passionflower
- 1/4 cup vodka

PREPARATION

1. Add passionflower to a small jar and cover with vodka.
2. Let it sit for 2 weeks, shaking daily.
3. Strain and store in a dark dropper bottle.

Benefits: Passionflower promotes relaxation by reducing anxiety and tension. It helps calm the nervous system and is beneficial for managing stress and insomnia.

Skullcap Nerve Calming Tea

INGREDIENTS

- 1 teaspoon dried skullcap
- 1 cup hot water

PREPARATION

1. Steep skullcap in hot water for 10 minutes.
2. Strain and drink warm.

Benefits: Skullcap has calming properties that soothe the nervous system. It is effective for reducing anxiety, nervous tension, and promoting restful sleep.

Lemon Verbena Stress Relief Infusion

INGREDIENTS

- 1 teaspoon dried lemon verbena leaves
- 1 cup boiling water

PREPARATION

1. Steep lemon verbena in boiling water for 10 minutes.
2. Strain and drink warm or cold.

Benefits: Lemon verbena is known for its calming effects, helping to ease stress and promote a sense of tranquility. It also supports digestive health, further reducing tension.

Kava Kava Tension Relief Elixir

INGREDIENTS

- 1 teaspoon kava kava powder
- 1 cup warm water

PREPARATION

1. Mix kava kava powder with warm water.
2. Stir until fully dissolved and drink immediately.

Benefits: Kava kava helps relax muscles and calm the mind, making it ideal for reducing stress and tension. It supports a state of relaxation without impairing mental clarity.

Blue Vervain Emotional Balance Drops

INGREDIENTS

- 1 teaspoon dried blue vervain
- 1/4 cup vodka

PREPARATION

1. Combine blue vervain and vodka in a jar.
2. Let it infuse for 2 weeks, shaking occasionally.
3. Strain and store in a dropper bottle.

Benefits: Blue vervain is beneficial for managing emotional stress and tension. It helps restore balance, calm nerves, and improve mood.

Chamomile and Lavender Bath Soak

INGREDIENTS

- 1/2 cup dried chamomile flowers
- 1/2 cup dried lavender buds

PREPARATION

1. Mix chamomile and lavender in a muslin bag.
2. Place the bag in a warm bath and soak for 20 minutes.

Benefits: The combination of chamomile and lavender promotes relaxation, relieves muscle tension, and reduces stress, making it perfect for a calming bath experience.

Rhodiola Adaptogenic Tonic

INGREDIENTS

- 1 teaspoon dried rhodiola root
- 1 cup boiling water

PREPARATION

1. Steep rhodiola root in boiling water for 10 minutes.
2. Strain and drink warm.

Benefits: Rhodiola is an adaptogen that helps the body adapt to stress. It improves energy levels, supports mental clarity, and reduces fatigue.

Hops Restful Sleep Tea

INGREDIENTS

- 1 teaspoon dried hops flowers
- 1 cup hot water

PREPARATION

1. Steep hops flowers in hot water for 10 minutes.
2. Strain and drink before bedtime.

Benefits: Hops flowers have sedative properties that promote restful sleep. They help relax the body and mind, making them ideal for managing insomnia and stress.

Magnolia Bark Stress Reduction Capsules

INGREDIENTS

- 1 teaspoon powdered magnolia bark
- Empty capsules

PREPARATION

1. Fill capsules with powdered magnolia bark.
2. Take 1-2 capsules daily as needed.

Benefits: Magnolia bark helps reduce stress and anxiety by lowering cortisol levels. It promotes relaxation and supports overall emotional well-being.

Holy Basil (Tulsi) Mood Stabilizer Tea

INGREDIENTS

- 1 teaspoon dried holy basil leaves
- 1 cup boiling water

PREPARATION

1. Steep holy basil leaves in boiling water for 10 minutes.
2. Strain and drink warm.

Benefits: Holy basil is known for its adaptogenic properties that help balance mood, reduce anxiety, and enhance overall mental clarity.

Catnip Calming Tea Blend

INGREDIENTS

- 1 teaspoon dried catnip leaves
- 1 cup hot water

PREPARATION

1. Steep catnip leaves in hot water for 10 minutes.
2. Strain and drink warm.

Benefits: Catnip is effective for calming the nervous system and reducing anxiety. It helps alleviate stress and promotes a sense of relaxation.

Ashwagandha Mind-Soothing Paste

INGREDIENTS

- 1 teaspoon ashwagandha powder
- 1 tablespoon honey

PREPARATION

1. Mix ashwagandha powder with honey to form a paste.
2. Take before bedtime.

Benefits: Ashwagandha is an adaptogen that reduces stress and anxiety. It promotes mental clarity and supports better sleep.

Linden Flower Anxiety Ease Tea

INGREDIENTS

- 1 teaspoon dried linden flowers
- 1 cup hot water

PREPARATION

1. Steep linden flowers in hot water for 10 minutes.
2. Strain and drink warm.

Benefits: Linden flower tea helps calm the mind and reduce anxiety. It promotes a sense of relaxation and helps ease emotional tension.

Rose Petal Heart-Soothing Syrup

INGREDIENTS

- 1 cup dried rose petals
- 1 cup water
- 1/2 cup honey

PREPARATION

1. Simmer rose petals in water for 15 minutes.
2. Strain and mix the liquid with honey.
3. Store in a bottle and take 1 teaspoon as needed.

Benefits: Rose petals are known for their soothing properties. This syrup helps calm emotions, reduce anxiety, and promote a balanced mood.

California Poppy Tranquility Tincture

INGREDIENTS

- 1 teaspoon dried California poppy
- 1/4 cup vodka

PREPARATION

1. Combine California poppy and vodka in a small jar.
2. Infuse for 2 weeks, shaking occasionally.
3. Strain and store in a dropper bottle.

Benefits: California poppy is effective for promoting relaxation and reducing anxiety. It supports sleep and helps manage stress.

Gotu Kola Cognitive Clarity Elixir

INGREDIENTS

- 1 teaspoon dried gotu kola
- 1 cup hot water

PREPARATION

1. Steep gotu kola in hot water for 10 minutes.
2. Strain and drink warm.

Benefits: Gotu kola enhances cognitive function and mental clarity. It supports focus and reduces stress, making it ideal for mental clarity and concentration.

Eleuthero Energy Balancer Infusion

INGREDIENTS

- 1 teaspoon dried eleuthero root
- 1 cup hot water

PREPARATION

1. Steep eleuthero root in hot water for 15 minutes.
2. Strain and drink warm.

Benefits: Eleuthero is an adaptogen that helps balance energy levels and reduce fatigue. It supports mental clarity and resilience against stress.

Reishi Mushroom Calming Decoction

INGREDIENTS

- 1 teaspoon dried reishi mushroom slices
- 2 cups water

PREPARATION

1. Simmer reishi mushroom slices in water for 30 minutes.
2. Strain and drink warm.

Benefits: Reishi mushrooms support the nervous system and help reduce anxiety. They promote relaxation and balance, making them beneficial for managing stress.

Mimosa Bark Uplifting Tea

INGREDIENTS

- 1 teaspoon dried mimosa bark
- 1 cup hot water

PREPARATION

1. Steep mimosa bark in hot water for 10 minutes.
2. Strain and drink warm.

Benefits: Mimosa bark is known for its uplifting properties, helping to relieve depression and anxiety. It promotes emotional balance and a sense of well-being.

Schisandra Berry Stress Management Drops

INGREDIENTS

- 1 teaspoon dried schisandra berries
- 1/4 cup vodka

PREPARATION

1. Combine schisandra berries and vodka in a jar.
2. Infuse for 2 weeks, shaking daily.
3. Strain and store in a dropper bottle.

Benefits: Schisandra berries are adaptogenic, enhancing the body's resistance to stress and improving energy levels. They help manage stress and boost cognitive function.

Motherwort Emotional Comfort Tea

INGREDIENTS

- 1 teaspoon dried motherwort leaves
- 1 cup boiling water

PREPARATION

1. Steep motherwort leaves in boiling water for 10 minutes.
2. Strain and drink warm.

Benefits: Motherwort is effective for relieving anxiety and emotional stress. It supports the nervous system and promotes a calming effect, making it useful for managing emotional turmoil.

Wild Oat Nervous System Tonic

INGREDIENTS

- 1 teaspoon dried wild oat tops
- 1 cup boiling water

PREPARATION

1. Steep wild oat tops in boiling water for 10 minutes.
2. Strain and drink warm.

Benefits: Wild oats nourish the nervous system, helping to relieve stress and tension. They are beneficial for individuals experiencing exhaustion or burnout.

Lemon Balm and Rosemary Infusion

INGREDIENTS

- 1 teaspoon dried lemon balm leaves
- 1/2 teaspoon dried rosemary
- 1 cup boiling water

PREPARATION

1. Combine lemon balm and rosemary in boiling water.
2. Steep for 10 minutes, then strain and drink warm.

Benefits: This blend enhances mood and reduces anxiety, while rosemary supports mental clarity and focus. It is ideal for those seeking both relaxation and concentration.

Bacopa Brain Clarity Capsules

INGREDIENTS

- 1 teaspoon bacopa powder
- Empty capsules

PREPARATION

1. Fill capsules with bacopa powder.
2. Take 1 capsule daily for cognitive support.

Benefits: Bacopa supports brain function and clarity. It enhances memory, reduces stress, and is particularly effective for improving focus and mental performance.

Valerian and Passionflower Sleep Aid

INGREDIENTS

- 1/2 teaspoon dried valerian root
- 1/2 teaspoon dried passionflower
- 1 cup boiling water

PREPARATION

1. Steep valerian root and passionflower in boiling water for 15 minutes.
2. Strain and drink 30 minutes before bedtime.

Benefits: This combination promotes deep relaxation and restful sleep. It is effective for reducing anxiety and nervous tension, aiding in improved sleep quality.

Borage Nerve-Soothing Tea

INGREDIENTS

- 1 teaspoon dried borage leaves
- 1 cup hot water

PREPARATION

1. Steep borage leaves in hot water for 10 minutes.
2. Strain and drink warm.

Benefits: Borage tea is excellent for calming the nervous system, providing relief from stress and anxiety. It also supports adrenal health, helping the body adapt to stress.

Chrysanthemum Flower Mental Clarity Tea

INGREDIENTS

- 1 teaspoon dried chrysanthemum flowers
- 1 cup boiling water

PREPARATION

1. Steep chrysanthemum flowers in boiling water for 10 minutes.
2. Strain and drink warm.

Benefits: Chrysanthemum flower tea enhances mental clarity and soothes tension headaches. It is also beneficial for reducing eye strain and calming the mind.

Peony Root Anxiety Relief Capsules

INGREDIENTS

- 1 teaspoon peony root powder
- Empty capsules

PREPARATION

1. Fill capsules with peony root powder.
2. Take 1 capsule daily to reduce anxiety.

Benefits: Peony root helps balance emotions and reduce anxiety. It supports overall mental well-being and provides relief from stress-related symptoms.

Yerba Mate Cognitive Energizer

INGREDIENTS

- 1 teaspoon yerba mate leaves
- 1 cup hot water

PREPARATION

1. Steep yerba mate leaves in hot water for 5 minutes.
2. Strain and drink warm.

Benefits: Yerba mate boosts energy levels and enhances mental clarity, making it ideal for those experiencing mental fatigue or stress. It supports concentration and cognitive performance.

Wood Betony Calming Digestive Tonic

INGREDIENTS

- 1 teaspoon dried wood betony leaves
- 1 cup boiling water

PREPARATION

1. Steep wood betony leaves in boiling water for 10 minutes.
2. Strain and drink warm.

Benefits: Wood betony supports both the digestive and nervous systems, helping to relieve tension, indigestion, and stress-related digestive issues.

Cacao and Maca Mood-Boosting Drink

INGREDIENTS

- 1 teaspoon raw cacao powder
- 1 teaspoon maca powder
- 1 cup hot almond milk

PREPARATION

1. Mix cacao and maca powder in hot almond milk.
2. Stir until fully blended and drink warm.

Benefits: This drink is rich in adaptogens and mood-enhancing compounds, helping to boost energy, reduce stress, and enhance mental clarity and focus.

Fennel and Lavender Anti-Anxiety Blend

INGREDIENTS

- 1 teaspoon dried fennel seeds
- 1 teaspoon dried lavender buds
- 1 cup boiling water

PREPARATION

1. Steep fennel seeds and lavender in boiling water for 10 minutes.
2. Strain and drink warm.

Benefits: This blend supports relaxation and reduces anxiety. Fennel aids digestion, while lavender promotes calm and mental clarity, making it a comprehensive anti-anxiety remedy.

Angelica Root Emotional Balance Elixir

INGREDIENTS

- 1 teaspoon dried angelica root
- 1/4 cup vodka

PREPARATION

1. Combine angelica root and vodka in a jar.
2. Infuse for 2 weeks, shaking daily.
3. Strain and store in a dark bottle.

Benefits: Angelica root helps balance emotions and reduce feelings of tension. It supports the nervous system, making it a powerful ally for managing stress and promoting mental clarity.

Violet Leaf Stress Relief Salve

INGREDIENTS

- 1/2 cup dried violet leaves
- 1/2 cup coconut oil

PREPARATION

1. Simmer violet leaves in coconut oil for 30 minutes on low heat.
2. Strain and pour into a jar to cool.
3. Apply to the temples or wrists for relaxation.

Benefits: Violet leaves have soothing properties that help alleviate stress and tension. This salve is perfect for topical application to promote relaxation and emotional balance.

BOOK 3

Immune System Support

How Herbs Boost Immunity Naturally

THE NATURAL POWER OF HERBS IN ENHANCING IMMUNITY

Herbs have long been used in traditional medicine to support and strengthen the immune system. Unlike synthetic medications, which often target specific symptoms, herbs work holistically, enhancing the body's natural defenses and promoting balance. By stimulating immune responses, reducing inflammation, and providing essential nutrients, herbs offer a comprehensive approach to immunity that aligns with the body's innate healing abilities. For individuals like Emma, seeking natural and sustainable solutions, understanding how these herbs work can empower them to incorporate these powerful allies into their wellness routines effectively.

Modulating the Immune Response

One of the ways herbs boost immunity is through immune modulation, a process that helps regulate the immune system's response. Immune modulation is essential because it ensures that the body can effectively respond to pathogens without overreacting, which can lead to inflammation or autoimmune conditions. Adaptogenic herbs like **astragalus** and **reishi mushroom** are particularly effective in this regard. They balance the immune system, enhancing its responsiveness when needed while preventing overactivity.

Astragalus, commonly used in Traditional Chinese Medicine (TCM), helps to stimulate the production of white blood cells, the body's primary defenders against infection. This herb not only supports immune function but also protects cells from damage, making it ideal for building resilience over time. For someone like Emma, who may be exposed to various stressors and environmental challenges, astragalus offers a preventive approach that keeps her immune system adaptable and strong.

Reishi mushroom, another potent adaptogen, also plays a significant role in immune modulation. It enhances the body's ability to fight off viruses and bacteria while reducing inflammation. Reishi's effects extend beyond immunity, as it also supports overall vitality, making it a versatile herb that can be incorporated into daily routines through teas or tinctures.

Providing Antioxidant Support

Herbs are rich sources of antioxidants, which are crucial for neutralizing free radicals that can damage cells and weaken the immune system. By providing antioxidant support, herbs such as **elderberry**, **echinacea**, and **turmeric** help protect the body from oxidative stress, which is often a byproduct of environmental toxins and stressors.

Elderberry is a well-known herb for its antiviral properties and high antioxidant content. The anthocyanins found in elderberries not only give them their deep purple color but also enhance immune function by reducing oxidative stress. Elderberry has been shown to reduce the duration and severity of cold and flu symptoms, making it a practical addition to Emma's wellness toolkit, particularly during cold seasons.

Turmeric, containing the active compound curcumin,

is another powerful herb with immune-boosting properties. Curcumin is known for its anti-inflammatory and antioxidant effects, which help to fortify the immune system. Turmeric can be easily integrated into diets through golden milk or cooking, offering Emma and others a simple and effective way to support immune health daily.

Antimicrobial and Antiviral Properties

Several herbs possess natural antimicrobial and antiviral properties that directly enhance the immune system's ability to fight off infections. **Garlic**, **oregano**, and **thyme** are examples of herbs that not only support immunity but also actively combat pathogens.

Garlic is particularly noteworthy for its antimicrobial capabilities, thanks to its sulfur-containing compounds like allicin. These compounds have been shown to enhance the body's immune response and reduce the severity of common infections, such as colds and flu. For Emma, incorporating garlic into meals not only enhances flavor but also serves as a preventive measure against seasonal illnesses.

Oregano, often used as an essential oil or dried herb, is another potent antimicrobial. It contains carvacrol, a compound effective against bacteria and viruses. Oregano oil can be taken as drops in water or applied topically for its immune-supporting effects, providing Emma with versatile options for both prevention and treatment.

Thyme is another powerful herb that supports respiratory health, making it particularly beneficial during cold and flu season. Its antibacterial and antiviral properties help clear infections, while its anti-inflammatory effects soothe respiratory pathways. A thyme steam inhalation or tea can be a practical way for Emma to keep her immune system strong and her respiratory health in check.

Nutrient-Rich Support for Immune Health

In addition to their active compounds, many herbs provide essential vitamins and minerals that support overall immune health. **Nettle** and **rose hips** are prime examples of nutrient-dense herbs that offer additional benefits for the immune system.

Nettle is rich in vitamins A, C, and K, as well as iron and magnesium, all of which are vital for maintaining a healthy immune response. It also contains flavonoids, which have anti-inflammatory and antioxidant properties. Nettle tea or infusions can be an effective and nourishing way for Emma to boost her immunity naturally while also addressing other health needs like energy levels and inflammation.

Rose hips, the fruit of the wild rose plant, are one of the richest sources of vitamin C available, surpassing even citrus fruits. Vitamin C is essential for the immune system, as it promotes the production of white blood cells and enhances the body's ability to fight off infections. By incorporating rose hip tea or powder into her daily routine, Emma can provide her body with a potent dose of immune-boosting nutrients.

These herbs not only enhance immune function but also provide a holistic approach that supports the body's ability to defend itself naturally.

Seasonal and Preventive Herbal Approaches

COMPREHENSIVE IMMUNE-BOOSTING REMEDIES FOR EVERY LIFE STAGE

A robust immune system is essential for everyone, regardless of age. Whether it's a child developing their immunity, an adult navigating daily stressors, or an elderly individual seeking to maintain vitality, herbs offer versatile solutions tailored to different life stages. Immune-boosting remedies that are safe and effective for all ages not only strengthen the body's defenses but also promote overall health. Understanding these age-appropriate remedies allows individuals, like Emma, to implement them for herself, her clients, and her family with confidence.

Immune Support for Children

Children's immune systems are still developing, making them more susceptible to common illnesses such as colds, flu, and other infections. Herbal remedies for children must be gentle yet effective, providing the support needed to build resilience without overwhelming their bodies. Two particularly child-friendly herbs are **elderberry** and **chamomile**.

Elderberry syrup is a staple remedy for children due to its antiviral properties and high antioxidant content. It's not only effective in reducing the duration of cold and flu symptoms but also has a pleasant taste, making it easy for children to take. Elderberries are rich in vitamins A and C, both of which are essential for immune function. A teaspoon of elderberry syrup daily, especially during cold seasons, can help fortify a child's immune system naturally.

Chamomile tea is another gentle option for children. Known for its calming properties, chamomile also has mild antibacterial and anti-inflammatory effects. It is ideal for children experiencing mild fevers or digestive upsets, which are common when their immune systems are compromised. A mild infusion of chamomile flowers can be given to children as a comforting and supportive remedy that addresses both physical and emotional needs, ensuring they feel calm and cared for during times of illness.

Immune Support for Adults

For adults, immune support must often balance the demands of a busy lifestyle while addressing stress and environmental factors that can compromise immunity. Adaptogenic herbs, such as **astragalus** and **echinacea**, are excellent choices for adults looking to maintain their health and resilience.

Astragalus, an adaptogenic herb used extensively in Traditional Chinese Medicine, helps to enhance the immune system by stimulating white blood cell production. It is also effective in reducing inflammation and protecting against seasonal illnesses. For Emma, who manages multiple responsibilities, incorporating astragalus into her daily routine through tinctures or capsules can provide a preventive boost that keeps her immune system prepared for the challenges of modern life.

Echinacea is another powerful immune booster suitable

for adults. Often used as a tincture or tea, echinacea enhances the immune response by activating key immune cells. It is most effective when used at the onset of symptoms, such as the early stages of a cold, helping to shorten the duration and severity of illness. For adults like Emma, who might face periods of increased exposure to germs, echinacea serves as a reliable ally in their immune toolkit.

Immune Support for the Elderly

As individuals age, their immune systems naturally weaken, making them more vulnerable to infections and illnesses. For the elderly, herbs must be not only effective but also gentle and supportive to avoid any potential strain on the body. **Ginseng** and **reishi mushroom** are excellent herbs for maintaining vitality and boosting immunity in older adults.

Ginseng, particularly American ginseng, is known for its adaptogenic properties that help the body adapt to stressors and support immune function. It also boosts energy levels and overall vitality, making it ideal for elderly individuals looking to enhance their immune response while staying active and energized. For seniors, a ginseng tea or capsule can be a practical addition to their wellness routine, providing sustained support that helps maintain health and resilience.

Reishi mushroom is another superb option for older adults. This adaptogen works to modulate the immune system, ensuring that it functions efficiently without becoming overactive, which is particularly important for individuals at risk of inflammation or autoimmune conditions. Reishi is also known for its anti-inflammatory and antioxidant properties, supporting longevity and overall health. A reishi extract taken as a tincture or tea can provide older adults with the support needed to maintain a balanced and resilient immune system.

Safe Remedies for Pregnant and Breastfeeding Women

For pregnant and breastfeeding women, immune support must be carefully chosen to ensure safety for both mother and child. **Nettle** and **ginger** are two safe and nourishing herbs suitable for this stage of life.

Nettle is a highly nutritious herb rich in vitamins and minerals such as iron, calcium, and magnesium. It helps to boost the immune system while also supporting overall health, making it particularly beneficial for pregnant and breastfeeding women who require additional nutrients. Nettle tea or infusions can be consumed regularly to enhance immunity and provide the body with essential nourishment.

Ginger is another safe option for this demographic, offering immune-boosting and anti-inflammatory effects while being gentle on the system. Ginger tea can help alleviate nausea, a common symptom during pregnancy, while also supporting the immune system. For Emma or her clients who are in these life stages, ginger's dual role in providing relief and boosting immunity makes it a valuable herbal remedy.

Versatility for the Whole Family

Herbs like **turmeric** and **lemon balm** are versatile and can be used safely across different age groups, making them ideal for family-wide immune support.

Turmeric, with its anti-inflammatory and antioxidant properties, is suitable for children, adults, and the elderly alike. It can be added to meals as a spice or consumed as golden milk, offering a warming and immune-boosting effect for all ages.

Lemon balm, known for its antiviral and calming properties, can also be used safely by most family members. It supports the immune system while reducing stress, making it a beneficial herb for Emma's entire family. A lemon balm tea or tincture provides a simple and soothing way to promote relaxation and immunity simultaneously.

By tailoring remedies to the needs of each life stage, individuals and families can create comprehensive, natural strategies for immune support, ensuring resilience and health throughout life's many changes.

Immune-Boosting Remedies for All Ages

Astragalus Root Immune Tonic

INGREDIENTS

- 1 tablespoon dried astragalus root
- 2 cups water

PREPARATION

1. Simmer astragalus root in water for 20 minutes.
2. Strain and drink warm.

Benefits: Astragalus is known for its immune-boosting properties, enhancing the body's defenses and helping to prevent colds and flu. It is particularly beneficial for long-term immune system support.

Elderflower Immune Support Tea

INGREDIENTS

- 1 teaspoon dried elderflowers
- 1 cup boiling water

PREPARATION

1. Steep elderflowers in boiling water for 10 minutes.
2. Strain and drink warm.

Benefits: Elderflower tea is a traditional remedy for enhancing the immune system and reducing symptoms of colds. It has anti-inflammatory and antiviral properties that provide effective support against respiratory infections.

Eucalyptus Cold Relief Steam

INGREDIENTS

- 5 drops eucalyptus essential oil
- 1 bowl of hot water

PREPARATION

1. Add eucalyptus oil to the hot water.
2. Inhale the steam for 10 minutes with a towel over your head.

Benefits: Eucalyptus steam helps to clear nasal passages, reduce congestion, and support respiratory health. It is effective for relieving cold symptoms and boosting immunity.

Olive Leaf Antiviral Extract

INGREDIENTS

- 1 tablespoon dried olive leaves
- 1/4 cup vodka

PREPARATION

1. Combine olive leaves and vodka in a jar.
2. Infuse for 2 weeks, shaking daily.
3. Strain and store in a dropper bottle.

Benefits: Olive leaf extract has potent antiviral properties that enhance immune function and help fight infections, making it a valuable remedy for maintaining overall health.

Andrographis Herbal Defense Capsules

INGREDIENTS

- 1 teaspoon andrographis powder
- Empty capsules

PREPARATION

1. Fill capsules with andrographis powder.
2. Take one capsule daily for immune support.

Benefits: Andrographis is a powerful herb that supports the immune system and reduces inflammation. It is effective for preventing and treating upper respiratory infections.

Maitake Mushroom Immune-Enhancing Decoction

INGREDIENTS

- 1 tablespoon dried maitake mushrooms
- 2 cups water

PREPARATION

1. Simmer maitake mushrooms in water for 30 minutes.
2. Strain and drink warm.

Benefits: Maitake mushrooms enhance immune response by stimulating white blood cells. They are also rich in antioxidants, which help the body fight infections.

Pine Needle Vitamin C Infusion

INGREDIENTS

- 1 tablespoon dried pine needles
- 1 cup hot water

PREPARATION

1. Steep pine needles in hot water for 10 minutes.
2. Strain and drink warm.

Benefits: Pine needles are rich in vitamin C, boosting immunity and aiding in the prevention of colds and flu. This infusion also has antioxidant properties that support overall health.

Goldenseal Antimicrobial Tincture

INGREDIENTS

- 1 tablespoon dried goldenseal root
- 1/4 cup vodka

PREPARATION

1. Combine goldenseal root and vodka in a jar.
2. Infuse for 2 weeks, shaking daily.
3. Strain and store in a dark bottle.

Benefits: Goldenseal tincture supports the immune system with its antibacterial and antimicrobial properties. It is effective for fighting infections and supporting overall immune health.

Hyssop Immune Strength Tea

INGREDIENTS

- 1 teaspoon dried hyssop leaves
- 1 cup boiling water

PREPARATION

1. Steep hyssop leaves in boiling water for 10 minutes.
2. Strain and drink warm.

Benefits: Hyssop tea strengthens the immune system and helps to reduce symptoms of respiratory illnesses. It is also useful for soothing coughs and sore throats.

Black Cumin Seed Oil Elixir

INGREDIENTS

- 1 teaspoon black cumin seed oil
- 1/2 cup warm water

PREPARATION

1. Mix black cumin seed oil in warm water.
2. Drink immediately.

Benefits: Black cumin seed oil has immune-boosting properties and is rich in antioxidants, which help protect the body from infections and inflammation. It is particularly effective for respiratory and digestive health.

Red Clover Detoxifying Tea

INGREDIENTS

- 1 teaspoon dried red clover flowers
- 1 cup hot water

PREPARATION

1. Steep red clover flowers in hot water for 10 minutes.
2. Strain and drink warm.

Benefits: Red clover tea aids in detoxification and supports the immune system. It is beneficial for cleansing the blood and maintaining overall health, making it an excellent tonic for immune support.

Elecampane Respiratory Support Syrup

INGREDIENTS

- 1 tablespoon dried elecampane root
- 1 cup water
- 1/4 cup honey

PREPARATION

1. Simmer elecampane root in water for 15 minutes.
2. Strain and add honey, stirring until dissolved.
3. Store in a jar and take a spoonful as needed.

Benefits: Elecampane syrup supports respiratory health and helps to clear mucus. It is particularly effective for boosting the immune system and fighting respiratory infections.

Angelica Root Immune-Boosting Capsules

INGREDIENTS

- 1 teaspoon angelica root powder
- Empty capsules

PREPARATION

1. Fill capsules with angelica root powder.
2. Take one capsule daily for immune support.

Benefits: Angelica root enhances immune function and helps the body resist infections. It is also known for its anti-inflammatory properties, supporting overall wellness.

Mullein Leaf Lung Support Infusion

INGREDIENTS

- 1 teaspoon dried mullein leaves
- 1 cup hot water

PREPARATION

1. Steep mullein leaves in hot water for 10 minutes.
2. Strain and drink warm.

Benefits: Mullein leaf infusion supports lung health and helps to clear congestion. It is a gentle remedy that is effective for respiratory issues, making it ideal for immune support.

Echinacea and Peppermint Throat Spray

INGREDIENTS

- 1 teaspoon echinacea tincture
- 5 drops peppermint essential oil
- 1/4 cup water

PREPARATION

1. Combine all ingredients in a spray bottle.
2. Shake well before each use.
3. Spray directly onto the throat as needed.

Benefits: This throat spray combines the immune-boosting properties of echinacea with the soothing effects of peppermint, providing relief for sore throats and enhancing overall immune defense.

Reishi and Shiitake Mushroom Immune Blend

INGREDIENTS

- 1 teaspoon dried reishi mushrooms
- 1 teaspoon dried shiitake mushrooms
- 2 cups water

PREPARATION

1. Simmer the mushrooms in water for 30 minutes.
2. Strain and drink warm.

Benefits: This mushroom blend supports the immune system and boosts overall vitality. Reishi and shiitake mushrooms are rich in polysaccharides that enhance immune function, making them effective for long-term wellness.

Bee Propolis Throat Elixir

INGREDIENTS

- 1 teaspoon bee propolis tincture
- 1/4 cup warm water

PREPARATION

1. Mix bee propolis tincture with warm water.
2. Gargle for 30 seconds, then swallow.

Benefits: Bee propolis is a powerful natural antimicrobial and immune booster. This elixir soothes the throat while protecting against infections, supporting respiratory health and overall immunity.

Licorice Root Immune Balancing Tea

INGREDIENTS

- 1 teaspoon dried licorice root
- 1 cup boiling water

PREPARATION

1. Steep licorice root in boiling water for 10 minutes.
2. Strain and drink warm.

Benefits: Licorice root tea helps balance the immune response and reduce inflammation. It is particularly effective in supporting respiratory health and soothing coughs, making it a valuable addition to immune support routines.

Burdock and Dandelion Detox Decoction

INGREDIENTS

- 1 teaspoon dried burdock root
- 1 teaspoon dried dandelion root
- 2 cups water

PREPARATION

1. Simmer burdock and dandelion roots in water for 20 minutes.
2. Strain and drink warm.

Benefits: This decoction supports detoxification and liver health, enhancing the body's ability to maintain a strong immune system. Burdock and dandelion are known for their cleansing properties, which help remove toxins and improve overall vitality.

Japanese Knotweed Immune Capsules

INGREDIENTS

- 1 teaspoon Japanese knotweed powder
- Empty capsules

PREPARATION

1. Fill capsules with Japanese knotweed powder.
2. Take one capsule daily for immune support.

Benefits: Japanese knotweed is rich in resveratrol, a compound that supports immune health and reduces inflammation. It is particularly effective for enhancing resilience against infections and improving overall immune function.

Oregon Grape Root Antimicrobial Drops

INGREDIENTS

- 1 tablespoon Oregon grape root tincture
- 1/4 cup water

PREPARATION

1. Mix Oregon grape root tincture with water.
2. Take a few drops under the tongue twice daily.

Benefits: Oregon grape root has strong antimicrobial properties that boost the immune system and protect against bacterial and viral infections. It is particularly useful for enhancing digestive and respiratory health.

Lemon Myrtle Antioxidant Tea

INGREDIENTS

- 1 teaspoon dried lemon myrtle leaves
- 1 cup boiling water

PREPARATION

1. Steep lemon myrtle leaves in boiling water for 10 minutes.
2. Strain and drink warm.

Benefits: Lemon myrtle is rich in antioxidants and has powerful antimicrobial properties, making it an excellent tea for supporting the immune system and protecting against colds and infections.

Plantain Leaf Wound Healing Poultice

INGREDIENTS

- Fresh plantain leaves
- Mortar and pestle

PREPARATION

1. Crush plantain leaves into a paste using the mortar and pestle.
2. Apply the poultice directly to wounds and cover with a bandage.

Benefits: Plantain leaves are known for their wound-healing and anti-inflammatory properties. This poultice helps speed up the healing process, reduce swelling, and prevent infection.

Horehound Cough Relief Syrup

INGREDIENTS

- 1 tablespoon dried horehound leaves
- 1 cup water
- 1/4 cup honey

PREPARATION

1. Simmer horehound leaves in water for 15 minutes.
2. Strain and add honey, stirring until dissolved.
3. Store in a jar and take a spoonful as needed.

Benefits: Horehound syrup is effective for relieving coughs and supporting respiratory health. It soothes the throat and helps expel mucus, making it a valuable remedy for colds and bronchial infections.

Spilanthes Immune Activation Tincture

INGREDIENTS

- 1 tablespoon spilanthes leaves
- 1/4 cup vodka

PREPARATION

1. Combine spilanthes leaves and vodka in a jar.
2. Infuse for 2 weeks, shaking daily.
3. Strain and store in a dropper bottle.

Benefits: Spilanthes, known as the "toothache plant," has immune-boosting and antimicrobial properties. This tincture supports the immune system and helps prevent infections, particularly in the oral cavity.

Baikal Skullcap Antiviral Tea

INGREDIENTS

- 1 teaspoon dried Baikal skullcap root
- 1 cup hot water

PREPARATION

1. Steep Baikal skullcap root in hot water for 10 minutes.
2. Strain and drink warm.

Benefits: Baikal skullcap is a powerful antiviral herb that supports the immune system and reduces inflammation. It is effective for preventing and managing viral infections, enhancing overall immunity.

Elderberry and Hibiscus Immune Tonic

INGREDIENTS

- 1 teaspoon dried elderberries
- 1 teaspoon dried hibiscus flowers
- 1 cup boiling water

PREPARATION

1. Steep elderberries and hibiscus flowers in boiling water for 15 minutes.
2. Strain and drink warm.

Benefits: This immune tonic combines the antiviral properties of elderberries with the antioxidant benefits of hibiscus, making it a powerful remedy for boosting the immune system and fighting infections.

Yarrow Fever Management Infusion

INGREDIENTS

- 1 teaspoon dried yarrow leaves
- 1 cup hot water

PREPARATION

1. Steep yarrow leaves in hot water for 10 minutes.
2. Strain and drink warm.

Benefits: Yarrow is traditionally used to manage fevers and boost immunity. This infusion helps reduce fever and inflammation, supporting the body's natural defenses during illness.

Alfalfa Immune-Nourishing Capsules

INGREDIENTS

- 1 teaspoon alfalfa powder
- Empty capsules

PREPARATION

1. Fill capsules with alfalfa powder.
2. Take one capsule daily for immune support.

Benefits: Alfalfa is rich in nutrients and antioxidants that nourish the immune system. It helps build resilience and provides long-term immune support.

Ginger and Lemongrass Immunity Tea

INGREDIENTS

- 1 teaspoon fresh grated ginger
- 1 teaspoon dried lemongrass
- 1 cup hot water

PREPARATION

1. Steep ginger and lemongrass in hot water for 10 minutes.
2. Strain and drink warm.

Benefits: This tea combines ginger's anti-inflammatory properties with lemongrass's immune-boosting effects, making it an excellent remedy for strengthening the immune system and protecting against infections.

Pine Bark Extract Antioxidant Boost

INGREDIENTS

- 1 teaspoon pine bark extract powder
- 1 cup water

PREPARATION

1. Mix pine bark extract with water and stir well.
2. Drink once daily.

Benefits: Pine bark extract is rich in antioxidants that support the immune system and protect cells from oxidative stress, enhancing overall immunity and reducing inflammation.

Nettles and Mint Iron-Rich Tea

INGREDIENTS

- 1 teaspoon dried nettle leaves
- 1 teaspoon dried mint leaves
- 1 cup hot water

PREPARATION

1. Steep nettle and mint leaves in hot water for 10 minutes.
2. Strain and drink warm.

Benefits: This tea combines nettles, which are rich in iron and nutrients, with mint to enhance digestion and immune support. It is beneficial for overall health and vitality.

Calendula Flower Antiseptic Wash

INGREDIENTS

- 1 tablespoon dried calendula flowers
- 1 cup boiling water

PREPARATION

1. Steep calendula flowers in boiling water for 15 minutes.
2. Strain and cool. Use as a wash for wounds.

Benefits: Calendula has antiseptic and anti-inflammatory properties, making it an excellent remedy for cleansing wounds and supporting the immune system during the healing process.

Bee Balm Herbal Respiratory Steam

INGREDIENTS

- 1 tablespoon dried bee balm leaves
- 1 bowl of hot water

PREPARATION

1. Add bee balm leaves to the hot water.
2. Inhale the steam for 10 minutes with a towel over your head.

Benefits: Bee balm is a powerful herb for respiratory health. This steam helps clear nasal passages, supports the lungs, and enhances immune function, making it effective for relieving cold symptoms.

BOOK 4

Digestive Health and Detoxification

Herbs for Optimal Digestive Function

NATURAL ALLIES FOR DIGESTIVE WELLNESS

A well-functioning digestive system is the cornerstone of overall health, as it enables the absorption of essential nutrients and the elimination of toxins. Herbs have long been used to support digestive health, offering natural solutions that enhance digestive function, reduce inflammation, and alleviate discomfort. For those like Emma, who seek natural and effective remedies to maintain balance in their digestive systems, incorporating these herbs can provide substantial benefits. Below, we explore some of the most effective herbs that promote optimal digestive function and their specific applications.

Peppermint: A Soothing Digestive Aid

Peppermint is a well-known herb for its soothing properties, particularly beneficial for individuals experiencing digestive discomfort. Its active compound, menthol, has an antispasmodic effect, which helps relax the muscles in the gastrointestinal tract, making it effective for alleviating bloating, gas, and cramping. Peppermint tea is a popular choice for immediate relief from such symptoms, as its cooling and calming effect eases tension and promotes smooth digestion.

For Emma, or anyone managing a busy schedule, peppermint tea offers a simple and quick remedy that can be consumed throughout the day. Additionally, peppermint oil capsules are available as an alternative, providing a convenient solution for on-the-go support. This adaptability makes peppermint a versatile ally for those aiming to maintain digestive balance naturally.

Ginger: Stimulating Digestion and Reducing Inflammation

Ginger is another potent herb for digestive health, widely recognized for its warming properties and ability to stimulate digestion. It enhances digestive enzyme activity, promoting efficient breakdown and absorption of food. Ginger is particularly beneficial for individuals experiencing sluggish digestion, nausea, or inflammation in the gut, as it supports overall digestive function while reducing irritation.

A simple preparation of fresh ginger tea, made by simmering sliced ginger root in hot water, can be an effective way to incorporate this herb into daily routines. Ginger's versatility allows it to be used in both food and beverages, making it an easily adaptable remedy for digestive health. For Emma, who might seek efficient and easy-to-integrate remedies, ginger offers a flavorful and therapeutic option that fits seamlessly into meals and snacks.

Fennel: Relieving Bloating and Gas

Fennel seeds are another traditional remedy for digestive discomfort, particularly effective in reducing bloating and gas. The seeds contain compounds such as anethole, which have antispasmodic and anti-inflammatory effects, relaxing the muscles of the gastrointestinal tract and easing digestive distress. Chewing a small amount of fennel seeds after meals or preparing a fennel tea can help alleviate post-meal bloating and promote digestive comfort.

For those, like Emma, who may frequently dine out or have irregular eating patterns, carrying a small supply of fennel seeds provides a convenient solution for managing digestive issues. Fennel's mild, licorice-like flavor is also appealing, making it a pleasant addition to digestive health routines.

Dandelion: Supporting Liver and Digestive Health

Dandelion is an herb often associated with detoxification, but it also plays a significant role in supporting digestive health, particularly through liver support. The liver is crucial for digestion, as it produces bile necessary for breaking down fats. Dandelion root stimulates bile production, enhancing the body's ability to digest and absorb fats efficiently.

Consuming dandelion root tea before meals can be an effective way to stimulate digestive function and support liver health. This herb not only aids digestion but also acts as a gentle diuretic, promoting the elimination of toxins and excess fluid. For Emma, who may look for holistic solutions that cover multiple health benefits, dandelion offers a dual approach that supports both the digestive and detoxification systems.

Chamomile: Calming Digestive Inflammation

Chamomile is widely known for its calming effects, making it a valuable herb for addressing digestive issues, especially those triggered by stress or inflammation. Its anti-inflammatory and antispasmodic properties help soothe the digestive tract, reducing symptoms such as bloating, cramps, and indigestion. Chamomile tea is a gentle yet effective remedy that can be used regularly to maintain digestive health and promote relaxation.

For individuals like Emma, who may experience stress-related digestive discomfort, chamomile provides both physical and emotional relief, making it an ideal option for holistic digestive care. Drinking chamomile tea before or after meals can help ease tension and create a calming routine that supports overall wellness.

Slippery Elm: Protecting the Digestive Lining

Slippery elm is an excellent herb for individuals who suffer from irritation or inflammation in the digestive tract. The inner bark of slippery elm contains mucilage, a gel-like substance that coats and soothes the lining of the stomach and intestines. This protective layer not only alleviates discomfort but also promotes healing, making it especially beneficial for conditions like acid reflux or gastritis.

Slippery elm powder can be prepared as a tea or mixed into water to create a soothing drink that provides immediate relief for digestive irritation. This gentle approach makes slippery elm a suitable remedy for a wide range of digestive issues, including those experienced by individuals with sensitive stomachs.

Licorice Root: Balancing Stomach Acid and Reducing Inflammation

Licorice root, particularly in its deglycyrrhizinated form (DGL), is another powerful herb for digestive health. DGL licorice is known to balance stomach acid and protect the stomach lining, making it effective for treating heartburn and acid reflux. It also has anti-inflammatory properties that help reduce irritation and promote healing in the digestive tract.

Consuming DGL licorice tablets before meals can provide protection and relief for those experiencing frequent heartburn or discomfort after eating. For Emma, incorporating DGL licorice into her regimen could offer a preventative approach, ensuring that digestive health is maintained without the need for more invasive treatments.

Herbs like peppermint, ginger, fennel, dandelion, chamomile, slippery elm, and licorice root offer a comprehensive and natural approach to digestive wellness. By using these herbs appropriately, individuals can support their digestive systems, alleviate discomfort, and promote overall balance and health.

The Role of Detox in Gut Health

UNDERSTANDING THE IMPACT OF DETOXIFICATION ON GUT HEALTH

Detoxification is an essential process for maintaining a healthy digestive system and overall well-being. The gut plays a crucial role in the body's natural detox processes, as it is responsible for breaking down food, absorbing nutrients, and eliminating waste. However, when toxins accumulate due to poor diet, stress, or environmental exposure, the gut can become sluggish, leading to various health issues such as inflammation, bloating, and fatigue. By supporting the body's detox pathways, particularly those related to the gut, individuals like Emma can promote better digestive function, enhance nutrient absorption, and maintain overall health.

The Connection Between Detoxification and Gut Function

The gut serves as the body's first line of defense against toxins, working alongside the liver to filter and eliminate harmful substances. The liver processes toxins and releases them into bile, which is then transported into the digestive system for excretion. However, when the liver or gut is overwhelmed by toxins or stress, these processes can become less efficient, leading to a build-up of waste in the body. This stagnation affects gut motility, the balance of gut bacteria, and the integrity of the gut lining, making detoxification vital for maintaining gut health.

Detoxification supports gut health by:

- **Stimulating Bile Production**: Bile is crucial for digesting fats and removing toxins from the liver. Herbs like dandelion root and milk thistle are known to enhance bile flow, ensuring that the digestive system efficiently breaks down food and eliminates waste.
- **Balancing Gut Flora**: A healthy balance of gut bacteria is essential for optimal digestion and detoxification. Certain herbs, such as oregano and garlic, have antimicrobial properties that help eliminate harmful bacteria, while others like licorice root and marshmallow support beneficial microbes and gut lining integrity.
- **Reducing Inflammation**: Toxins can trigger inflammation in the gut, leading to conditions like leaky gut syndrome. Anti-inflammatory herbs like turmeric and ginger not only reduce gut inflammation but also promote healing, ensuring that the gut remains an effective barrier against toxins.

Key Herbs for Supporting Gut Detoxification

Several herbs are particularly effective for enhancing the gut's detoxification functions. These herbs not only aid in the elimination of toxins but also promote digestive health, ensuring that the gut remains balanced and functional.

1. Dandelion Root

Dandelion root is a well-known detoxifying herb that supports both liver and gut health. By stimulating bile production, it aids in the breakdown and absorption of fats while ensuring the efficient removal of waste products. Dandelion root also has mild diuretic properties, helping to flush out excess fluids and toxins through the urinary system. For Emma, incorporating dandelion root tea into her routine can provide a gentle and effective way to support her digestive and detox systems, particularly after periods of stress or dietary indulgence.

2. **Milk Thistle**

Milk thistle is another powerful herb that supports liver detoxification, indirectly benefiting the gut. The active compound in milk thistle, silymarin, protects liver cells from damage while enhancing their ability to process and remove toxins. When the liver functions efficiently, the digestive system receives cleaner bile, promoting better digestion and toxin elimination. For individuals seeking to maintain gut health, milk thistle can be taken as a tincture or capsule, offering a convenient way to enhance liver and digestive function simultaneously.

3. **Turmeric**

Turmeric is widely recognized for its anti-inflammatory and antioxidant properties. These attributes make it an excellent herb for gut detoxification, as it helps reduce inflammation caused by toxins or an imbalanced gut microbiome. Turmeric supports liver health and aids in bile production, ensuring that the digestive system remains effective in breaking down and eliminating waste. A turmeric infusion or golden milk can be easily added to a daily routine, offering both digestive and systemic benefits.

4. **Ginger**

Ginger is a warming herb that stimulates digestion and enhances gut motility, making it valuable for detoxification. It helps reduce inflammation in the digestive tract and promotes the breakdown of food, preventing stagnation that can lead to toxin accumulation. Ginger tea is an accessible and effective way to use this herb for gut health, particularly for those like Emma who seek efficient solutions to digestive discomfort and toxin build-up.

Supporting the Gut Microbiome During Detox

A balanced gut microbiome is essential for optimal digestive health and effective detoxification. Beneficial bacteria in the gut aid in breaking down food, producing vitamins, and protecting against harmful pathogens. However, toxins, poor diet, and stress can disrupt this balance, leading to digestive issues and compromised immunity.

Marshmallow Root

Marshmallow root is an herb that soothes the digestive tract and supports the gut lining. Its mucilaginous properties create a protective barrier, which helps prevent leaky gut syndrome, a condition where toxins pass through the gut lining into the bloodstream. By promoting gut integrity, marshmallow root ensures that the gut remains an effective barrier against harmful substances, making it an excellent addition to detox routines.

Licorice Root (DGL)

Deglycyrrhizinated licorice (DGL) is another herb that supports gut health during detoxification. It soothes inflammation in the gut lining and promotes healing, making it particularly useful for individuals with digestive issues related to toxin exposure. DGL can be consumed in tablet form before meals, offering a simple way to protect and heal the gut.

Herbs that support detoxification do more than just cleanse; they help build a resilient, balanced, and functional digestive system. Incorporating these herbs thoughtfully ensures that the body's detox pathways remain open and efficient, promoting long-term gut health and overall well-being.

Remedies for Cleansing and Digestive Balance

Fennel Seed Digestive Tea

INGREDIENTS

- 1 teaspoon fennel seeds
- 1 cup boiling water

PREPARATION

1. Steep fennel seeds in boiling water for 10 minutes.
2. Strain and drink warm.

Benefits: Fennel seeds help relax the digestive muscles, reducing bloating and gas. This tea soothes the digestive system, supports nutrient absorption, and promotes a healthy gut.

Dandelion Root Liver Cleanse Decoction

INGREDIENTS

- 1 teaspoon dried dandelion root
- 2 cups water

PREPARATION

1. Simmer dandelion root in water for 15 minutes.
2. Strain and drink warm.

Benefits: Dandelion root is a powerful liver cleanser that aids digestion and detoxification. It stimulates bile production, enhancing the breakdown of fats and supporting a healthy digestive process.

Milk Thistle Gut Detox Capsules

INGREDIENTS

- 1 teaspoon milk thistle powder
- Empty capsules

PREPARATION

1. Fill capsules with milk thistle powder.
2. Take one capsule daily for gut detox support.

Benefits: Milk thistle is known for its liver-protective properties, which aid in detoxification and promote gut health. It supports liver regeneration and helps cleanse the body of toxins.

Chicory Root Digestive Support Infusion

INGREDIENTS

- 1 teaspoon dried chicory root
- 1 cup boiling water

PREPARATION

1. Steep chicory root in boiling water for 10 minutes.
2. Strain and drink warm.

Benefits: Chicory root is rich in inulin, a prebiotic that supports healthy gut bacteria. This infusion aids digestion, reduces inflammation, and improves overall digestive balance.

Artichoke Leaf Gallbladder Tonic

INGREDIENTS

- 1 teaspoon dried artichoke leaves
- 1 cup hot water

PREPARATION

1. Steep artichoke leaves in hot water for 10 minutes.
2. Strain and drink warm.

Benefits: Artichoke leaf supports bile production and gallbladder function, promoting healthy fat digestion. It also aids in reducing symptoms of indigestion and bloating.

Marshmallow Root Soothing Digestive Syrup

INGREDIENTS

- 1 tablespoon dried marshmallow root
- 1 cup water
- 1/4 cup honey

PREPARATION

1. Simmer marshmallow root in water for 20 minutes.
2. Strain and add honey, stirring until dissolved.
3. Take a spoonful as needed.

Benefits: Marshmallow root soothes the digestive tract, reducing inflammation and irritation. This syrup helps with conditions like gastritis and acid reflux, promoting digestive comfort.

Burdock and Yellow Dock Detox Elixir

INGREDIENTS

- 1 teaspoon dried burdock root
- 1 teaspoon dried yellow dock root
- 2 cups water

PREPARATION

1. Simmer burdock and yellow dock roots in water for 20 minutes.
2. Strain and drink warm.

Benefits: This elixir supports liver detoxification and enhances bowel function, aiding in the elimination of toxins. Burdock and yellow dock also help improve digestion and skin health.

Gentian Root Appetite Stimulant Tea

INGREDIENTS

- 1 teaspoon dried gentian root
- 1 cup boiling water

PREPARATION

1. Steep gentian root in boiling water for 5 minutes.
2. Strain and drink 30 minutes before meals.

Benefits: Gentian root stimulates appetite and digestive enzymes, enhancing nutrient absorption. It is particularly effective for individuals with poor digestion or low appetite.

Celandine Liver Support Drops

INGREDIENTS

- 1 tablespoon celandine tincture
- 1/4 cup water

PREPARATION

1. Mix celandine tincture with water.
2. Take a few drops before meals.

Benefits: Celandine supports liver function and bile flow, aiding in digestion and detoxification. It helps reduce symptoms of indigestion and promotes overall digestive health.

Cardamom and Ginger Digestive Bitters

INGREDIENTS

- 1 teaspoon dried cardamom pods
- 1 teaspoon fresh grated ginger
- 1/2 cup vodka

PREPARATION

1. Combine cardamom, ginger, and vodka in a jar.
2. Let it infuse for 2 weeks, shaking daily.
3. Strain and store in a dropper bottle.

Benefits: This digestive bitters blend stimulates digestive juices, aiding in the breakdown of food and improving gut function. It helps alleviate bloating, gas, and indigestion.

Anise Seed Digestive Ease Drops

INGREDIENTS

- 1 teaspoon anise seeds
- 1 cup boiling water

PREPARATION

1. Steep anise seeds in boiling water for 10 minutes.
2. Strain and take a teaspoon as needed.

Benefits: Anise seed drops are effective for reducing bloating, gas, and indigestion. They relax digestive muscles and promote a comfortable and balanced digestive system.

Barberry Bark Digestive Cleanse Tincture

INGREDIENTS

- 1 tablespoon dried barberry bark
- 1/2 cup vodka

PREPARATION

1. Combine barberry bark and vodka in a jar.
2. Let it infuse for 2 weeks, shaking daily.
3. Strain and store in a dropper bottle.

Benefits: Barberry bark supports liver function and bile production, aiding digestion and detoxification. It is particularly useful for cleansing the digestive system and promoting gut health.

Slippery Elm Gut Repair Infusion

INGREDIENTS

- 1 teaspoon slippery elm powder
- 1 cup warm water

PREPARATION

1. Mix slippery elm powder with warm water and stir well.
2. Let it sit for 5 minutes before drinking.

Benefits: Slippery elm coats the digestive tract, reducing inflammation and promoting healing. It is beneficial for conditions such as leaky gut, gastritis, and ulcers.

Goldenseal and Licorice Root Gut Balance Capsules

INGREDIENTS

- 1/2 teaspoon goldenseal powder
- 1/2 teaspoon licorice root powder
- Empty capsules

PREPARATION

1. Fill capsules with the goldenseal and licorice root powder mixture.
2. Take one capsule daily for gut balance support.

Benefits: This combination of goldenseal and licorice root promotes gut health by reducing inflammation and supporting the immune response in the digestive system. It helps restore balance and reduce symptoms of indigestion.

Cascara Sagrada Colon Cleanse Tea

INGREDIENTS

- 1 teaspoon cascara sagrada bark
- 1 cup hot water

PREPARATION

1. Steep cascara sagrada bark in hot water for 10 minutes.
2. Strain and drink before bedtime.

Benefits: Cascara sagrada is a natural laxative that stimulates bowel movements, supporting colon health and promoting regularity. It helps cleanse the digestive tract effectively.

Black Walnut Parasite Cleanse Tincture

INGREDIENTS

- 1 tablespoon black walnut hulls
- 1/2 cup vodka

PREPARATION

1. Combine black walnut hulls and vodka in a jar.
2. Let it infuse for 2 weeks, shaking daily.
3. Strain and store in a dropper bottle.

Benefits: Black walnut tincture is effective for cleansing the digestive system of parasites. It also supports overall digestive health and promotes a balanced gut environment.

Aloe Vera Digestive Soothing Drink

INGREDIENTS

- 1 tablespoon fresh aloe vera gel
- 1 cup water
- 1 teaspoon honey (optional)

PREPARATION

1. Blend aloe vera gel with water until smooth.
2. Add honey if desired, and stir well.
3. Drink immediately.

Benefits: Aloe vera soothes the digestive tract, reducing inflammation and irritation. It is effective for relieving symptoms of acid reflux, ulcers, and indigestion. Aloe also supports the healing of the gut lining.

Cinnamon and Clove Digestive Fire Tea

INGREDIENTS

- 1 cinnamon stick
- 3 cloves
- 1 cup boiling water

PREPARATION

1. Steep cinnamon stick and cloves in boiling water for 10 minutes.
2. Strain and drink warm.

Benefits: This tea stimulates digestive enzymes and improves circulation within the digestive system. It is particularly helpful for enhancing metabolism and reducing bloating.

Holy Basil Gut-Calming Infusion

INGREDIENTS

- 1 teaspoon dried holy basil leaves
- 1 cup hot water

PREPARATION

1. Steep holy basil leaves in hot water for 10 minutes.
2. Strain and drink warm.

Benefits: Holy basil is an adaptogen that calms the digestive system and reduces stress-related digestive issues. It supports overall gut health and promotes balance.

Meadowsweet Acid Reflux Relief Tea

INGREDIENTS

- 1 teaspoon dried meadowsweet leaves
- 1 cup boiling water

PREPARATION

1. Steep meadowsweet leaves in boiling water for 10 minutes.
2. Strain and drink warm.

Benefits: Meadowsweet helps balance stomach acid levels, providing relief from acid reflux and heartburn. It also reduces inflammation in the digestive tract, promoting comfort.

Lemon Balm Bloating Relief Elixir

INGREDIENTS

- 1 teaspoon dried lemon balm leaves
- 1 cup hot water

PREPARATION

1. Steep lemon balm leaves in hot water for 10 minutes.
2. Strain and drink warm.

Benefits: Lemon balm has carminative properties that relieve bloating and gas. It also supports a calm digestive process, reducing stress-related digestive discomfort.

Peppermint and Dill Carminative Tea

INGREDIENTS

- 1 teaspoon dried peppermint leaves
- 1/2 teaspoon dill seeds
- 1 cup boiling water

PREPARATION

1. Steep peppermint and dill seeds in boiling water for 10 minutes.
2. Strain and drink warm.

Benefits: This tea helps reduce gas and bloating, easing digestive discomfort. The combination of peppermint and dill promotes smooth digestion and prevents spasms.

Triphala Ayurvedic Digestive Cleanse Capsules

INGREDIENTS

- 1 teaspoon triphala powder
- Empty capsules

PREPARATION

1. Fill capsules with triphala powder.
2. Take one capsule before bedtime.

Benefits: Triphala is a traditional Ayurvedic blend that promotes digestion and detoxification. It balances the digestive system and supports bowel regularity and gut health.

Wormwood Gut Health Tonic

INGREDIENTS

- 1 teaspoon dried wormwood
- 1 cup boiling water

PREPARATION

1. Steep wormwood in boiling water for 5 minutes.
2. Strain and drink before meals.

Benefits: Wormwood helps stimulate digestive secretions, improving nutrient absorption and overall digestion. It is also effective for maintaining gut balance and preventing bloating.

Catnip and Chamomile Digestive Relaxer

INGREDIENTS

- 1 teaspoon dried catnip leaves
- 1 teaspoon dried chamomile flowers
- 1 cup hot water

PREPARATION

1. Steep catnip and chamomile in hot water for 10 minutes.
2. Strain and drink warm.

Benefits: This blend calms the digestive tract, reducing spasms and discomfort. It is particularly effective for relieving stress-induced digestive issues and promoting relaxation.

Psyllium Husk Fiber Support Drink

INGREDIENTS

- 1 tablespoon psyllium husk
- 1 cup water

PREPARATION

1. Mix psyllium husk with water, stirring well.
2. Drink immediately before it thickens.

Benefits: Psyllium husk is a rich source of fiber that supports bowel regularity. It helps cleanse the digestive system and promotes overall gut health.

Cranberry Gut Detox Juice

INGREDIENTS

- 1/2 cup fresh cranberries
- 1 cup water
- 1 teaspoon honey (optional)

PREPARATION

1. Blend cranberries and water until smooth.
2. Strain and add honey if desired.
3. Drink fresh.

Benefits: Cranberry juice detoxifies the digestive system and supports urinary health. It is rich in antioxidants, promoting a healthy gut environment.

Coriander Seed Digestive Aid Capsules

INGREDIENTS

- 1 teaspoon ground coriander seeds
- Empty capsules

PREPARATION

1. Fill capsules with ground coriander seeds.
2. Take one capsule before meals.

Benefits: Coriander seeds enhance digestion by reducing bloating and gas. They also have anti-inflammatory properties that support a healthy gut environment.

Angelica Root Digestive Comfort Tincture

INGREDIENTS

- 1 tablespoon dried angelica root
- 1/2 cup vodka

PREPARATION

1. Combine angelica root and vodka in a jar.
2. Let it infuse for 2 weeks, shaking daily.
3. Strain and store in a dropper bottle.

Benefits: Angelica root supports digestion by stimulating stomach acids and enzymes. It helps reduce bloating and discomfort, making it ideal for digestive balance.

Licorice and Peppermint Leaky Gut Tea

INGREDIENTS

- 1 teaspoon dried licorice root
- 1 teaspoon dried peppermint leaves
- 1 cup boiling water

PREPARATION

1. Steep licorice root and peppermint in boiling water for 10 minutes.
2. Strain and drink warm.

Benefits: This tea soothes and repairs the gut lining, making it beneficial for leaky gut syndrome. The combination of licorice and peppermint reduces inflammation and promotes gut healing.

Ginger and Turmeric Anti-Inflammatory Shot

INGREDIENTS

- 1 teaspoon grated ginger
- 1 teaspoon turmeric powder
- 1/2 cup water

PREPARATION

1. Blend ginger, turmeric, and water until smooth.
2. Strain and drink immediately.

Benefits: This shot reduces inflammation in the digestive tract, supports digestion, and boosts immune function. It is effective for relieving digestive discomfort and promoting gut health.

Hibiscus and Rosehip Detox Water

INGREDIENTS

- 1 teaspoon dried hibiscus flowers
- 1 teaspoon dried rosehips
- 1 cup cold water

PREPARATION

1. Steep hibiscus and rosehips in cold water for 1 hour.
2. Strain and drink chilled.

Benefits: Hibiscus and rosehip detox water is rich in antioxidants, helping cleanse the digestive system. It supports liver health and promotes a balanced gut.

Blue Flag Root Gallbladder Support Elixir

INGREDIENTS

- 1 teaspoon dried blue flag root
- 1/2 cup vodka

PREPARATION

1. Combine blue flag root and vodka in a jar.
2. Let it infuse for 2 weeks, shaking daily.

Strain and store in a dropper

3. bottle.

Benefits: Blue flag root stimulates bile production and supports gallbladder function, improving fat digestion and overall digestive health.

Cascara Sagrada Gentle Bowel Stimulant Tea

INGREDIENTS

- 1 teaspoon dried cascara sagrada bark
- 1 cup boiling water

PREPARATION

1. Steep cascara sagrada bark in boiling water for 10 minutes.
2. Strain and drink before bedtime.

Benefits: Cascara sagrada is a natural laxative that gently stimulates the bowels, promoting regularity and supporting colon health. It is beneficial for those with constipation.

BOOK 5

Respiratory Health

Supporting Lung Health Naturally

NATURAL WAYS TO ENHANCE LUNG HEALTH

The lungs play a critical role in overall health by supplying oxygen and removing carbon dioxide from the body. Supporting lung health naturally involves enhancing lung function, protecting against environmental pollutants, and reducing inflammation. For individuals like Emma, who prioritize natural and holistic solutions, incorporating lung-supportive herbs and practices into daily life offers a way to maintain respiratory health and enhance vitality. This approach is especially relevant in today's environment, where pollutants and allergens are increasingly common.

Protecting the Lungs from Environmental Toxins

One of the primary ways to support lung health naturally is by protecting the respiratory system from environmental toxins such as air pollution, cigarette smoke, and allergens. Herbs like **mullein**, **thyme**, and **nettle** provide essential support for cleansing and fortifying the lungs, ensuring they remain resilient in the face of these challenges.

Mullein, a traditional respiratory herb, is known for its ability to soothe and protect the lung tissues. Its anti-inflammatory properties help reduce irritation in the respiratory tract, making it effective for both chronic and acute conditions. Mullein leaf tea is a simple and effective way to incorporate this herb into daily routines, providing a gentle remedy that supports long-term lung health. For Emma, who values practical, everyday solutions, adding mullein tea can serve as a preventive measure against respiratory stress.

Thyme, another powerful herb, offers antibacterial and antiviral properties that help clear the lungs of pathogens and toxins. Thyme's natural compounds, such as thymol, work to open up airways and promote clearer breathing, making it particularly beneficial for those exposed to pollutants or experiencing congestion. Consuming thyme as a tea or using it in steam inhalations can provide immediate and effective relief, ensuring that the lungs remain free from harmful build-up.

Nettle is an anti-inflammatory herb that supports respiratory health by reducing the body's allergic response. Allergens are a common cause of respiratory issues, leading to inflammation and congestion in the lungs. Nettle's antihistamine properties make it an excellent choice for individuals prone to seasonal allergies, offering a natural way to reduce symptoms and protect lung function. For Emma, who may encounter allergens during her work and outdoor activities, nettle tea can be a proactive measure to support her respiratory system.

Enhancing Lung Function and Breathing Capacity

Optimizing lung function is essential for maintaining respiratory health. Herbs that enhance lung capacity, support oxygen uptake, and clear mucus build-up play a vital role in keeping the lungs functioning efficiently. **Licorice root**, **peppermint**, and **ginger** are particularly beneficial in this regard.

Licorice root is an adaptogen that soothes the mucous membranes of the respiratory tract, making it effective for reducing inflammation and improving breathing. It also has antiviral and antibacterial properties that protect the lungs from infections, ensuring they remain resilient. Licorice root tea or tinctures are accessible ways for Emma to incorporate this herb into her routine, particularly during cold or flu seasons when respiratory health is more vulnerable.

Peppermint contains menthol, a compound that opens the airways, making it easier to breathe and improving lung capacity. The cooling effect of menthol also helps reduce irritation in the respiratory system. Peppermint tea or inhaling steam infused with peppermint oil can provide immediate relief from congestion and promote better airflow. For someone like Emma, who might need quick and effective solutions during busy periods, peppermint offers an efficient and accessible remedy.

Ginger is well-known for its anti-inflammatory and antioxidant properties, making it an excellent herb for supporting lung function. It works by reducing inflammation in the respiratory tract and thinning mucus, which helps clear the airways and improves breathing. Ginger tea or fresh ginger added to meals can be a simple yet powerful way to maintain lung health. For Emma, ginger's versatility and ease of use align well with her need for practical, effective solutions.

Reducing Inflammation and Supporting Lung Repair

Inflammation is a common issue in the respiratory system, often caused by exposure to allergens, pollutants, or infections. Supporting the body's natural ability to reduce inflammation and repair lung tissue is key to maintaining long-term lung health. Herbs like **turmeric**, **eucalyptus**, and **marshmallow root** offer targeted benefits for reducing inflammation and supporting the lungs.

Turmeric, with its active compound curcumin, is a powerful anti-inflammatory agent. It not only reduces inflammation in the lungs but also acts as an antioxidant, protecting lung tissue from damage. Consuming turmeric in the form of golden milk or adding it to meals provides an accessible way to support lung health daily. For Emma, who seeks to integrate wellness into her lifestyle effortlessly, turmeric offers a versatile and beneficial option.

Eucalyptus is another potent herb for lung support, particularly effective in clearing mucus and reducing inflammation. Eucalyptus oil, used in steam inhalations, helps open the airways and allows for deeper breathing. Its antimicrobial properties also protect against respiratory infections, making it a valuable ally for lung health. For Emma, using eucalyptus during cold and allergy seasons can help maintain respiratory clarity and prevent congestion.

Marshmallow root supports lung repair by coating and soothing the mucous membranes. Its mucilaginous properties create a protective barrier in the respiratory tract, reducing irritation and promoting healing. Marshmallow root tea is a gentle and effective way to incorporate this herb into a daily routine, providing consistent support for respiratory health. This aligns with Emma's preference for simple, nurturing remedies that can be easily integrated into her day.

By using these herbs, individuals can naturally enhance lung function, protect against environmental toxins, and reduce inflammation, ensuring that their respiratory systems remain strong and resilient.

Herbs for Common Respiratory Conditions

EFFECTIVE HERBS FOR TREATING RESPIRATORY AILMENTS

Herbs have been used for centuries to treat various respiratory conditions, offering natural, effective alternatives to conventional medicines. From clearing congestion to soothing inflammation, these herbs work in synergy with the body to promote respiratory health. For individuals like Emma, who prefer holistic and sustainable solutions, understanding these herbs and their applications can provide practical ways to manage common respiratory issues such as colds, asthma, and bronchitis. Below, we explore some of the most effective herbs for supporting respiratory health, each targeting specific conditions.

Mullein: Clearing Congestion and Soothing the Airways

Mullein is a powerful herb traditionally used to treat respiratory congestion and inflammation. Its demulcent and expectorant properties make it highly effective for clearing mucus from the lungs, providing relief for conditions like bronchitis and chronic coughs. The herb's leaves and flowers contain saponins that help break down mucus, while its mucilage component coats and soothes the respiratory tract.

For Emma, who may seek simple and effective solutions, mullein tea is a practical option. It not only provides immediate relief by reducing inflammation but also aids in loosening phlegm, making it easier to expel. Additionally, mullein can be used in steam inhalations to further open up the airways, offering a versatile approach to respiratory care that fits seamlessly into daily routines.

Licorice Root: Aiding in Asthma and Inflammatory Conditions

Licorice root is a well-known herb for its anti-inflammatory and soothing properties, making it ideal for treating asthma and other inflammatory respiratory conditions. The glycyrrhizin found in licorice root helps reduce inflammation in the airways, promoting easier breathing and lessening the severity of asthma symptoms. It also acts as an expectorant, clearing mucus and reducing congestion.

Licorice root tea or tinctures can be incorporated into daily regimens to provide consistent support for those managing chronic respiratory conditions. For individuals like Emma, who may experience periods of heightened respiratory stress or exposure to allergens, using licorice root offers a preventive approach, ensuring the respiratory system remains resilient and functional.

Eucalyptus: Combatting Colds and Opening Airways

Eucalyptus is a potent herb widely used to treat respiratory infections like colds and sinusitis. Its essential oil, rich in eucalyptol, is known for its antibacterial, antiviral, and anti-inflammatory properties. Eucalyptus helps clear nasal and chest congestion, making it easier to breathe, while also reducing inflammation in the airways.

Inhaling steam infused with eucalyptus oil is a quick and effective remedy for clearing blocked sinuses and relieving coughs. Eucalyptus can also be used as an ingredient in chest rubs, providing relief for colds and other respiratory issues. For Emma, who values fast-acting and efficient remedies, eucalyptus serves as a practical addition to her respiratory care toolkit, particularly during cold seasons or times of increased exposure to respiratory pathogens.

Thyme: Supporting Bronchial Health

Thyme is another herb recognized for its ability to support respiratory health, particularly in cases of bronchitis and chronic coughs. It contains thymol, a powerful compound with antibacterial and antifungal properties that helps protect the respiratory system from infections. Thyme also acts as a bronchodilator, relaxing the bronchial tubes and promoting easier breathing, making it effective for individuals dealing with asthma or bronchitis.

Thyme tea or tincture can be taken regularly to maintain respiratory health and reduce symptoms of chronic conditions. Additionally, thyme steam inhalations can help clear mucus and open airways, offering an accessible method for respiratory relief. For Emma, who might manage respiratory issues in herself or her clients, thyme provides a versatile and effective option that fits into various forms, whether as tea, tincture, or inhalation.

Peppermint: Relieving Sinus Congestion and Coughs

Peppermint is commonly used to alleviate sinus congestion and soothe coughs, thanks to its high menthol content. Menthol acts as a natural decongestant, opening up the airways and easing breathing. It also has anti-inflammatory and antimicrobial properties that support respiratory health, making it a useful herb for managing colds and sinus issues.

Peppermint tea, steam inhalations, or using peppermint oil in a diffuser are all effective ways to utilize this herb. For Emma, who may need quick relief during busy or stressful periods, peppermint offers a convenient and potent remedy. Its versatility ensures that it can be used in different forms, making it easy to integrate into her lifestyle.

Marshmallow Root: Protecting and Healing the Respiratory Tract

Marshmallow root is another effective herb for respiratory health, particularly for conditions involving irritation or inflammation of the respiratory tract. Its mucilage content creates a protective layer over the mucous membranes, reducing inflammation and soothing the airways. This makes it an ideal herb for treating dry coughs, asthma, and sore throats.

Marshmallow root tea or syrup provides a gentle yet effective way to incorporate this herb into respiratory care routines. For Emma, who may value remedies that are gentle enough for various ages and conditions, marshmallow root offers a nurturing option that is both effective and safe for long-term use.

By using these herbs, individuals can manage and treat common respiratory conditions naturally, ensuring their respiratory systems remain robust and adaptable in various environmental conditions.

Remedies for Breathing and Respiratory Support

Coltsfoot Lung Support Tea

INGREDIENTS

- 1 teaspoon dried coltsfoot leaves
- 1 cup boiling water

PREPARATION

1. Steep coltsfoot leaves in boiling water for 10 minutes.
2. Strain and drink warm.

Benefits: Coltsfoot helps soothe the respiratory system, reducing inflammation and irritation in the lungs. It is beneficial for easing coughs and promoting lung health.

Lobelia Respiratory Relaxant Tincture

INGREDIENTS

- 1 tablespoon dried lobelia leaves
- 1/2 cup vodka

PREPARATION

1. Combine lobelia leaves and vodka in a jar.
2. Let it infuse for 2 weeks, shaking daily.
3. Strain and store in a dropper bottle.

Benefits: Lobelia acts as a natural bronchodilator, easing respiratory tension and aiding in breathing. It is particularly helpful for asthma relief and supporting lung function.

Mullein and Thyme Chest Rub

INGREDIENTS

- 1 tablespoon dried mullein leaves
- 1 teaspoon dried thyme
- 1/2 cup olive oil

PREPARATION

1. Heat olive oil and add mullein and thyme.
2. Simmer on low heat for 20 minutes.
3. Strain and store in a jar for chest rub application.

Benefits: This chest rub helps to clear the lungs and relieve congestion. Mullein and thyme work together to soothe the respiratory system and ease breathing difficulties.

Wild Cherry Bark Cough Syrup

INGREDIENTS

- 1 tablespoon dried wild cherry bark
- 1 cup water
- 1 tablespoon honey

PREPARATION

1. Simmer wild cherry bark in water for 15 minutes.
2. Strain and add honey.
3. Store in a bottle and take as needed for cough relief.

Benefits: Wild cherry bark has antitussive properties that help to calm coughs. This syrup soothes the throat and reduces irritation in the respiratory system.

Pleurisy Root Lung Tonic

INGREDIENTS

- 1 teaspoon dried pleurisy root
- 1 cup boiling water

PREPARATION

1. Steep pleurisy root in boiling water for 10 minutes.
2. Strain and drink warm.

Benefits: Pleurisy root is known for its expectorant properties, making it effective in clearing mucus from the lungs. It also supports lung function and reduces inflammation.

Horehound Cough Relief Tea

INGREDIENTS

- 1 teaspoon dried horehound leaves
- 1 cup boiling water

PREPARATION

1. Steep horehound leaves in boiling water for 10 minutes.
2. Strain and drink warm.

Benefits: Horehound helps to clear phlegm and ease coughing. It supports respiratory health by soothing irritation in the throat and lungs.

Lungwort Respiratory Strength Infusion

INGREDIENTS

- 1 teaspoon dried lungwort leaves
- 1 cup boiling water

PREPARATION

1. Steep lungwort leaves in boiling water for 10 minutes.
2. Strain and drink warm.

Benefits: Lungwort strengthens lung function and aids in respiratory issues, promoting clear breathing. It is beneficial for managing chronic lung conditions.

Elecampane Expectorant Syrup

INGREDIENTS

- 1 tablespoon dried elecampane root
- 1 cup water
- 1 tablespoon honey

PREPARATION

1. Simmer elecampane root in water for 15 minutes.
2. Strain and add honey.
3. Store in a bottle for use.

Benefits: Elecampane is an expectorant that helps clear mucus from the lungs. This syrup relieves congestion and supports respiratory health.

Pine Needle Respiratory Support Steam

INGREDIENTS

- 1 handful fresh pine needles
- 1 bowl boiling water

PREPARATION

1. Place pine needles in a bowl of boiling water.
2. Inhale the steam for 10 minutes.

Benefits: Pine needle steam opens airways, supports lung function, and clears respiratory passages. It is effective for colds and respiratory discomfort.

Osha Root Bronchial Aid Capsules

INGREDIENTS

- 1 teaspoon ground osha root
- Empty capsules

PREPARATION

1. Fill capsules with ground osha root.
2. Take one capsule daily for respiratory support.

Benefits: Osha root has bronchodilator properties that support lung function and ease breathing difficulties. It is particularly useful for bronchial support.

Eucalyptus and Peppermint Chest Balm

INGREDIENTS

- 1 tablespoon eucalyptus oil
- 1 tablespoon peppermint oil
- 1/2 cup coconut oil

PREPARATION

1. Melt coconut oil and mix in eucalyptus and peppermint oils.
2. Let the mixture cool and solidify.
3. Apply to the chest for respiratory relief.

Benefits: This balm opens airways and provides relief from congestion. Eucalyptus and peppermint work synergistically to promote clear breathing and ease respiratory discomfort.

Fenugreek and Honey Respiratory Soothing Syrup

INGREDIENTS

- 1 tablespoon fenugreek seeds
- 1 cup water
- 1 tablespoon honey

PREPARATION

1. Simmer fenugreek seeds in water for 15 minutes.
2. Strain and add honey.
3. Store in a bottle and use as needed for respiratory relief.

Benefits: Fenugreek soothes the respiratory system, reducing inflammation and irritation. This syrup is beneficial for easing coughs and promoting lung health.

Anise Seed Respiratory Relief Drops

INGREDIENTS

- 1 teaspoon anise seeds
- 1 cup boiling water

PREPARATION

1. Steep anise seeds in boiling water for 10 minutes.
2. Strain and use as drops when needed for respiratory relief.

Benefits: Anise seeds provide relief from respiratory discomfort by reducing inflammation and promoting clear airways. It is particularly effective for easing breathing issues.

Angelica Root Bronchial Dilator Tincture

INGREDIENTS

- 1 tablespoon dried angelica root
- 1/2 cup vodka

PREPARATION

1. Combine angelica root and vodka in a jar.
2. Let it infuse for 2 weeks, shaking daily.
3. Strain and store in a dropper bottle.

Benefits: Angelica root acts as a bronchodilator, opening airways and easing breathing difficulties. It supports lung health and is effective for managing asthma symptoms.

Grindelia Asthma Relief Tea

INGREDIENTS

- 1 teaspoon dried grindelia leaves
- 1 cup boiling water

PREPARATION

1. Steep grindelia leaves in boiling water for 10 minutes.
2. Strain and drink warm.

Benefits: Grindelia helps open the airways and reduce respiratory spasms. This tea is beneficial for asthma relief and general respiratory support.

Sweet Violet Respiratory Soothing Infusion

INGREDIENTS

- 1 teaspoon dried sweet violet leaves
- 1 cup boiling water

PREPARATION

1. Steep sweet violet leaves in boiling water for 10 minutes.
2. Strain and drink warm.

Benefits: Sweet violet is known for its soothing effects on the respiratory system. It helps reduce irritation and inflammation in the lungs, promoting easier breathing and relief from congestion.

Hyssop Lung Clear Tea

INGREDIENTS

- 1 teaspoon dried hyssop leaves
- 1 cup boiling water

PREPARATION

1. Steep hyssop leaves in boiling water for 10 minutes.
2. Strain and drink warm.

Benefits: Hyssop has expectorant properties that help to clear mucus from the lungs, making it effective for respiratory congestion and lung health support.

Licorice and Ginger Cough Lozenge

INGREDIENTS

- 1 teaspoon powdered licorice root
- 1 teaspoon powdered ginger
- 1/2 cup honey

PREPARATION

1. Mix licorice and ginger powder into honey.
2. Simmer the mixture on low heat until it thickens.
3. Drop small amounts onto parchment paper to form lozenges.
4. Let them cool and harden.

Benefits: Licorice and ginger soothe the throat and reduce inflammation, making these lozenges effective for cough relief and respiratory support.

Yarrow Respiratory Steam

INGREDIENTS

- 1 tablespoon dried yarrow leaves
- 1 bowl boiling water

PREPARATION

1. Place yarrow leaves in the bowl of boiling water.
2. Inhale the steam for 10 minutes to clear the respiratory passages.

Benefits: Yarrow steam opens airways and reduces respiratory congestion. It is effective for easing breathing difficulties and supporting lung health.

Balm of Gilead Respiratory Balm

INGREDIENTS

- 1 tablespoon balm of Gilead buds
- 1/2 cup olive oil
- 1 tablespoon beeswax

PREPARATION

1. Simmer balm of Gilead buds in olive oil for 20 minutes.
2. Strain and add beeswax to the warm oil.
3. Pour into a jar and let it solidify.

Benefits: Balm of Gilead provides relief for respiratory discomfort, soothing inflammation and easing congestion. It is beneficial when applied to the chest for respiratory support.

Sage and Thyme Respiratory Tonic

INGREDIENTS

- 1 teaspoon dried sage
- 1 teaspoon dried thyme
- 1 cup boiling water

PREPARATION

1. Steep sage and thyme in boiling water for 10 minutes.
2. Strain and drink warm.

Benefits: Sage and thyme work together to open airways, reduce inflammation, and support overall lung health, making this tonic effective for respiratory conditions.

Evening Primrose Bronchial Relief Capsules

INGREDIENTS

- 1 teaspoon ground evening primrose root
- Empty capsules

PREPARATION

1. Fill capsules with ground evening primrose root.
2. Take one capsule daily to support bronchial health.

Benefits: Evening primrose helps reduce inflammation in the bronchial tubes, easing breathing difficulties and supporting lung health, especially for asthma sufferers.

Marshmallow Root Lung Soothing Syrup

INGREDIENTS

- 1 tablespoon dried marshmallow root
- 1 cup water
- 1 tablespoon honey

PREPARATION

1. Simmer marshmallow root in water for 15 minutes.
2. Strain and add honey.
3. Store in a bottle for use when needed.

Benefits: Marshmallow root soothes and coats the respiratory system, reducing inflammation and irritation, making it effective for cough relief and lung support.

Elderberry and Mullein Respiratory Tonic

INGREDIENTS

- 1 tablespoon dried elderberries
- 1 teaspoon dried mullein leaves
- 1 cup boiling water

PREPARATION

1. Steep elderberries and mullein leaves in boiling water for 10 minutes.
2. Strain and drink warm.

Benefits: This tonic combines elderberry's immune-boosting properties with mullein's lung-soothing effects, providing comprehensive support for respiratory health.

Plantain Leaf Mucus-Clearing Tea

INGREDIENTS

- 1 teaspoon dried plantain leaves
- 1 cup boiling water

PREPARATION

1. Steep plantain leaves in boiling water for 10 minutes.
2. Strain and drink warm.

Benefits: Plantain is effective in reducing mucus build-up and soothing respiratory passages, promoting easier breathing and lung health.

Horehound and Licorice Expectorant Elixir

INGREDIENTS

- 1 teaspoon dried horehound leaves
- 1 teaspoon licorice root
- 1 cup water

PREPARATION

1. Simmer horehound and licorice root in water for 15 minutes.
2. Strain and store the elixir in a bottle for use.

Benefits: Horehound and licorice work together to clear mucus and ease coughing, making this elixir effective for respiratory congestion relief.

Red Clover Respiratory Detox Tea

INGREDIENTS

- 1 teaspoon dried red clover flowers
- 1 cup boiling water

PREPARATION

1. Steep red clover flowers in boiling water for 10 minutes.
2. Strain and drink warm.

Benefits: Red clover helps detoxify the respiratory system, clearing toxins and supporting lung function, which is particularly beneficial for those with respiratory conditions.

Peppermint and Lemon Respiratory Relief Drops

INGREDIENTS

- 1 teaspoon dried peppermint leaves
- 1 lemon slice
- 1 cup boiling water

PREPARATION

1. Steep peppermint leaves and lemon in boiling water for 10 minutes.
2. Strain and store in a dropper bottle for use.

Benefits: Peppermint and lemon provide relief from respiratory discomfort, helping to open airways and soothe the lungs. It is effective for sinus relief as well.

Nettle and Thyme Respiratory Strength Infusion

INGREDIENTS

- 1 teaspoon dried nettle leaves
- 1 teaspoon dried thyme
- 1 cup boiling water

PREPARATION

1. Steep nettle and thyme in boiling water for 10 minutes.
2. Strain and drink warm.

Benefits: Nettle and thyme provide antioxidant and anti-inflammatory benefits, strengthening the respiratory system and supporting lung health.

Catnip and Fenugreek Chest Rub

INGREDIENTS

- 1 tablespoon dried catnip leaves
- 1 teaspoon fenugreek seeds
- 1/2 cup coconut oil

PREPARATION

1. Heat coconut oil and add catnip and fenugreek seeds.
2. Simmer on low for 15 minutes.
3. Strain and store for use as a chest rub.

Benefits: This chest rub soothes respiratory passages and reduces congestion, making it effective for cough relief and lung support.

Comfrey and Elecampane Bronchial Syrup

INGREDIENTS

- 1 tablespoon dried comfrey leaves
- 1 teaspoon dried elecampane root
- 1 cup water
- 1 tablespoon honey

PREPARATION

1. Simmer comfrey and elecampane in water for 20 minutes.
2. Strain and add honey.
3. Store in a bottle for use.

Benefits: This syrup helps to clear bronchial congestion and supports respiratory health, easing symptoms associated with respiratory distress.

Cinnamon and Clove Respiratory Comfort Tea

INGREDIENTS

- 1 teaspoon cinnamon bark
- 2 whole cloves
- 1 cup boiling water

PREPARATION

1. Steep cinnamon and cloves in boiling water for 10 minutes.
2. Strain and drink warm.

Benefits: Cinnamon and clove work to open airways and reduce inflammation, providing relief for respiratory discomfort and promoting easier breathing.

Goldenrod Lung Support Capsules

INGREDIENTS

- 1 teaspoon dried goldenrod flowers
- Empty capsules

PREPARATION

1. Fill capsules with dried goldenrod powder.
2. Take one capsule daily for lung support.

Benefits: Goldenrod strengthens lung health and provides anti-inflammatory support, promoting clearer breathing and respiratory resilience.

Wild Lettuce Respiratory Aid Tincture

INGREDIENTS

- 1 tablespoon dried wild lettuce leaves
- 1/2 cup vodka

PREPARATION

1. Combine wild lettuce leaves and vodka in a jar.
2. Let it infuse for 2 weeks, shaking daily.
3. Strain and store in a dropper bottle.

Benefits: Wild lettuce supports respiratory health and acts as a natural expectorant, helping to clear airways and ease breathing difficulties.

BOOK 6

Women's Health and Hormonal Balance

Herbal Remedies for Menstrual Health

NATURAL HERBAL SUPPORT FOR MENSTRUAL HEALTH

Managing menstrual health with herbal remedies offers a gentle and effective approach to balance the body and alleviate discomfort associated with menstruation. Herbs have been used for centuries to regulate cycles, reduce cramping, and address hormonal imbalances. For women like Emma, who may seek natural and holistic solutions for their health, understanding these remedies provides a toolkit for better menstrual health, improving overall well-being and daily comfort. By integrating specific herbs into her lifestyle, Emma can find balance and relief naturally.

Regulating the Menstrual Cycle

Irregular periods or disruptions in the menstrual cycle can be challenging, affecting not only physical health but emotional well-being. Several herbs, including **chasteberry** and **black cohosh**, have proven effective in regulating cycles and balancing hormones.

Chasteberry, also known as vitex, is a powerful herb used to balance hormones and regulate menstrual cycles. It works by influencing the pituitary gland, which controls the production of reproductive hormones such as estrogen and progesterone. Chasteberry is particularly helpful for women experiencing irregular periods, PMS, or symptoms of polycystic ovary syndrome (PCOS). For Emma, taking chasteberry in the form of capsules or tinctures can support hormone regulation and improve cycle regularity, providing a natural method for achieving menstrual balance.

Black cohosh is another effective herb that supports menstrual health, especially in cases of hormonal imbalances that cause irregular or painful cycles. It has phytoestrogenic properties, meaning it can mimic the effects of estrogen in the body, helping to regulate cycles and reduce symptoms like cramping. This herb is often used as a tea or tincture, making it a versatile option for women seeking to regulate their menstrual health naturally. Emma could incorporate black cohosh as part of her monthly routine, using it during phases when her symptoms are most intense.

Alleviating Menstrual Cramps

Menstrual cramps, or dysmenorrhea, are a common issue for many women. Herbal remedies like **cramp bark**, **ginger**, and **raspberry leaf** offer effective, natural pain relief, helping to ease cramps and reduce inflammation without the need for pharmaceutical options.

Cramp bark is specifically named for its ability to relieve menstrual cramps. The herb acts as a muscle relaxant, helping to ease the contractions of the uterus that cause discomfort during menstruation. A simple cramp bark tea or tincture taken at the onset of symptoms can provide relief quickly. For someone like Emma, who may prefer quick and accessible remedies, cramp bark offers a straightforward solution to manage menstrual pain effectively.

Ginger is another powerful anti-inflammatory herb

that not only reduces menstrual pain but also supports digestion and reduces nausea, which can sometimes accompany menstruation. A warm ginger tea made from fresh ginger root can help relax the muscles and reduce inflammation, providing a soothing and effective remedy. Ginger's versatility and ease of use make it an ideal option for women looking for an all-around remedy to support their menstrual health.

Raspberry leaf is often called the "women's herb" due to its broad applications for reproductive health. It contains fragarine, a compound that tones and relaxes the muscles of the uterus, helping to alleviate menstrual cramps and discomfort. Drinking raspberry leaf tea throughout the menstrual cycle can not only reduce cramping but also support overall reproductive health. For Emma, integrating raspberry leaf tea into her daily routine could provide both immediate relief and long-term benefits, making it an essential part of her natural health toolkit.

Supporting Hormonal Balance and PMS Relief

Premenstrual syndrome (PMS) is a common challenge, affecting mood, physical comfort, and overall well-being. Herbal remedies such as **evening primrose oil**, **St. John's wort**, and **dandelion** offer natural ways to manage symptoms and promote hormonal balance.

Evening primrose oil is rich in gamma-linolenic acid (GLA), a fatty acid that supports hormonal balance and reduces PMS symptoms like breast tenderness and mood swings. Taking evening primrose oil supplements regularly can help stabilize hormone levels and alleviate discomfort, providing long-term benefits. For women like Emma, who may experience cyclical mood changes or physical discomfort, this oil can be a valuable addition to her wellness routine.

St. John's wort is another herb that supports mood stability, particularly in cases of PMS-related mood swings or mild depression. It works by enhancing serotonin levels, improving mood and reducing irritability. St. John's wort can be taken as a tea, tincture, or capsule, offering multiple ways to incorporate it into daily life. For Emma, who might prefer holistic solutions that enhance both physical and emotional well-being, St. John's wort provides an effective and natural option.

Dandelion is often used to alleviate water retention and bloating, common symptoms of PMS. Its diuretic properties help flush excess fluids from the body while providing essential minerals like potassium, which help reduce cramping. Dandelion tea is an easy and effective way to consume this herb, supporting menstrual health by managing bloating and maintaining hydration. Emma could easily integrate dandelion tea into her monthly regimen, especially in the days leading up to her period, to prevent and reduce discomfort.

By using these herbs, women can effectively manage and support their menstrual health, ensuring both physical and emotional well-being throughout their cycles. This natural approach empowers individuals to take control of their health, aligning with holistic practices that promote balance and harmony within the body.

Support for Pregnancy, Postpartum, and Menopause

NATURAL HERBAL SUPPORT DURING PREGNANCY, POSTPARTUM, AND MENOPAUSE

Navigating the various stages of womanhood—from pregnancy to postpartum and into menopause—requires thoughtful and effective support. Herbs have long been used to offer relief and balance during these transformative phases, providing natural solutions tailored to the unique needs of each stage. Understanding how to use these herbs safely and effectively empowers women like Emma to manage their health holistically, ensuring well-being and balance throughout each phase of life. Below, we explore specific herbal remedies and their applications during pregnancy, postpartum recovery, and menopause.

Herbs for Pregnancy: Supporting Health and Balance

During pregnancy, the body undergoes numerous changes, requiring gentle support to maintain balance and address common discomforts. While not all herbs are safe during pregnancy, several, including **red raspberry leaf**, **ginger**, and **nettles**, have been traditionally used to provide safe and effective support.

Red Raspberry Leaf is widely recognized as a pregnancy-supportive herb due to its high nutrient content and toning properties for the uterus. Rich in vitamins A, C, and E, as well as magnesium, calcium, and iron, red raspberry leaf strengthens the uterine muscles, potentially easing labor and improving outcomes. Drinking red raspberry leaf tea during the second and third trimesters can be an excellent way for Emma to prepare her body for childbirth naturally while also ensuring she receives essential nutrients.

Ginger is another essential herb for pregnancy, particularly for managing nausea and morning sickness. Its anti-inflammatory properties help soothe the digestive system, reducing nausea and discomfort commonly experienced in early pregnancy. A simple ginger tea made from fresh ginger slices can offer fast relief, making it an easy and effective remedy for Emma to incorporate into her daily routine.

Nettles, or stinging nettle, provide a rich source of vitamins and minerals crucial for both mother and developing baby. It supports overall vitality, helping to prevent iron deficiency and boosting energy levels. Nettle tea is a safe and nourishing option that can be consumed throughout pregnancy, particularly in the later stages when the body requires more support. For Emma, nettle tea offers a simple way to maintain health and energy levels as her body prepares for childbirth.

Postpartum Support: Healing and Recovery

The postpartum period, or the "fourth trimester," is a crucial time for recovery and nourishment. The body undergoes significant changes as it heals from childbirth, and specific herbs like **motherwort**, **fenugreek**, and **calendula** can provide essential support for this transition.

Motherwort is known for its calming and restorative

effects, making it a valuable ally for new mothers. It helps reduce postpartum anxiety and supports uterine recovery by promoting contraction and reducing bleeding. Consuming motherwort tea or tincture can help ease emotional stress while supporting physical recovery, ensuring a balanced and holistic approach to postpartum health. For Emma, who values natural remedies for both emotional and physical support, motherwort offers a comprehensive solution.

Fenugreek is another beneficial herb in the postpartum period, particularly for promoting lactation. It has long been used as a galactagogue to enhance milk production in breastfeeding mothers. Fenugreek seeds can be taken as capsules or infused in tea to support lactation naturally, providing Emma with a simple yet effective method to ensure her breastfeeding journey is successful.

Calendula is often used externally during the postpartum period for its soothing and anti-inflammatory properties. It is effective for healing perineal tears or cesarean incisions and can be used as a poultice or infused in sitz baths. Calendula's gentle yet powerful healing properties make it an essential herb for promoting skin repair and reducing inflammation. For Emma, calendula-infused sitz baths provide a nurturing way to support physical healing while ensuring comfort during recovery.

Herbal Remedies for Menopause: Balance and Relief

As women transition into menopause, they often experience a range of symptoms, including hot flashes, mood swings, and hormonal imbalances. Herbs like **black cohosh**, **sage**, and **dong quai** are particularly beneficial during this phase, offering natural relief and balance.

Black Cohosh is one of the most well-researched herbs for managing menopausal symptoms, especially hot flashes and night sweats. Its phytoestrogenic properties help balance hormones naturally, reducing the intensity and frequency of symptoms. Black cohosh is commonly taken as a tincture or capsule, providing an accessible and effective option for managing menopausal discomfort. For Emma, incorporating black cohosh into her daily routine could help ease her transition, ensuring she maintains balance and comfort.

Sage is another valuable herb for menopause, known for its ability to reduce hot flashes and excessive sweating. Sage's cooling properties make it ideal for managing the heat and night sweats that often accompany menopause. Drinking sage tea or using sage tincture can provide quick relief, allowing women like Emma to continue their daily activities comfortably.

Dong Quai, often referred to as the "female ginseng," is an herb traditionally used in Chinese medicine to balance hormones and support reproductive health during menopause. It works by improving blood flow and supporting hormonal balance, helping to reduce symptoms such as fatigue and mood swings. For women transitioning through menopause, taking dong quai as part of a holistic wellness routine can support overall vitality and emotional balance. Emma, who might appreciate remedies that offer both physical and emotional support, can benefit from its comprehensive effects.

Incorporating these herbs thoughtfully into routines during pregnancy, postpartum, and menopause ensures that women have the support they need to navigate these significant life transitions naturally. Each herb offers a unique set of benefits, providing a holistic and nurturing approach to maintaining health and balance at every stage.

Remedies for Women's Hormonal Wellness

Red Raspberry Leaf Menstrual Tonic Tea

INGREDIENTS

- 1 teaspoon dried red raspberry leaves
- 1 cup boiling water

PREPARATION

1. Steep the red raspberry leaves in boiling water for 10 minutes.
2. Strain and drink warm.

Benefits: This tonic is rich in nutrients and helps to tone the uterine muscles, easing menstrual cramps and supporting overall reproductive health. It is often recommended for women to regulate menstrual cycles and enhance fertility.

Chaste Tree (Vitex) Hormonal Balance Capsules

INGREDIENTS

- 1 teaspoon ground chaste tree berries
- Empty capsules

PREPARATION

1. Fill the capsules with ground chaste tree berries.
2. Take one capsule daily for hormonal balance support.

Benefits: Vitex is known to balance hormone levels by regulating the pituitary gland. It helps alleviate PMS symptoms, reduce acne, and support a healthy menstrual cycle. It is particularly beneficial for women with irregular periods or hormonal imbalances.

Dong Quai Hormone Regulating Tincture

INGREDIENTS

- 1 tablespoon dried dong quai root
- 1/2 cup vodka

PREPARATION

1. Combine dong quai root and vodka in a jar.
2. Let it infuse for 2 weeks, shaking daily.
3. Strain and store in a dropper bottle.

Benefits: Dong quai is a traditional Chinese herb used to regulate hormones, improve circulation, and reduce menstrual discomfort. It is especially helpful for balancing estrogen levels and enhancing reproductive health.

Black Cohosh Menopause Support Elixir

INGREDIENTS

- 1 teaspoon dried black cohosh root
- 1 cup water
- 1 tablespoon honey

PREPARATION

1. Simmer black cohosh root in water for 15 minutes.
2. Strain and add honey.
3. Store in a bottle and take as needed.

Benefits: Black cohosh is effective for alleviating menopause symptoms, such as hot flashes and mood swings, by supporting hormone balance and providing anti-inflammatory benefits.

Evening Primrose Oil PMS Relief Capsules

INGREDIENTS

- Evening primrose oil
- Empty capsules

PREPARATION

1. Fill the capsules with evening primrose oil.
2. Take one capsule daily to alleviate PMS symptoms.

Benefits: Evening primrose oil is rich in essential fatty acids that help reduce PMS symptoms such as bloating, breast tenderness, and mood swings. It also supports overall hormonal health.

Shatavari Reproductive Health Infusion

INGREDIENTS

- 1 teaspoon dried shatavari root
- 1 cup boiling water

PREPARATION

1. Steep shatavari root in boiling water for 10 minutes.
2. Strain and drink warm.

Benefits: Shatavari is an adaptogenic herb that supports reproductive health by balancing hormones and enhancing fertility. It is also known for its soothing properties, making it ideal for easing menstrual discomfort.

Cramp Bark Menstrual Pain Relief Tea

INGREDIENTS

- 1 teaspoon dried cramp bark
- 1 cup boiling water

PREPARATION

1. Steep cramp bark in boiling water for 10 minutes.
2. Strain and drink warm.

Benefits: Cramp bark is a natural antispasmodic that helps alleviate menstrual cramps by relaxing the uterine muscles. It is effective for reducing pain and discomfort during menstruation.

Lady's Mantle Fertility Support Tea

INGREDIENTS

- 1 teaspoon dried lady's mantle leaves
- 1 cup boiling water

PREPARATION

1. Steep lady's mantle leaves in boiling water for 10 minutes.
2. Strain and drink warm.

Benefits: Lady's mantle is known for its astringent and anti-inflammatory properties, supporting fertility and overall reproductive health. It helps to regulate menstrual cycles and tone the uterus.

Wild Yam Hormone Balancing Cream

INGREDIENTS

- 1 teaspoon wild yam root extract
- 1/2 cup shea butter

PREPARATION

1. Melt the shea butter in a double boiler.
2. Add the wild yam extract and mix well.
3. Store in a jar and apply to the skin daily.

Benefits: Wild yam is commonly used to balance hormones, especially progesterone levels. It is beneficial for women experiencing menopause symptoms or hormonal imbalances related to menstruation.

Blue Cohosh Pregnancy Preparation Capsules

INGREDIENTS

- 1 teaspoon ground blue cohosh root
- Empty capsules

PREPARATION

1. Fill capsules with ground blue cohosh root.
2. Take one capsule daily when preparing for pregnancy.

Benefits: Blue cohosh supports reproductive health and prepares the uterus for pregnancy. It is traditionally used to strengthen the reproductive system and support a regular menstrual cycle.

Motherwort Calming Menstrual Tea

INGREDIENTS

- 1 teaspoon dried motherwort leaves
- 1 cup boiling water

PREPARATION

1. Steep motherwort leaves in boiling water for 10 minutes.
2. Strain and drink warm.

Benefits: Motherwort helps to calm the nervous system and alleviate anxiety related to menstruation. It is also effective for reducing menstrual cramps and supporting overall hormonal balance.

Yarrow Menstrual Flow Regulation Drops

INGREDIENTS

- 1 teaspoon dried yarrow flowers
- 1/2 cup vodka

PREPARATION

1. Combine yarrow flowers and vodka in a jar.
2. Let it infuse for 2 weeks, shaking daily.
3. Strain and store in a dropper bottle.

Benefits: Yarrow is known for its ability to regulate menstrual flow, making it effective for women with heavy periods or irregular cycles. It also supports overall reproductive health.

Stinging Nettle Postpartum Iron Support Tonic

INGREDIENTS

- 1 teaspoon dried stinging nettle leaves
- 1 cup boiling water

PREPARATION

1. Steep stinging nettle leaves in boiling water for 10 minutes.
2. Strain and drink warm.

Benefits: Stinging nettle is rich in iron and other essential nutrients, making it ideal for postpartum recovery. It supports overall energy levels and replenishes iron lost during childbirth.

Ashwagandha Hormonal Balance Adaptogen

INGREDIENTS

- 1 teaspoon dried ashwagandha root powder
- 1 cup warm milk

PREPARATION

1. Mix ashwagandha powder into warm milk.
2. Stir until well combined and drink before bedtime.

Benefits: Ashwagandha is an adaptogen that helps balance hormones and reduce stress, making it effective for women experiencing hormonal imbalances or stress-related menstrual issues.

Calendula Breast Health Salve

INGREDIENTS

- 1 tablespoon dried calendula petals
- 1/2 cup olive oil
- 1 tablespoon beeswax

PREPARATION

1. Simmer calendula petals in olive oil for 20 minutes.
2. Strain and add beeswax to the warm oil.
3. Pour into a jar and let it solidify.

Benefits: Calendula is effective for breast health, reducing inflammation and supporting lymphatic drainage. It can be applied as a salve to promote overall breast wellness.

Fenugreek Milk Production Capsules

INGREDIENTS

- 1 tablespoon fenugreek seeds
- Capsule shells

PREPARATION

1. Grind fenugreek seeds into a fine powder.
2. Fill capsule shells with the fenugreek powder.
3. Take 1-2 capsules daily with water, preferably with meals.

Benefits: Fenugreek is a well-known galactagogue that helps promote milk production in nursing mothers. It contains phytoestrogens that mimic estrogen, stimulating the milk ducts and enhancing milk supply. This remedy is particularly useful during the early stages of breastfeeding when milk production may need a boost.

Lemon Balm Mood Balancing Infusion

INGREDIENTS

- 1 teaspoon dried lemon balm leaves
- 1 cup hot water

PREPARATION

1. Steep lemon balm leaves in hot water for 5-7 minutes.
2. Strain and drink warm or at room temperature.

Benefits: Lemon balm has calming effects on the nervous system, making it an excellent herb for reducing anxiety and mood swings, particularly related to hormonal changes such as PMS or menopause. It promotes relaxation and helps in managing stress, which often exacerbates hormonal imbalances.

Sage Hot Flash Relief Tea

INGREDIENTS

- 1 teaspoon dried sage leaves
- 1 cup boiling water

PREPARATION

1. Steep sage leaves in boiling water for 5-10 minutes.
2. Strain and drink 1-2 times a day.

Benefits: Sage is a natural remedy for menopausal symptoms, especially hot flashes. Its estrogen-like properties help balance hormone levels, providing relief from excessive sweating and heat surges during menopause. Regular consumption can reduce the frequency and intensity of hot flashes.

Maca Root Hormonal Support Powder

INGREDIENTS

- 1 teaspoon maca root powder
- Smoothie or water for mixing

PREPARATION

1. Mix 1 teaspoon of maca powder into a smoothie, juice, or water.
2. Consume daily, preferably in the morning.

Benefits: Maca root is an adaptogen known for its ability to support hormonal balance, particularly in women experiencing menopause or PMS. It helps stabilize estrogen and progesterone levels, improving mood, energy, and overall hormonal health. Maca is also beneficial for enhancing fertility and boosting libido.

Schisandra Berry Energy Boosting Elixir

INGREDIENTS

- 1 teaspoon schisandra berries
- 1 cup water

PREPARATION

1. Simmer schisandra berries in water for 15 minutes.
2. Strain and consume warm or cold.

Benefits: Schisandra berries are a powerful adaptogen that enhances energy, endurance, and stamina. They also help modulate hormonal imbalances and alleviate symptoms of fatigue caused by stress or hormonal shifts, making this elixir ideal for women experiencing hormonal changes.

Rose Hip Uterine Tonic Infusion

INGREDIENTS

- 1 teaspoon dried rose hips
- 1 cup boiling water

PREPARATION

1. Steep rose hips in boiling water for 10 minutes.
2. Strain and drink warm.

Benefits: Rose hips are rich in vitamin C and bioflavonoids, which support uterine health. They help tone and strengthen the uterine walls, making them useful for postpartum recovery and overall reproductive health. The antioxidants also combat inflammation and support hormonal balance.

Sarsaparilla Hormonal Detox Tea

INGREDIENTS

- 1 teaspoon dried sarsaparilla root
- 1 cup water

PREPARATION

1. Simmer sarsaparilla root in water for 10–15 minutes.
2. Strain and drink up to twice daily.

Benefits: Sarsaparilla root has natural detoxifying properties that help cleanse the liver, aiding in the removal of excess hormones from the body. This tea is especially beneficial for clearing estrogen dominance, promoting hormonal balance, and improving skin health.

Dandelion Root PMS Bloating Relief Tea

INGREDIENTS

- 1 teaspoon dried dandelion root
- 1 cup boiling water

PREPARATION

1. Steep dandelion root in boiling water for 10 minutes.
2. Strain and drink warm.

Benefits: Dandelion root acts as a natural diuretic, helping to reduce water retention and bloating associated with PMS. It supports liver function, which is essential for breaking down excess hormones, thus easing PMS symptoms such as breast tenderness and bloating.

Black Haw Cramp Relief Tincture

INGREDIENTS

- 1 teaspoon black haw root tincture
- Water or juice for dilution

PREPARATION

1. Add the tincture to a small amount of water or juice.
2. Take 1-2 times a day, as needed.

Benefits: Black haw is renowned for its ability to relieve menstrual cramps and uterine spasms. It works by relaxing the smooth muscles of the uterus, reducing pain and discomfort associated with menstruation or uterine contractions. This tincture provides fast-acting relief.

Burdock Root Hormonal Detox Capsules

INGREDIENTS

- 1 tablespoon dried burdock root powder
- Capsule shells

PREPARATION

1. Grind burdock root into a fine powder.
2. Fill capsules with the burdock root powder.
3. Take 1-2 capsules daily with water.

Benefits: Burdock root supports the body's natural detoxification processes, particularly through the liver. It helps cleanse excess hormones from the system, especially estrogen, aiding in hormonal balance. This makes it an ideal remedy for women experiencing hormonal imbalances due to PMS or menopause.

Blessed Thistle Lactation Support Tea

INGREDIENTS

- 1 teaspoon dried blessed thistle leaves
- 1 cup boiling water

PREPARATION

1. Steep the blessed thistle leaves in boiling water for 10 minutes.
2. Strain and drink up to 3 times daily.

Benefits: Blessed thistle is a well-known galactagogue that helps increase milk production in nursing mothers. It also supports overall breast health and can soothe digestive discomfort. Regular consumption of this tea helps boost lactation and ensure a steady milk supply.

Marigold (Calendula) Hormone Balance Elixir

INGREDIENTS

- 1 teaspoon dried calendula flowers
- 1 cup boiling water

PREPARATION

1. Steep calendula flowers in boiling water for 10 minutes.
2. Strain and drink once a day.

Benefits: Calendula is known for its hormone-balancing properties. It supports liver function, which plays a key role in metabolizing hormones, helping to balance estrogen levels. This elixir also has anti-inflammatory properties that can alleviate PMS and menstrual discomfort.

Oatstraw Rejuvenating Infusion for Women

INGREDIENTS

- 1 tablespoon dried oatstraw
- 1 cup boiling water

PREPARATION

1. Steep oatstraw in boiling water for 10-15 minutes.
2. Strain and drink daily.

Benefits: Oatstraw is an excellent tonic for the nervous system and helps rejuvenate the body, especially during times of hormonal stress. It provides essential nutrients like calcium and magnesium, which are crucial for managing PMS, menopause, and overall hormonal health.

Hibiscus Menstrual Flow Regulation Tea

INGREDIENTS

- 1 teaspoon dried hibiscus flowers
- 1 cup boiling water

PREPARATION

1. Steep hibiscus flowers in boiling water for 5-10 minutes.
2. Strain and drink warm.

Benefits: Hibiscus is known for regulating menstrual flow. It helps balance estrogen levels, which can reduce heavy or irregular bleeding. The high vitamin C content also promotes uterine health and provides an anti-inflammatory effect, easing menstrual discomfort.

Dong Quai and Ginger Menstrual Support Syrup

INGREDIENTS

- 1 tablespoon dried dong quai root
- 1 teaspoon grated ginger
- 1 cup water
- 1/2 cup honey

PREPARATION

1. Simmer dong quai and ginger in water for 20 minutes.
2. Strain and add honey to the liquid.

3. Store in a jar and take 1 tablespoon daily during menstruation.

Benefits: Dong quai, often referred to as "female ginseng," supports overall reproductive health and helps regulate menstrual cycles. Combined with ginger, it alleviates menstrual cramps, reduces inflammation, and promotes blood circulation, making this syrup highly beneficial for menstrual discomfort.

Vitex and Licorice Hormonal Balancer Capsules

INGREDIENTS

- 1 tablespoon vitex powder
- 1 tablespoon licorice root powder
- Capsule shells

PREPARATION

1. Mix vitex and licorice root powders together.
2. Fill capsule shells with the powder mixture.
3. Take 1-2 capsules daily.

Benefits: Vitex (chasteberry) is renowned for its ability to regulate the menstrual cycle and balance hormone levels, particularly progesterone. Licorice root helps modulate estrogen levels and reduces inflammation. Together, they create a powerful remedy for hormonal imbalances, particularly for women experiencing PMS, irregular periods, or menopausal symptoms.

Eleuthero Menstrual Cycle Regulation Tea

INGREDIENTS

- 1 teaspoon dried eleuthero root
- 1 cup water

PREPARATION

1. Simmer eleuthero root in water for 15 minutes.
2. Strain and drink warm.

Benefits: Eleuthero is an adaptogen that helps the body respond to stress and promotes overall hormonal balance. It is particularly effective for regulating menstrual cycles and easing the effects of stress on the body, which can disrupt hormonal rhythms. Regular consumption helps create stability in the menstrual cycle.

Alfalfa Postpartum Recovery Tonic

INGREDIENTS

- 1 teaspoon dried alfalfa leaves
- 1 cup boiling water

PREPARATION

1. Steep alfalfa leaves in boiling water for 10 minutes.
2. Strain and drink warm.

Benefits: Alfalfa is rich in vitamins and minerals, particularly calcium, magnesium, and vitamin K, which are crucial for postpartum recovery. It helps support the body's healing process after childbirth, replenishing nutrients and boosting energy levels, while also aiding in lactation.

Tribulus Hormonal Wellness Capsules

INGREDIENTS

- 1 tablespoon tribulus powder
- Capsule shells

PREPARATION

1. Fill capsule shells with tribulus powder.
2. Take 1-2 capsules daily with meals.

Benefits: Tribulus terrestris supports the endocrine system by regulating hormone production, particularly testosterone and estrogen. It helps improve libido, balance mood, and enhance overall hormonal wellness. This makes it especially beneficial for women dealing with hormonal imbalances, including those related to menopause and fertility.

BOOK 7

Skin Care and Beauty

Understanding the Skin's Needs

THE ESSENTIAL ASPECTS OF SKIN HEALTH

The skin is the body's largest organ, acting as a protective barrier while also playing a key role in regulating temperature and sensation. Understanding its needs is crucial for maintaining healthy, radiant skin. The skin is affected by a variety of factors, including environmental elements, diet, hydration, and lifestyle choices. For individuals like Emma, who seek natural and effective skincare solutions, understanding these needs allows them to create a skincare routine that is not only holistic but also deeply nourishing. To achieve optimal skin health, it's important to consider several core aspects: hydration, protection, nourishment, and balance.

Hydration: The Foundation of Skin Health

Hydration is fundamental for healthy skin, as it helps maintain elasticity, texture, and overall appearance. When the skin is well-hydrated, it appears plump and smooth, reducing the appearance of fine lines and dryness. Dehydrated skin, on the other hand, can become rough, flaky, and more prone to irritation. Drinking plenty of water is the first step in keeping the skin hydrated, but external hydration through skincare is equally important.

Natural moisturizers like **aloe vera** and **rose water** are excellent for maintaining skin hydration. Aloe vera, known for its soothing properties, not only hydrates but also calms inflammation, making it suitable for all skin types, including sensitive skin. Rose water, another hydrating agent, is rich in antioxidants and has anti-inflammatory properties, providing a gentle way to lock in moisture and refresh the skin. Incorporating these natural remedies into Emma's skincare routine can help maintain her skin's hydration levels, ensuring it stays soft and supple.

Protection: Shielding the Skin from Environmental Stressors

The skin is constantly exposed to environmental stressors such as UV rays, pollution, and harsh weather conditions. These elements can damage the skin barrier, leading to premature aging, dryness, and pigmentation issues. Protecting the skin from these external factors is crucial for long-term health and radiance.

One of the most effective ways to protect the skin naturally is by using **herbal sunscreens** and **antioxidant-rich serums.** Ingredients like **carrot seed oil** and **green tea extract** provide natural sun protection while delivering antioxidants that fight free radicals, reducing the damage caused by UV exposure. Carrot seed oil is particularly beneficial as it contains SPF properties and nourishes the skin with vitamins A and E. Green tea extract, on the other hand, is rich in polyphenols, which protect the skin cells from oxidative stress. For Emma, who may spend time outdoors or work in environments exposed to pollutants, incorporating these protective herbs into her daily skincare regimen can help her shield her skin from damage and maintain its youthful appearance.

Nourishment: Feeding the Skin Essential Nutrients

Just like the body, the skin requires a variety of nutrients to function optimally. Vitamins, minerals, and essential fatty acids are crucial for keeping the skin healthy, as they support cell regeneration, collagen production, and barrier function. A lack of these nutrients can lead to dullness, loss of elasticity, and an increased susceptibility to irritation.

Herbs such as **calendula**, **chamomile**, and **sea buckthorn** provide the skin with essential nourishment. **Calendula** is rich in antioxidants and flavonoids, promoting skin repair and reducing inflammation. It's especially effective for healing minor cuts, burns, and acne scars. **Chamomile** soothes irritation and provides anti-inflammatory support, making it ideal for sensitive or reactive skin types. Meanwhile, **sea buckthorn** is packed with omega-3 and omega-7 fatty acids, which support skin regeneration and hydration. For Emma, using products or DIY remedies infused with these herbs can nourish her skin from the outside, ensuring it gets the vitamins and minerals it needs to remain healthy and resilient.

Balance: Maintaining the Skin's Natural Microbiome

The skin has its own ecosystem known as the microbiome, consisting of beneficial bacteria that protect against pathogens and help maintain a balanced pH level. When this microbiome is disrupted—by harsh products, pollution, or diet—skin issues like acne, eczema, and sensitivity can arise. Therefore, maintaining the skin's microbiome balance is crucial for overall skin health.

Probiotic-rich herbs and ingredients like **yogurt**, **honey**, and **tea tree oil** can help restore and maintain the skin's natural balance. **Yogurt** contains lactic acid and probiotics that support the skin barrier and maintain its pH. Applying a yogurt mask can provide mild exfoliation while nourishing the microbiome. **Honey** is another powerful natural remedy, offering antimicrobial and moisturizing benefits. It helps maintain skin hydration while protecting against infections. **Tea tree oil**, known for its antibacterial properties, can be used as a spot treatment to balance oil production and reduce acne without disrupting the skin's microbiome. For someone like Emma, who values both effectiveness and simplicity, these natural remedies provide a balanced approach to maintaining her skin's health.

Herbs for Radiant and Healthy Skin

NATURAL HERBS FOR GLOWING, HEALTHY SKIN

Achieving radiant and healthy skin requires more than just external care; it involves using natural, holistic remedies that nourish the skin from within and without. Herbs are powerful allies in skincare, offering antioxidants, vitamins, and anti-inflammatory properties that promote a glowing complexion and improve skin health. For individuals like Emma, who seek effective and natural solutions, understanding how to use these herbs allows them to incorporate beneficial practices into their daily skincare routines. Below, we explore some of the most effective herbs for achieving vibrant, healthy skin, each providing unique properties that target different skin needs.

Calendula: The Skin Healer

Calendula, also known as marigold, is a versatile herb that has long been valued for its healing properties. It contains flavonoids and carotenoids, which offer anti-inflammatory and antioxidant benefits, making it particularly effective for soothing irritated or sensitive skin. Calendula supports skin repair, reduces redness, and promotes a smooth, even complexion.

A calendula-infused oil or cream can be used as a daily moisturizer to provide hydration and calm inflammation. For Emma, who may have a busy schedule but values simple, effective skincare, using calendula oil after cleansing her face can keep her skin soft and radiant while reducing the risk of irritation. Additionally, calendula tea can be used as a facial rinse to further enhance its calming effects.

Aloe Vera: The Ultimate Moisturizer

Aloe vera is well-known for its hydrating and cooling properties, making it a staple for anyone seeking radiant skin. Rich in vitamins A, C, and E, aloe vera promotes skin regeneration and repair while providing deep moisture that keeps the skin plump and supple. It also has antibacterial properties, which make it effective for treating acne and other skin irritations.

Applying fresh aloe vera gel directly from the plant offers the most benefits, providing an instant boost of hydration and a soothing effect that is ideal for all skin types, including sensitive skin. For Emma, who appreciates natural and accessible remedies, keeping an aloe vera plant at home allows her to use this herb whenever her skin needs a hydration boost or relief from irritation.

Chamomile: Calming and Anti-Inflammatory

Chamomile is another valuable herb for skincare, particularly for those with sensitive or reactive skin. Its anti-inflammatory and antioxidant properties make it effective for reducing redness, calming irritation, and soothing conditions like eczema or rosacea. Chamomile's gentle nature makes it suitable for all skin types, and it can be incorporated into skincare routines in various forms, such as chamomile-infused oils, creams, or teas.

A chamomile compress made by soaking chamomile flowers in warm water and applying it to the face is an excellent way to calm inflammation and refresh the skin. For Emma, who might face stressful situations that can trigger skin reactions, using chamomile as part of her evening routine can help her unwind while simultaneously caring for her skin.

Rosehip: Rich in Antioxidants and Essential Fatty Acids

Rosehip oil is a powerful herb-derived skincare ingredient, packed with vitamins A and C and essential fatty acids that are crucial for skin regeneration. It helps reduce signs of aging, fades scars, and improves overall skin texture. The high antioxidant content of rosehip oil protects against environmental damage and supports collagen production, promoting a more youthful and glowing complexion.

Rosehip oil can be used as a nightly facial serum, providing a concentrated dose of nutrients that penetrate deeply into the skin. For Emma, incorporating rosehip oil into her routine before bed offers a simple way to maintain her skin's health and prevent signs of aging, ensuring she wakes up with a fresh and nourished appearance.

Lavender: Balancing and Soothing

Lavender is not only known for its relaxing scent but also for its balancing and healing properties for the skin. It has antiseptic and anti-inflammatory effects, making it ideal for treating acne, soothing irritations, and balancing oily skin. Lavender's calming properties also make it effective for reducing stress-related skin issues, such as breakouts or flare-ups.

Lavender essential oil can be added to facial masks, creams, or used as a steam treatment to open pores and cleanse the skin. For Emma, who values routines that support both physical and emotional wellness, lavender provides dual benefits—helping her maintain clear skin while promoting a sense of calm and relaxation.

Turmeric: The Anti-Inflammatory Powerhouse

Turmeric, with its active compound curcumin, is a potent anti-inflammatory and antioxidant herb that supports skin health by reducing inflammation and brightening the complexion. It helps diminish dark spots, fights acne, and enhances the skin's natural glow. Turmeric is particularly effective for those experiencing hyperpigmentation or dullness, as it promotes an even skin tone.

A turmeric mask made with turmeric powder and honey can be applied to the face weekly to brighten and revitalize the skin. For Emma, using a turmeric mask is a simple and effective way to refresh her skin and maintain a glowing complexion, ensuring her skin remains vibrant despite her active lifestyle.

Gotu Kola: Enhancing Collagen Production

Gotu kola is an herb traditionally used in Ayurvedic medicine for its skin-healing properties. It supports collagen production, which is crucial for maintaining skin elasticity and reducing signs of aging such as fine lines and sagging. Gotu kola also aids in wound healing, making it beneficial for improving the appearance of scars and skin texture.

Applying gotu kola-infused oils or creams can boost the skin's firmness and smoothness, providing long-term benefits for skin health. For Emma, who might seek ways to naturally maintain her skin's youthful appearance, gotu kola offers a holistic solution that fits seamlessly into her skincare regimen.

By incorporating these herbs, individuals can create a comprehensive skincare routine that enhances skin health, promotes radiance, and provides natural solutions tailored to their needs. For Emma, integrating these remedies ensures her skincare aligns with her values, supporting both her skin's health and her overall wellness journey.

Remedies for Skincare and Natural Beauty

Rose Petal Hydrating Facial Toner

INGREDIENTS

- 1/2 cup fresh or dried rose petals
- 1 cup distilled water
- 2 tablespoons witch hazel

PREPARATION

1. Bring the distilled water to a boil and pour over the rose petals.
2. Allow the mixture to steep for 20-30 minutes, then strain.
3. Add witch hazel to the strained rose water and mix well.
4. Transfer to a spray bottle and use as a facial toner.

Benefits: This toner hydrates the skin while balancing its natural oils. Rose petals are rich in antioxidants, which help protect the skin from environmental damage, while witch hazel tightens pores and reduces inflammation. Regular use leaves the skin feeling refreshed and glowing.

Calendula Skin Healing Salve

INGREDIENTS

- 1/2 cup dried calendula flowers
- 1/2 cup olive oil
- 2 tablespoons beeswax

PREPARATION

1. Infuse the calendula flowers in olive oil by heating them in a double boiler for 30-60 minutes on low heat.
2. Strain the mixture and discard the flowers.
3. Melt the beeswax in the calendula-infused oil.
4. Pour the mixture into a small jar and let it cool completely.

Benefits: Calendula is known for its anti-inflammatory and antimicrobial properties, making this salve ideal for healing cuts, scrapes, and skin irritations. It also promotes skin regeneration, soothes dry skin, and reduces the appearance of scars.

Witch Hazel Astringent Toner

INGREDIENTS

- 1/2 cup witch hazel
- 1/4 cup distilled water
- 10 drops tea tree essential oil

PREPARATION

1. Mix witch hazel and distilled water in a small bottle.
2. Add tea tree essential oil and shake well.
3. Apply to the face using a cotton pad after cleansing.

Benefits: Witch hazel is a natural astringent that tightens pores and reduces excess oil production, making it excellent for acne-prone skin. Tea tree oil enhances the toner's antimicrobial effects, helping to prevent breakouts and soothe inflamed skin.

Aloe Vera Soothing Gel for Sunburn

INGREDIENTS

- 2 tablespoons fresh aloe vera gel
- 1 teaspoon coconut oil

PREPARATION

1. Mix fresh aloe vera gel with coconut oil.
2. Apply the mixture to sunburned skin and leave it on to absorb.
3. Reapply as needed.

Benefits: Aloe vera is renowned for its cooling and anti-inflammatory properties, which provide immediate relief for sunburned skin. It helps soothe redness, reduce swelling, and promote faster healing, while coconut oil adds moisture to prevent dryness and peeling.

Chamomile and Oat Facial Mask

INGREDIENTS

- 1 tablespoon dried chamomile flowers
- 1 tablespoon ground oats
- 1 teaspoon honey

PREPARATION

1. Grind the chamomile flowers into a fine powder.
2. Mix the chamomile powder with ground oats and honey to form a paste.
3. Apply to clean skin and leave on for 15-20 minutes.
4. Rinse off with warm water.

Benefits: Chamomile soothes irritated skin and reduces redness, while oats gently exfoliate and calm inflammation. Honey provides deep moisture and has antibacterial properties, leaving the skin soft, nourished, and radiant. This mask is ideal for sensitive skin prone to dryness and irritation.

Lavender Acne Relief Serum

INGREDIENTS

- 1 tablespoon jojoba oil
- 5 drops lavender essential oil
- 5 drops tea tree essential oil

PREPARATION

1. Combine jojoba oil with lavender and tea tree essential oils.
2. Apply a few drops to the affected areas of the skin.
3. Use once or twice daily.

Benefits: Lavender essential oil has anti-inflammatory properties that reduce redness and calm irritated skin, while tea tree oil helps fight acne-causing bacteria. Jojoba oil acts as a non-comedogenic moisturizer that balances the skin's natural oils. This serum is ideal for treating acne without drying out the skin.

Green Tea Antioxidant Facial Mist

INGREDIENTS

- 1 green tea bag
- 1 cup distilled water
- 1 teaspoon aloe vera gel

PREPARATION

1. Steep the green tea bag in boiling water for 10 minutes, then let it cool.
2. Mix in the aloe vera gel.
3. Transfer to a spray bottle and mist onto the face as needed.

Benefits: Green tea is rich in antioxidants that protect the skin from free radical damage, reducing signs of aging and inflammation. Aloe vera soothes and hydrates the skin, making this mist a refreshing and protective treatment for daily use.

Cucumber and Mint Cooling Eye Gel

INGREDIENTS

- 1/2 cucumber, peeled and chopped
- 1 tablespoon fresh mint leaves
- 1 tablespoon aloe vera gel

PREPARATION

1. Blend the cucumber and mint leaves until smooth.
2. Mix the puree with aloe vera gel.
3. Apply the gel under the eyes and leave it on for 10-15 minutes.
4. Rinse off with cool water.

Benefits: Cucumber reduces puffiness and dark circles under the eyes, while mint leaves provide a cooling effect that refreshes tired skin. Aloe vera hydrates and soothes the delicate eye area, leaving it looking bright and revitalized. This gel is perfect for reducing signs of fatigue and stress around the eyes.

Hibiscus Anti-Aging Facial Oil

INGREDIENTS

- 1 tablespoon hibiscus-infused oil
- 5 drops rosehip oil
- 5 drops frankincense essential oil

PREPARATION

1. Mix the hibiscus-infused oil with rosehip and frankincense essential oils.
2. Apply a few drops to the face and neck after cleansing.
3. Use daily for best results.

Benefits: Hibiscus, often called the "Botox plant," helps firm and lift the skin while minimizing the appearance of fine lines and wrinkles. Rosehip oil is packed with vitamin C and fatty acids that support skin regeneration, while frankincense essential oil promotes collagen production. This facial oil deeply nourishes and rejuvenates aging skin.

Burdock Root Skin Detox Tea

INGREDIENTS

- 1 teaspoon dried burdock root
- 1 cup boiling water

PREPARATION

1. Steep burdock root in boiling water for 10 minutes.
2. Strain and drink 1-2 times daily.

Benefits: Burdock root is a natural blood purifier that helps detoxify the skin from the inside out. It promotes clear, radiant skin by flushing out toxins and supporting liver function. Regular consumption can reduce acne, eczema, and other skin conditions caused by impurities in the blood.

Lemon Balm Brightening Face Wash

INGREDIENTS

- 1 tablespoon dried lemon balm leaves
- 1 cup distilled water
- 1 teaspoon castile soap

PREPARATION

1. Steep lemon balm leaves in distilled water for 10 minutes, then strain.
2. Mix the lemon balm tea with castile soap.
3. Use as a gentle face wash, massaging onto wet skin, then rinse off with cool water.

Benefits: Lemon balm has natural brightening properties that help to even out skin tone and reduce dullness. It also soothes irritated skin and provides mild antibacterial benefits, making it suitable for sensitive and acne-prone skin. Castile soap gently cleanses without stripping the skin of its natural oils.

Horsetail Hair and Nail Strengthening Rinse

INGREDIENTS

- 1 tablespoon dried horsetail leaves
- 1 cup boiling water

PREPARATION

1. Steep the horsetail leaves in boiling water for 15 minutes.
2. Strain and use the liquid as a final rinse after washing your hair or soaking your nails.

Benefits: Horsetail is rich in silica, which strengthens hair and nails, helping to prevent breakage and promote growth. It also provides minerals that nourish the scalp and improve hair texture, leaving hair shiny and nails resilient.

Marshmallow Root Moisturizing Cream

INGREDIENTS

- 1 tablespoon marshmallow root powder
- 1/4 cup shea butter
- 2 tablespoons coconut oil

PREPARATION

1. Melt shea butter and coconut oil in a double boiler.
2. Stir in the marshmallow root powder until fully combined.
3. Allow the mixture to cool and solidify before applying to the skin.

Benefits: Marshmallow root has strong moisturizing and anti-inflammatory properties, making this cream ideal for dry, irritated, or sensitive skin. Shea butter and coconut oil further enhance hydration, creating a protective barrier to lock in moisture and soothe the skin.

Red Clover Skin Renewal Elixir

INGREDIENTS

- 1 tablespoon dried red clover flowers
- 1 cup water

PREPARATION

1. Simmer red clover flowers in water for 10 minutes, then strain.
2. Apply the elixir to clean skin using a cotton pad or add to your bath.

Benefits: Red clover is rich in isoflavones that promote skin regeneration and improve elasticity, making it beneficial for mature skin. It helps reduce signs of aging, such as wrinkles and fine lines, and soothes inflammatory skin conditions like eczema and psoriasis.

Nettle Leaf Skin Purifying Infusion

INGREDIENTS

- 1 teaspoon dried nettle leaves
- 1 cup boiling water

PREPARATION

1. Steep nettle leaves in boiling water for 10 minutes, then strain.
2. Drink daily or use as a skin rinse.

Benefits: Nettle is a natural detoxifier that purifies the blood and skin. It helps clear up acne and other skin issues by reducing inflammation and promoting the elimination of toxins. Regular use improves overall skin clarity and radiance.

Sage and Rosemary Pore-Reducing Toner

INGREDIENTS

- 1 teaspoon dried sage leaves
- 1 teaspoon dried rosemary leaves
- 1 cup distilled water

PREPARATION

1. Steep sage and rosemary leaves in boiling water for 10 minutes, then strain.
2. Allow the mixture to cool and apply to the face using a cotton pad.

Benefits: Sage and rosemary have natural astringent properties that tighten the skin and reduce the appearance of pores. This toner helps control excess oil production, preventing acne and leaving the skin smooth and toned.

Thyme Antimicrobial Face Cleanser

INGREDIENTS

- 1 tablespoon dried thyme
- 1 cup distilled water
- 1 teaspoon castile soap

PREPARATION

1. Steep thyme in boiling water for 10 minutes, then strain.
2. Mix the thyme tea with castile soap.

3. Use the mixture to cleanse the face, then rinse off with warm water.

Benefits: Thyme is a powerful antimicrobial herb that helps fight bacteria and clear up acne. This face cleanser gently cleanses the skin, removing dirt and impurities while reducing inflammation and preventing future breakouts.

Dandelion Leaf Skin Clarifying Tea

INGREDIENTS

- 1 teaspoon dried dandelion leaves
- 1 cup boiling water

PREPARATION

1. Steep dandelion leaves in boiling water for 10 minutes, then strain.
2. Drink 1-2 times daily for clearer skin.

Benefits: Dandelion leaf tea is a natural detoxifier that helps flush toxins from the body, which in turn clears the skin. It is particularly beneficial for reducing acne, eczema, and other skin conditions caused by internal imbalances. This tea also supports liver health, which is crucial for maintaining clear and healthy skin.

Comfrey Healing Balm for Scars

INGREDIENTS

- 1 tablespoon dried comfrey root
- 1/4 cup olive oil
- 1 tablespoon beeswax

PREPARATION

1. Infuse comfrey root in olive oil by heating in a double boiler for 30 minutes.
2. Strain and discard the comfrey root.
3. Melt beeswax and mix into the infused oil.
4. Pour into a small jar and allow to cool before using.

Benefits: Comfrey is rich in allantoin, a compound that promotes cell regeneration and heals damaged skin. This balm is highly effective for reducing the appearance of scars, promoting wound healing, and soothing irritated skin. It helps restore the skin's natural texture and elasticity.

Yarrow Anti-Inflammatory Skin Spray

INGREDIENTS

- 1 teaspoon dried yarrow flowers
- 1 cup distilled water

PREPARATION

1. Steep yarrow flowers in boiling water for 10 minutes, then strain.
2. Allow to cool and transfer to a spray bottle.
3. Spritz onto irritated or inflamed skin as needed.

Benefits: Yarrow is well-known for its anti-inflammatory and wound-healing properties. This spray helps reduce redness, soothe irritation, and promote healing for minor cuts, rashes, and insect bites. It is particularly effective for sensitive skin prone to inflammation.

Peppermint Foot and Hand Scrub

INGREDIENTS

- 1/4 cup coarse sea salt
- 1 tablespoon coconut oil
- 5 drops peppermint essential oil

PREPARATION

1. Mix sea salt, coconut oil, and peppermint essential oil together to form a scrub.
2. Gently massage the scrub onto feet or hands, then rinse off with warm water.

Benefits: Peppermint essential oil has a cooling effect that refreshes tired feet and hands, while the sea salt exfoliates dead skin, leaving the skin smooth and rejuvenated. Coconut oil moisturizes and protects the skin, making this scrub perfect for dry or rough areas.

Licorice Root Pigmentation Balance Cream

INGREDIENTS

- 1 teaspoon licorice root powder
- 1/4 cup shea butter
- 2 tablespoons coconut oil

PREPARATION

1. Melt shea butter and coconut oil in a double boiler.
2. Stir in the licorice root powder.
3. Allow the mixture to cool and solidify before applying to areas of pigmentation.

Benefits: Licorice root contains glabridin, which helps reduce the appearance of dark spots and hyperpigmentation by inhibiting melanin production. Combined with shea butter and coconut oil, this cream nourishes and brightens the skin, evening out skin tone over time.

Gotu Kola Wrinkle Reducing Serum

INGREDIENTS

- 1 tablespoon gotu kola powder
- 1 tablespoon jojoba oil
- 5 drops rosehip oil

PREPARATION

1. Mix gotu kola powder with jojoba and rosehip oils.
2. Apply a few drops of the serum to the face and neck, massaging in circular motions.
3. Use daily for best results.

Benefits: Gotu kola is a powerful herb that stimulates collagen production, reducing the appearance of wrinkles and fine lines. Rosehip oil enhances the serum's anti-aging effects, providing essential nutrients that promote skin regeneration and elasticity. This serum leaves the skin looking youthful and firm.

Violet Leaf Skin Soothing Cream

INGREDIENTS

- 1 tablespoon dried violet leaves
- 1/4 cup coconut oil
- 2 tablespoons beeswax

PREPARATION

1. Infuse violet leaves in coconut oil by heating in a double boiler for 30 minutes.
2. Strain and discard the leaves.
3. Melt beeswax and stir into the infused oil.
4. Pour into a jar and let it cool before applying to the skin.

Benefits: Violet leaves have soothing and anti-inflammatory properties that calm irritated and sensitive skin. This cream is perfect for eczema, dry patches, and skin rashes. It provides deep moisture and relieves inflammation, leaving the skin soft and hydrated.

Turmeric and Honey Face Mask

INGREDIENTS

- 1 teaspoon turmeric powder
- 1 tablespoon honey

PREPARATION

1. Mix turmeric powder and honey to form a paste.
2. Apply the paste to clean skin and leave on for 10-15 minutes.
3. Rinse off with warm water.

Benefits: Turmeric has powerful anti-inflammatory and antioxidant properties that brighten the skin and reduce acne scars. Honey adds moisture and has antibacterial effects, making this mask a perfect combination for improving skin tone, treating acne, and giving the skin a radiant glow.

Basil Anti-Acne Spot Treatment

INGREDIENTS

- 1 tablespoon dried basil leaves
- 1 cup boiling water

PREPARATION

1. Steep basil leaves in boiling water for 15 minutes, then strain.
2. Apply the basil tea to acne spots using a cotton ball.
3. Use twice daily for best results.

Benefits: Basil has strong antibacterial and anti-inflammatory properties that help reduce acne breakouts and calm irritated skin. This spot treatment clears up pimples and prevents future blemishes by killing acne-causing bacteria and soothing inflammation.

Fennel Seed Rejuvenating Face Oil

INGREDIENTS

- 1 tablespoon fennel seed-infused oil
- 5 drops frankincense essential oil

PREPARATION

1. Mix fennel seed-infused oil with frankincense essential oil.
2. Apply a few drops to the face and neck, massaging in circular motions.
3. Use daily for rejuvenated skin.

Benefits: Fennel seeds are rich in antioxidants that protect the skin from free radical damage, while frankincense essential oil promotes cell regeneration and reduces the appearance of fine lines. This face oil deeply nourishes the skin, leaving it smooth, firm, and youthful.

Chamomile Lip Moisturizing Balm

INGREDIENTS

- 1 tablespoon dried chamomile flowers
- 2 tablespoons beeswax
- 1 tablespoon coconut oil

PREPARATION

1. Infuse chamomile flowers in coconut oil by heating in a double boiler for 30 minutes.

2. Strain and discard the flowers.
3. Melt beeswax and stir into the infused oil.
4. Pour into a small container and let it solidify before using.

Benefits: Chamomile soothes and hydrates dry, chapped lips, while beeswax creates a protective barrier to lock in moisture. Coconut oil adds deep hydration, making this balm ideal for healing and preventing cracked lips. It leaves the lips soft and moisturized.

Sandalwood Soothing Face Mist

INGREDIENTS

- 1 teaspoon sandalwood powder
- 1 cup distilled water

PREPARATION

1. Mix sandalwood powder with distilled water and transfer to a spray bottle.
2. Mist onto the face as needed for a cooling effect.

Benefits: Sandalwood is known for its calming and cooling properties, making this face mist perfect for soothing irritated or sunburned skin. It also helps reduce redness and leaves the skin feeling refreshed and hydrated throughout the day.

Grapeseed Oil Anti-Aging Serum

INGREDIENTS

- 1 tablespoon grapeseed oil
- 5 drops rosehip oil
- 5 drops lavender essential oil

PREPARATION

1. Mix grapeseed oil with rosehip and lavender essential oils.
2. Apply a few drops to the face and neck before bedtime.
3. Use daily for best results.

Benefits: Grapeseed oil is a lightweight oil rich in antioxidants and essential fatty acids, which protect the skin from environmental damage and reduce signs of aging. Rosehip oil promotes collagen production, while lavender essential oil soothes and regenerates the skin. This serum improves skin texture and reduces the appearance of wrinkles.

Lemon Peel Brightening Exfoliant

INGREDIENTS

- 1 tablespoon dried lemon peel powder
- 1 tablespoon sugar
- 1 teaspoon honey

PREPARATION

1. Mix lemon peel powder, sugar, and honey to form a paste.
2. Gently massage onto damp skin, then rinse off with warm water.
3. Use 2-3 times a week.

Benefits: Lemon peel powder is rich in vitamin C, which brightens the skin and helps reduce dark spots. Sugar gently exfoliates dead skin cells, while honey provides moisture, leaving the skin smooth, glowing, and more even-toned.

Elderflower and Honey Face Mask

INGREDIENTS

- 1 tablespoon dried elderflowers
- 1 tablespoon honey

PREPARATION

1. Grind elderflowers into a fine powder.
2. Mix the elderflower powder with honey to form a paste.
3. Apply the mask to clean skin and leave on for 10-15 minutes.
4. Rinse off with warm water.

Benefits: Elderflowers are rich in antioxidants that protect the skin from aging and environmental damage. Combined with honey's moisturizing and antibacterial properties, this mask leaves the skin soft, smooth, and radiant. It is perfect for soothing sensitive or mature skin.

Catnip Calming Face Spray

INGREDIENTS

- 1 teaspoon dried catnip leaves
- 1 cup distilled water

PREPARATION

1. Steep catnip leaves in boiling water for 10 minutes, then strain.
2. Transfer to a spray bottle and mist onto the face as needed.

Benefits: Catnip has natural calming properties that soothe irritated or inflamed skin. This spray helps reduce redness, calm sensitive skin, and provide relief from stress-induced breakouts or rashes. It is particularly beneficial for skin prone to inflammation or sensitivity.

Echinacea Skin Healing Lotion

INGREDIENTS

- 1 tablespoon dried echinacea root
- 1/4 cup shea butter
- 1/4 cup coconut oil

PREPARATION

1. Infuse echinacea root in coconut oil by heating in a double boiler for 30 minutes.
2. Strain and discard the root.
3. Melt shea butter and mix with the echinacea-infused oil.
4. Pour into a jar and let it cool before applying to the skin.

Benefits: Echinacea is known for its immune-boosting and anti-inflammatory properties, which promote healing of the skin. This lotion is ideal for soothing irritated or damaged skin, reducing redness, and speeding up the recovery of minor wounds, rashes, or acne. It also moisturizes and nourishes the skin deeply.

BOOK 8

Herbal Remedies for Pain Relief

Natural Approaches to Pain Management

HOLISTIC STRATEGIES FOR MANAGING PAIN NATURALLY

Pain is a complex and often debilitating condition that can affect various aspects of life, from physical activity to emotional well-being. While conventional pain relief methods like pharmaceuticals offer quick solutions, they often come with side effects and the risk of dependency. Natural approaches to pain management provide effective alternatives that not only alleviate discomfort but also address the root causes of pain, supporting overall health and balance. For individuals like Emma, who seek sustainable and holistic solutions, understanding these approaches offers a way to manage pain naturally and safely. Below, we explore several natural pain management strategies, each targeting different types of pain while promoting long-term wellness.

Anti-Inflammatory Herbs: Reducing Pain at Its Source

Inflammation is a common underlying cause of pain, especially in conditions such as arthritis, muscle soreness, and injuries. Reducing inflammation is a crucial step in managing pain naturally, and certain herbs like **turmeric**, **ginger**, and **willow bark** are particularly effective in this regard.

Turmeric, with its active compound curcumin, is one of the most powerful anti-inflammatory herbs available. It works by inhibiting inflammatory pathways in the body, reducing swelling and pain associated with chronic conditions like arthritis. Turmeric can be consumed as a tea, added to meals, or taken as a supplement, providing a versatile and effective way for individuals like Emma to integrate it into their daily routines. For Emma, using turmeric regularly can help manage joint pain and reduce stiffness, ensuring she maintains her active lifestyle without discomfort.

Ginger is another potent anti-inflammatory herb, known for its ability to reduce muscle pain and soreness, particularly after physical activity. It works by blocking inflammatory compounds and increasing circulation, promoting healing and relief. A simple ginger tea made from fresh ginger slices can provide immediate soothing effects, while incorporating ginger into meals ensures consistent anti-inflammatory support. For those like Emma who value natural and accessible remedies, ginger serves as a practical solution for managing both acute and chronic pain.

Willow Bark, often referred to as nature's aspirin, contains salicin, a compound that reduces pain and inflammation. It is particularly effective for headaches, lower back pain, and joint discomfort. Consuming willow bark as a tea or tincture offers a natural and gentle approach to pain relief, making it suitable for regular use without the risks associated with synthetic medications. For Emma, who might seek alternatives to over-the-counter painkillers, willow bark provides a holistic option that supports her goal of maintaining health naturally.

Relaxation Techniques and Muscle Soothers

Tension and stress are significant contributors to pain, particularly in the muscles and joints. Herbs like **lav-**

ender, **valerian**, and **peppermint** not only relieve pain but also promote relaxation, reducing the impact of stress on the body.

Lavender is widely used for its calming properties, making it effective for managing tension headaches and muscle spasms. The essential oil of lavender can be applied topically to sore areas or added to a warm bath, providing a soothing effect that relaxes both the muscles and the mind. For Emma, incorporating lavender oil into her evening routine, perhaps through a massage or bath, can help alleviate tension and promote restful sleep, which is essential for pain management.

Valerian, known as a natural muscle relaxant, is particularly effective for treating cramps and spasms. It contains compounds that help relax the central nervous system, making it useful for conditions like menstrual cramps or muscle pain related to stress and anxiety. Valerian tea or tinctures can be used during periods of pain, offering a gentle yet effective approach to relaxation. Emma, who might experience muscle tension due to long work hours or physical activity, can benefit from using valerian as part of her self-care regimen.

Peppermint, with its high menthol content, provides a cooling and relaxing effect on muscles. It is effective for treating both tension headaches and muscle pain when applied as an essential oil or consumed as tea. A peppermint-infused compress applied to the forehead or neck can provide immediate relief for headaches, while a warm peppermint tea supports relaxation from the inside out. For Emma, using peppermint in these forms offers quick and accessible relief, fitting seamlessly into her active lifestyle.

Adaptogenic Herbs for Long-Term Pain Management

Chronic pain is often linked to stress, fatigue, and overall imbalance in the body. Adaptogenic herbs, such as **ashwagandha**, **rhodiola**, and **holy basil**, help the body adapt to stress and restore balance, reducing the intensity of chronic pain over time.

Ashwagandha is a powerful adaptogen that supports the body's response to stress and inflammation, making it effective for managing chronic pain conditions like fibromyalgia or arthritis. It works by modulating the body's stress hormone levels, reducing inflammation, and improving energy levels. Consuming ashwagandha as a powder in smoothies or taking it in capsule form can provide long-term benefits, helping Emma maintain balance and manage pain naturally.

Rhodiola is another adaptogen known for its ability to boost energy and reduce pain associated with physical and mental fatigue. It supports the nervous system, improving resilience to stress and reducing the impact of chronic pain. For Emma, who may experience periods of exhaustion due to her demanding schedule, rhodiola offers a way to enhance her stamina while supporting her pain management goals.

Holy Basil, also known as tulsi, provides both anti-inflammatory and adaptogenic properties. It helps reduce joint pain and muscle soreness while enhancing the body's response to stress. Drinking holy basil tea or taking a tincture can offer daily support for those managing chronic pain. For Emma, using holy basil regularly ensures she receives consistent benefits, supporting her body's resilience to stress and inflammation naturally.

By integrating these natural approaches, individuals can effectively manage pain without relying on synthetic medications, promoting long-term health and wellness.

Herbs for Joint, Muscle, and Chronic Pain

POWERFUL HERBS FOR MANAGING JOINT, MUSCLE, AND CHRONIC PAIN

Managing joint, muscle, and chronic pain holistically involves utilizing herbs that not only alleviate discomfort but also support the body's natural healing processes. These herbs offer anti-inflammatory, analgesic, and muscle-relaxant properties, providing effective and sustainable alternatives to conventional pain relief methods. For individuals like Emma, who seek natural solutions to maintain an active and balanced lifestyle, understanding these herbs can empower them to manage pain while promoting overall wellness. Below are some of the most effective herbs for addressing joint, muscle, and chronic pain, each offering unique properties tailored to different types of discomfort.

Turmeric: A Potent Anti-Inflammatory for Joint Pain

Turmeric is one of the most well-known herbs for pain relief, particularly effective for joint pain caused by arthritis or inflammation. The active compound in turmeric, **curcumin**, has strong anti-inflammatory properties that help reduce swelling and stiffness in the joints. By blocking inflammatory pathways, curcumin alleviates pain and promotes mobility, making it an essential herb for anyone dealing with joint issues.

For Emma, who may experience occasional joint discomfort from physical activities, incorporating turmeric into her daily routine—whether through capsules, teas, or as an addition to meals—can provide long-term benefits. To enhance curcumin absorption, combining turmeric with black pepper (which contains piperine) increases its effectiveness, ensuring Emma gets the maximum relief and support for her joint health.

Boswellia: Reducing Chronic Inflammation

Boswellia, also known as Indian frankincense, is another powerful herb for managing chronic inflammation and joint pain. The active compounds in boswellia, called boswellic acids, inhibit the inflammatory enzymes that contribute to pain and swelling, making it effective for conditions like rheumatoid arthritis and osteoarthritis. Regular use of boswellia helps improve joint flexibility and reduce stiffness, supporting both short-term relief and long-term joint health.

For individuals like Emma who seek sustainable solutions for managing chronic joint pain, boswellia supplements or extracts offer an accessible option. Unlike synthetic medications, boswellia has fewer side effects, allowing for consistent use that supports overall well-being and joint function.

Arnica: Fast Relief for Muscle Pain and Bruises

Arnica is a highly effective herb for treating muscle pain, bruises, and inflammation caused by injuries or overexertion. It contains **sesquiterpene lactones**, compounds that reduce inflammation and stimulate blood circulation, accelerating the healing process. Arnica is often applied topically as a cream, gel, or oil, providing targeted relief directly to the affected area.

Emma, who may experience muscle soreness from exercise or physical strain, can benefit from using arnica gel after workouts or stressful activities. Applying arnica to sore muscles not only reduces pain but also prevents the development of stiffness and swelling, ensuring she remains active and comfortable throughout her daily routine.

Ginger: Muscle Relaxant and Pain Reliever

Ginger is another versatile herb with powerful anti-inflammatory and analgesic properties, making it suitable for both joint and muscle pain. It works by blocking pro-inflammatory compounds, reducing swelling, and providing natural pain relief. Ginger is particularly effective for muscle pain resulting from physical exertion, cramps, or chronic conditions such as fibromyalgia.

For those like Emma, who might seek accessible and effective remedies, ginger tea is a simple solution. Fresh ginger can be steeped in hot water to create a warming, anti-inflammatory tea that supports muscle relaxation and reduces pain. Ginger can also be used in compresses or added to baths, offering a versatile approach to muscle and joint care.

Devil's Claw: Long-Term Joint Support

Devil's claw is an herb native to southern Africa, traditionally used to treat pain and inflammation, especially in the joints. Its active compounds, **harpagosides**, have been shown to reduce pain and improve joint function, making it particularly effective for arthritis and chronic joint conditions. Devil's claw not only reduces pain but also supports joint health by enhancing mobility and flexibility over time.

For Emma, who may seek holistic approaches to support her long-term joint health, devil's claw capsules or tinctures offer an option that aligns with her natural wellness values. By integrating this herb into her daily routine, she can manage joint pain sustainably, ensuring mobility and comfort in her active lifestyle.

White Willow Bark: The Natural Aspirin

White willow bark is often referred to as nature's aspirin due to its high content of **salicin**, a compound that reduces pain and inflammation. It has been used for centuries to alleviate joint pain, muscle soreness, and chronic discomfort. White willow bark is particularly beneficial for those experiencing ongoing pain, as it provides consistent relief with fewer side effects compared to synthetic painkillers.

White willow bark can be consumed as a tea or taken in capsule form, making it accessible for daily use. For Emma, using white willow bark provides an alternative to over-the-counter medications, allowing her to manage pain naturally without the risks of long-term pharmaceutical use. This herb supports her goal of maintaining health and wellness through natural, sustainable means.

Cayenne Pepper: Warming Relief for Muscle and Joint Pain

Cayenne pepper, or **capsaicin**, is another effective herb for managing pain, particularly for conditions like muscle soreness, arthritis, and neuropathic pain. Capsaicin works by depleting **substance P**, a chemical that transmits pain signals to the brain. By reducing the intensity of these signals, cayenne offers significant pain relief, particularly when applied topically.

Cayenne-infused creams or ointments can be used on sore muscles or joints, providing a warming sensation that enhances blood circulation and reduces stiffness. For Emma, using a capsaicin cream after physical activities or during periods of joint discomfort offers quick and effective relief, ensuring she can maintain her active lifestyle with ease.

These herbs offer a comprehensive approach to managing joint, muscle, and chronic pain, providing natural alternatives that align with holistic health values. By incorporating these remedies into daily routines, individuals can achieve pain relief while supporting long-term wellness and mobility.

Remedies for Pain Relief and Inflammation Control

White Willow Bark Pain Relief Tea

INGREDIENTS

- 1 teaspoon dried white willow bark
- 1 cup boiling water

PREPARATION

1. Steep white willow bark in boiling water for 10-15 minutes.
2. Strain and drink 1-2 times a day as needed for pain relief.

Benefits: White willow bark contains salicin, which is a natural compound similar to aspirin. It is highly effective for reducing pain and inflammation, making it useful for headaches, back pain, and joint discomfort. Its anti-inflammatory properties also support long-term pain management.

Arnica Muscle Relief Gel

INGREDIENTS

- 1 tablespoon arnica oil
- 1 tablespoon aloe vera gel

PREPARATION

1. Mix arnica oil with aloe vera gel until well combined.
2. Apply to sore muscles, massaging gently into the skin.
3. Use as needed for muscle relief.

Benefits: Arnica is known for its ability to reduce inflammation and speed up healing of bruises and muscle strains. Combined with aloe vera, this gel helps soothe sore muscles, reduce swelling, and promote faster recovery after physical exertion or injury.

Devil's Claw Joint Support Capsules

INGREDIENTS

- 1 tablespoon devil's claw root powder
- Capsule shells

PREPARATION

1. Fill capsule shells with devil's claw root powder.

2. Take 1-2 capsules daily for joint support.

Benefits: Devil's claw is a powerful anti-inflammatory herb that is especially beneficial for reducing joint pain and stiffness. It has been shown to improve mobility and reduce discomfort in people with arthritis or other joint-related issues. Regular use helps manage chronic pain and improve quality of life.

St. John's Wort Nerve Pain Oil

INGREDIENTS

- 1/4 cup St. John's wort oil
- 5 drops lavender essential oil

PREPARATION

1. Mix St. John's wort oil with lavender essential oil.
2. Apply to areas of nerve pain and massage gently.
3. Use as needed for relief.

Benefits: St. John's wort is renowned for its ability to soothe nerve pain, including conditions like sciatica and neuropathy. It helps calm inflammation around the nerves, reducing pain and promoting healing. The addition of lavender essential oil enhances the calming and anti-inflammatory effects of this remedy.

Turmeric and Black Pepper Anti-Inflammatory Paste

INGREDIENTS

- 1 tablespoon turmeric powder
- 1/4 teaspoon black pepper
- 1 tablespoon coconut oil

PREPARATION

1. Mix turmeric powder, black pepper, and coconut oil to form a paste.
2. Apply the paste to inflamed areas and leave it on for 20-30 minutes.
3. Rinse off with warm water.

Benefits: Turmeric contains curcumin, a potent anti-inflammatory compound that helps reduce swelling and pain. Black pepper enhances the absorption of curcumin, making this paste highly effective for managing chronic pain caused by conditions like arthritis and muscle inflammation. Coconut oil moisturizes the skin while delivering the active ingredients.

Boswellia (Frankincense) Arthritis Relief Capsules

INGREDIENTS

- 1 tablespoon boswellia powder
- Capsule shells

PREPARATION

1. Fill capsule shells with boswellia powder.
2. Take 1-2 capsules daily for arthritis relief.

Benefits: Boswellia, also known as frankincense, is a powerful anti-inflammatory herb that has been used for centuries to treat arthritis. It helps reduce joint pain, swelling, and stiffness, improving mobility and overall joint function. Regular use can help alleviate symptoms of osteoarthritis and rheumatoid arthritis.

Meadowsweet Headache Relief Infusion

INGREDIENTS

- 1 teaspoon dried meadowsweet leaves
- 1 cup boiling water

PREPARATION

1. Steep meadowsweet leaves in boiling water for 10 minutes.
2. Strain and drink at the onset of a headache.

Benefits: Meadowsweet contains natural salicylates, which are similar to the active ingredient in aspirin. This makes it an effective remedy for relieving headaches and reducing inflammation. Meadowsweet also soothes the digestive system, making it a gentle option for those who experience headaches with nausea.

Cayenne Pepper Muscle Rub

INGREDIENTS

- 1/2 teaspoon cayenne pepper powder
- 1/4 cup coconut oil

PREPARATION

1. Melt coconut oil in a double boiler and stir in the cayenne pepper powder.
2. Allow the mixture to cool slightly, then apply to sore muscles, massaging gently.
3. Use as needed for muscle pain relief.

Benefits: Cayenne pepper contains capsaicin, a compound known for its ability to relieve pain by blocking pain signals to the brain. This muscle rub helps reduce soreness, improve circulation, and promote healing in overworked or strained muscles. The heat from the cayenne also provides a soothing sensation to relieve discomfort.

Ginger and Lemongrass Pain Relief Balm

INGREDIENTS

- 1 tablespoon grated ginger
- 1 tablespoon chopped lemongrass
- 1/4 cup coconut oil

PREPARATION

1. Melt coconut oil in a double boiler and add the ginger and lemongrass.
2. Simmer the mixture for 15 minutes, then strain and allow it to cool.
3. Apply to areas of pain and massage gently.

Benefits: Ginger and lemongrass are both known for their anti-inflammatory and analgesic properties. This balm helps relieve pain from sore muscles, joint inflammation, and tension headaches. Ginger improves circulation, while lemongrass adds a refreshing scent and enhances the pain-relieving effects.

Skullcap Tension Headache Tea

INGREDIENTS

- 1 teaspoon dried skullcap leaves
- 1 cup boiling water

PREPARATION

1. Steep skullcap leaves in boiling water for 10 minutes.
2. Strain and drink when experiencing a tension headache.

Benefits: Skullcap is an herb known for its calming effects on the nervous system. It helps relieve tension headaches by reducing muscle spasms and promoting relaxation. This tea is particularly effective for headaches caused by stress, anxiety, or muscle tension in the neck and shoulders.

Valerian Root Muscle Relaxant Capsules

INGREDIENTS

- 1 tablespoon valerian root powder
- Capsule shells

PREPARATION

1. Fill capsule shells with valerian root powder.
2. Take 1-2 capsules before bed for muscle relaxation.

Benefits: Valerian root is a natural sedative that helps relax muscles and relieve tension. It is particularly useful for people who experience muscle pain or spasms at night, as it promotes restful sleep while easing discomfort. Regular use can help reduce muscle tension and improve sleep quality.

Cat's Claw Joint Support Elixir

INGREDIENTS

- 1 teaspoon dried cat's claw bark
- 1 cup boiling water

PREPARATION

1. Steep cat's claw bark in boiling water for 15 minutes.
2. Strain and drink daily for joint support.

Benefits: Cat's claw is a powerful anti-inflammatory herb that helps reduce joint pain and improve mobility. It is particularly beneficial for people with arthritis, as it reduces swelling and stiffness in the joints. Regular consumption can help support overall joint health and flexibility.

Feverfew Migraine Relief Tincture

INGREDIENTS

- 1/4 cup dried feverfew leaves
- 1/2 cup vodka or glycerin

PREPARATION

1. Place feverfew leaves in a jar and cover with vodka or glycerin.
2. Seal the jar and let it sit for 2-4 weeks, shaking occasionally.
3. Strain the tincture and take 1 teaspoon at the onset of a migraine.

Benefits: Feverfew has been used for centuries to prevent and treat migraines. It works by reducing inflammation and relaxing blood vessels, helping to alleviate the pain and sensitivity associated with migraines. This tincture is a fast-acting remedy for people who suffer from chronic migraines.

Lemon Verbena Anti-Inflammatory Compress

INGREDIENTS

- 1 teaspoon dried lemon verbena leaves
- 1 cup boiling water

PREPARATION

1. Steep lemon verbena leaves in boiling water for 10 minutes, then strain.
2. Soak a clean cloth in the tea and apply it as a compress to inflamed areas.
3. Leave the compress on for 15-20 minutes.

Benefits: Lemon verbena is a gentle anti-inflammatory herb that helps reduce swelling and soothe inflamed tissues. This compress is particularly effective for easing muscle or joint pain caused by overexertion or injury. It also provides a refreshing and calming effect on the skin.

Birch Bark Joint Pain Tea

INGREDIENTS

- 1 teaspoon dried birch bark
- 1 cup boiling water

PREPARATION

1. Steep birch bark in boiling water for 10 minutes.
2. Strain and drink once or twice daily for joint pain relief.

Benefits: Birch bark contains salicylates, which are similar to the active ingredient in aspirin. This makes it an effective remedy for relieving joint pain and inflammation, particularly in people with arthritis. Regular consumption helps improve joint mobility and reduce stiffness.

Eucalyptus Pain Relief Steam

INGREDIENTS

- 5-10 drops eucalyptus essential oil
- 1 bowl of hot water

PREPARATION

1. Add eucalyptus essential oil to the bowl of hot water.
2. Lean over the bowl and cover your head with a towel to trap the steam.
3. Inhale deeply for 10-15 minutes.

Benefits: Eucalyptus oil has strong anti-inflammatory and analgesic properties that help relieve pain and reduce swelling. This steam treatment is particularly effective for respiratory-related pain, headaches, and muscle tension. Inhaling the steam helps open airways and soothe inflamed tissues.

Wild Lettuce Pain Relief Drops

INGREDIENTS

- 1 teaspoon wild lettuce extract
- 1/4 cup water

PREPARATION

1. Dilute the wild lettuce extract in water.
2. Take the mixture 1-2 times daily as needed for pain relief.

Benefits: Wild lettuce is known as "nature's opium" for its strong pain-relieving properties. It works as a natural sedative, helping to reduce pain and promote relaxation without the side effects of pharmaceutical painkillers.

This remedy is particularly useful for chronic pain, muscle spasms, and insomnia caused by pain.

Marjoram Muscle Soothing Oil

INGREDIENTS

- 1 tablespoon marjoram-infused oil
- 5 drops lavender essential oil

PREPARATION

1. Mix marjoram-infused oil with lavender essential oil.
2. Apply to sore muscles and massage gently into the skin.
3. Use as needed for muscle relaxation.

Benefits: Marjoram is a natural muscle relaxant that helps ease tension and soreness. Combined with lavender, this oil provides a soothing effect that relieves muscle pain, promotes relaxation, and reduces stress. It is particularly beneficial after exercise or physical activity.

Yarrow Wound Healing Poultice

INGREDIENTS

- 1 tablespoon dried yarrow leaves
- 1 tablespoon water

PREPARATION

1. Mix dried yarrow leaves with water to form a paste.
2. Apply the paste directly to the wound or inflamed area.
3. Cover with a clean cloth and leave on for 20-30 minutes.

Benefits: Yarrow is known for its wound-healing properties, reducing inflammation and promoting tissue regeneration. It helps stop bleeding and disinfects minor cuts or scrapes, making this poultice an ideal remedy for first aid. The anti-inflammatory compounds also reduce swelling and pain in the affected area.

Nettle Joint Pain Relief Infusion

INGREDIENTS

- 1 teaspoon dried nettle leaves
- 1 cup boiling water

PREPARATION

1. Steep nettle leaves in boiling water for 10 minutes.
2. Strain and drink up to 3 times daily.

Benefits: Nettle has strong anti-inflammatory properties, making it effective in relieving joint pain and arthritis. It supports the body's natural detoxification process, helping to reduce swelling and stiffness in the joints. Regular consumption can improve mobility and reduce chronic pain.

Horsetail Bone and Joint Strength Tea

INGREDIENTS

- 1 teaspoon dried horsetail leaves
- 1 cup boiling water

PREPARATION

1. Steep horsetail leaves in boiling water for 10-15 minutes.
2. Strain and drink once or twice daily.

Benefits: Horsetail is rich in silica, which helps strengthen bones, joints, and connective tissues. This tea supports bone health and reduces inflammation in joints, making it beneficial for people with arthritis, osteoporosis, or recovering from bone injuries. Regular use can improve joint flexibility and bone density.

Clove Toothache Relief Oil

INGREDIENTS

- 5 drops clove essential oil
- 1 tablespoon coconut oil

PREPARATION

1. Mix clove essential oil with coconut oil.
2. Apply a small amount to the affected tooth using a cotton swab.
3. Repeat as needed to relieve pain.

Benefits: Clove oil is a powerful natural analgesic and antiseptic, commonly used to relieve toothaches. Its active compound, eugenol, numbs the area and reduces pain, while also helping to fight infection. This oil provides fast relief from toothache and gum pain.

Juniper Berry Muscle Pain Relief Salve

INGREDIENTS

- 1 tablespoon juniper berry-infused oil
- 2 tablespoons beeswax

PREPARATION

1. Melt beeswax in a double boiler and stir in juniper berry-infused oil.
2. Pour into a small jar and let it cool before applying to sore muscles.
3. Massage gently into the skin as needed for muscle pain relief.

Benefits: Juniper berries contain natural anti-inflammatory and pain-relieving properties, making this salve effective for sore muscles and joint pain. The warming effect of the juniper helps improve circulation and speed up recovery, providing soothing relief from aches and tension.

Celery Seed Inflammation Reduction Tea

INGREDIENTS

- 1 teaspoon dried celery seeds
- 1 cup boiling water

PREPARATION

1. Steep celery seeds in boiling water for 10 minutes.
2. Strain and drink once daily to reduce inflammation.

Benefits: Celery seeds are known for their anti-inflammatory and diuretic properties, helping to reduce swelling and discomfort associated with joint pain or arthritis. This tea promotes the elimination of excess fluids, reducing pressure on joints and improving overall mobility.

Chamomile Joint Pain Bath Soak

INGREDIENTS

- 1/2 cup dried chamomile flowers
- 1/4 cup Epsom salt

PREPARATION

1. Mix chamomile flowers and Epsom salt together.
2. Add the mixture to warm bathwater and soak for 20-30 minutes.

Benefits: Chamomile is a gentle anti-inflammatory herb that helps reduce pain and swelling in the joints. Combined with Epsom salts, which provide magnesium to relax muscles and ease discomfort, this bath soak is perfect for relieving joint pain, especially after a long day or physical exertion.

Black Cohosh Back Pain Capsules

INGREDIENTS

- 1 tablespoon black cohosh root powder
- Capsule shells

PREPARATION

1. Fill capsule shells with black cohosh root powder.
2. Take 1-2 capsules daily for back pain relief.

Benefits: Black cohosh is a powerful anti-inflammatory herb often used to treat muscle and joint pain, particularly in the back. It helps relax tense muscles and reduce inflammation, providing relief from chronic back pain and discomfort associated with conditions like sciatica.

Peppermint and Eucalyptus Cooling Pain Gel

INGREDIENTS

- 1 tablespoon aloe vera gel
- 5 drops peppermint essential oil
- 5 drops eucalyptus essential oil

PREPARATION

1. Mix aloe vera gel with peppermint and eucalyptus essential oils.
2. Apply to sore muscles or joints and massage gently.
3. Use as needed for pain relief.

Benefits: Peppermint and eucalyptus essential oils have cooling and anti-inflammatory properties that help soothe sore muscles and joints. This gel provides fast relief from pain and reduces inflammation, making it ideal for muscle strains, sprains, and general body aches.

Plantain Leaf Bruise Healing Poultice

INGREDIENTS

- 1 tablespoon fresh plantain leaves
- 1 tablespoon water

PREPARATION

1. Crush fresh plantain leaves and mix with water to form a paste.
2. Apply the paste directly to the bruise and cover with a clean cloth.
3. Leave on for 20-30 minutes.

Benefits: Plantain leaves are known for their wound-healing and anti-inflammatory properties. This poultice helps reduce swelling and discoloration from bruises, speeding up the healing process. It also provides relief from pain and prevents further tissue damage.

Helichrysum Pain Relief Cream

INGREDIENTS

- 1 tablespoon helichrysum-infused oil
- 2 tablespoons shea butter

PREPARATION

1. Melt shea butter in a double boiler and stir in the helichrysum-infused oil.
2. Pour into a jar and let it cool before applying to painful areas.
3. Massage gently into the skin as needed for pain relief.

Benefits: Helichrysum is a powerful anti-inflammatory and analgesic herb that helps relieve pain and reduce swelling. This cream is effective for treating sore muscles, joint pain, and even minor injuries. The shea butter provides moisture, helping to soothe and nourish the skin.

Ginger and Arnica Inflammation Relief Balm

INGREDIENTS

- 1 tablespoon grated ginger
- 1 tablespoon arnica oil
- 2 tablespoons coconut oil

PREPARATION

1. Melt coconut oil in a double boiler and add the grated ginger and arnica oil.
2. Simmer for 10 minutes, then strain and let the mixture cool.
3. Apply the balm to inflamed areas and massage gently.

Benefits: Ginger is a natural anti-inflammatory, and arnica helps reduce swelling and speed up healing. This balm is highly effective for relieving inflammation caused by muscle injuries, arthritis, or overexertion. It helps soothe pain, improve circulation, and promote recovery.

Rosemary and Olive Oil Joint Rub

INGREDIENTS

- 1 tablespoon dried rosemary leaves
- 1/4 cup olive oil

PREPARATION

1. Heat olive oil in a double boiler and add the dried rosemary leaves.
2. Simmer for 20 minutes, then strain and let the mixture cool.
3. Massage into sore joints for pain relief.

Benefits: Rosemary is a natural anti-inflammatory and analgesic herb that helps reduce joint pain and stiffness. Combined with olive oil, which provides deep moisture and nourishment, this joint rub improves flexibility and reduces discomfort associated with arthritis and other joint conditions.

Ashwagandha Anti-Inflammatory Decoction

INGREDIENTS

- 1 teaspoon dried ashwagandha root powder
- 1 cup water

PREPARATION

1. Simmer ashwagandha root powder in water for 10 minutes.
2. Strain and drink once daily for inflammation relief.

Benefits: Ashwagandha is an adaptogen that helps the body manage stress and reduces inflammation. This decoction is particularly useful for people with chronic inflammatory conditions like arthritis or autoimmune disorders, as it helps balance the immune response and reduce pain and swelling.

Mugwort Pain Relief Compress

INGREDIENTS

- 1 tablespoon dried mugwort leaves
- 1 cup boiling water

PREPARATION

1. Steep mugwort leaves in boiling water for 10 minutes, then strain.
2. Soak a clean cloth in the tea and apply as a compress to areas of pain.
3. Leave on for 15-20 minutes.

Benefits: Mugwort is a natural analgesic and anti-inflammatory herb that helps relieve pain and swelling. This compress is particularly effective for menstrual cramps, joint pain, and muscle soreness. It also helps calm the nervous system, making it beneficial for tension-related pain.

Wintergreen Muscle Ache Massage Oil

INGREDIENTS

- 1 tablespoon wintergreen-infused oil
- 1 tablespoon coconut oil

PREPARATION

1. Mix wintergreen-infused oil with coconut oil.
2. Massage into sore muscles and joints as needed for pain relief.

Benefits: Wintergreen oil contains methyl salicylate, a compound similar to aspirin that provides powerful pain relief. This massage oil is perfect for soothing muscle aches, joint pain, and inflammation. The cooling sensation of wintergreen also helps relax tight muscles and improve circulation.

BOOK 9

Sleep and Relaxation

The Importance of Sleep for Overall Wellness

WHY QUALITY SLEEP IS ESSENTIAL FOR OPTIMAL HEALTH

Sleep is a fundamental pillar of health, playing a critical role in physical, mental, and emotional well-being. It is not merely a time of rest; it is a period during which the body performs vital processes such as tissue repair, hormone regulation, and memory consolidation. For individuals like Emma, who may lead busy and demanding lifestyles, prioritizing quality sleep is crucial for maintaining overall health and ensuring daily vitality. Below, we explore the multifaceted importance of sleep and its impact on various aspects of wellness, emphasizing why it must be regarded as an essential component of any holistic health regimen.

The Role of Sleep in Physical Health

During sleep, the body enters a state of restoration, repairing tissues and muscles that have been stressed or damaged throughout the day. The production of growth hormone increases during deep sleep, which is essential for cell regeneration and muscle repair. For active individuals like Emma, who may engage in physical activities or have demanding work schedules, sufficient sleep ensures the body recovers properly, preventing muscle fatigue and injury.

Sleep is also integral to maintaining a healthy immune system. Studies have shown that during sleep, the body produces cytokines, proteins that help fight infection and inflammation. A lack of sleep can weaken the immune response, making the body more susceptible to illnesses such as colds and other infections. Emma, who values staying healthy to keep up with her responsibilities, benefits from prioritizing restful sleep as a natural way to enhance her immunity and resilience against daily stressors.

The Connection Between Sleep and Mental Wellness

Sleep is not only important for physical recovery but also for mental health and cognitive function. During deep and REM (Rapid Eye Movement) sleep stages, the brain processes and consolidates information, converting short-term memories into long-term storage. This function is crucial for maintaining memory, learning new skills, and ensuring cognitive clarity throughout the day.

Insufficient sleep, on the other hand, can impair cognitive function, leading to difficulties in concentration, decision-making, and memory retention. Over time, chronic sleep deprivation has been linked to increased risks of anxiety and depression. For Emma, who may juggle various responsibilities, ensuring adequate sleep helps maintain her mental sharpness, emotional balance, and ability to manage daily challenges effectively.

Sleep and Hormonal Balance

Another critical aspect of sleep is its impact on hormonal regulation. Hormones such as cortisol, insulin, and ghrelin are directly influenced by sleep cycles, playing significant roles in metabolism, stress management, and appetite control. During quality sleep, cortisol levels—

known as the body's primary stress hormone—are balanced, preparing the body for energy production in the morning. When sleep is disrupted, cortisol levels may remain elevated, leading to feelings of stress and fatigue throughout the day.

Additionally, sleep regulates ghrelin and leptin, hormones responsible for controlling hunger and fullness. Poor sleep can disrupt the balance of these hormones, leading to increased appetite and cravings, which may contribute to weight gain or other metabolic issues. For Emma, maintaining hormonal balance through restful sleep supports her in managing stress naturally and maintaining a healthy lifestyle, aligning with her preference for natural wellness practices.

Emotional Regulation and Sleep

The connection between sleep and emotional regulation is profound. The amygdala, a part of the brain responsible for emotional processing, is highly influenced by sleep quality. During REM sleep, the brain processes emotions, helping individuals manage and react to stressful situations with clarity and calmness. When sleep is insufficient, the amygdala becomes overactive, leading to heightened emotional responses and reduced control over mood and impulses.

For individuals like Emma, who may encounter stressful situations or need to balance professional and personal demands, achieving quality sleep helps her maintain emotional resilience and manage stress with composure. Prioritizing sleep allows her to stay emotionally balanced, ensuring she can navigate challenges effectively while supporting her overall well-being.

The Impact of Sleep on Skin and Beauty

Beyond internal health, sleep also plays a significant role in skin health and appearance. Often called "beauty sleep," quality rest allows the skin to repair itself, producing new collagen and preventing the development of fine lines and wrinkles. Blood flow to the skin increases during sleep, ensuring the skin receives the nutrients and oxygen needed for a healthy, glowing complexion.

Lack of sleep, conversely, can result in dull skin, dark circles, and inflammation, impacting one's overall appearance and self-confidence. For Emma, who may value maintaining her appearance alongside her health, ensuring consistent sleep supports her skin's natural repair processes, promoting a youthful and vibrant look that reflects her holistic lifestyle.

Creating a Sleep-Friendly Environment

To maximize the benefits of sleep, it is essential to create an environment conducive to rest. Factors like room temperature, light exposure, and noise levels significantly influence sleep quality. A cool, dark, and quiet room promotes deeper sleep cycles, allowing the body and mind to fully relax and recover.

For Emma, establishing a consistent sleep schedule and developing a nighttime routine that includes relaxing activities like reading, herbal teas, or meditation can enhance sleep quality. Incorporating natural sleep aids such as lavender essential oil or chamomile tea into her bedtime ritual further supports relaxation and ensures restorative sleep, aligning with her preference for natural, effective solutions.

Understanding the importance of sleep is a vital step in maintaining a holistic approach to health. For those like Emma, who aim for balanced and natural wellness, sleep serves as a cornerstone that supports physical, mental, and emotional health in a comprehensive and sustainable manner.

Herbs That Promote Restful Sleep and Relaxation

NATURAL HERBS FOR DEEP SLEEP AND RELAXATION

Achieving restful sleep and relaxation naturally can be greatly supported by the use of herbs. These plants have been used for centuries in traditional medicine to calm the nervous system, promote relaxation, and prepare the body for restorative sleep. For individuals like Emma, who seek holistic solutions to improve their sleep quality without relying on pharmaceuticals, understanding these herbs provides a pathway to achieving balance and tranquility. Below, we explore some of the most effective herbs for promoting restful sleep and relaxation, each offering unique properties tailored to different aspects of the sleep cycle and stress management.

Valerian Root: Nature's Sedative

Valerian root is one of the most well-known herbs for promoting sleep, often referred to as nature's sedative. It works by increasing gamma-aminobutyric acid (GABA) levels in the brain, a neurotransmitter that helps calm the nervous system and reduce anxiety. Valerian's ability to relax the body and mind makes it particularly effective for individuals who struggle with insomnia or restlessness at night.

Valerian root is commonly taken as a tea, tincture, or capsule before bedtime. For Emma, who may have a demanding schedule and could experience stress or anxiety that interferes with her sleep, incorporating valerian into her nightly routine offers a natural way to prepare her body for rest. By calming the nervous system, valerian helps transition the body into a relaxed state, promoting a deeper, more restorative sleep cycle.

Chamomile: The Classic Relaxant

Chamomile is another popular herb used to support relaxation and improve sleep quality. It contains apigenin, an antioxidant that binds to receptors in the brain, promoting a sense of calm and reducing insomnia. Chamomile tea is one of the most traditional ways to consume this herb, offering a gentle and soothing effect that can be easily incorporated into an evening ritual.

For Emma, who values natural and accessible remedies, a warm cup of chamomile tea an hour before bed serves as a simple yet effective way to unwind and prepare for sleep. Chamomile not only relaxes the body but also soothes the digestive system, making it a versatile herb that supports overall nighttime wellness. Its mild, floral flavor also provides a comforting experience, encouraging consistent use as part of a relaxing bedtime habit.

Passionflower: Calming the Mind

Passionflower is particularly effective for individuals who struggle with overthinking or anxiety, which can disrupt sleep patterns. It works similarly to valerian by increasing GABA levels in the brain, but it also has mild sedative effects that help quiet the mind and ease the transition into sleep. Passionflower is beneficial for those who experience racing thoughts at night, making it a valuable herb for promoting mental relaxation.

Passionflower can be consumed as a tea or tincture, offering flexibility in how it is used. For Emma, who may need additional support to calm her mind after a busy day, passionflower tea could be a practical solution. By integrating it into her nightly routine, Emma can reduce mental stress and achieve a more peaceful state before sleep, aligning with her holistic approach to health.

Lavender: A Multisensory Approach to Relaxation

Lavender is renowned for its soothing and calming properties, and it offers a multisensory approach to promoting sleep. The scent of lavender has been shown to reduce anxiety and improve sleep quality by slowing the heart rate and relaxing the nervous system. Lavender can be used as an essential oil in diffusers, added to baths, or applied topically as part of a massage oil.

For Emma, using lavender oil in her evening routine—whether diffusing it in her bedroom or adding a few drops to her pillow—creates a calming environment that supports her body's natural relaxation processes. The gentle aroma not only promotes physical relaxation but also enhances mood, helping Emma release the day's stress and prepare for restorative sleep.

Lemon Balm: Gentle Sedation for Stress Relief

Lemon balm is a gentle, yet powerful, herb that helps reduce anxiety and improve sleep. It belongs to the mint family and has mild sedative properties, making it effective for individuals who experience stress-related sleep disruptions. Lemon balm works by increasing GABA levels, promoting a calm state and easing the tension that can build up throughout the day.

Lemon balm tea is an excellent way to consume this herb, as it provides a light, refreshing flavor that pairs well with other sleep-promoting herbs like chamomile or passionflower. For Emma, combining lemon balm with other herbs in a tea blend can create a customized sleep aid that fits her specific needs, ensuring she receives a well-rounded approach to relaxation and stress relief before bed.

Hops: Supporting Deep Sleep Cycles

Hops, commonly associated with beer, also have significant benefits for sleep and relaxation. The herb contains compounds called **alpha acids** that promote sedation and relieve tension, making it particularly effective for those who have difficulty falling or staying asleep. Hops can be combined with valerian root to enhance their effects, offering a potent herbal remedy for deep sleep.

For Emma, who might need a more robust solution for occasional sleep disturbances, hops-infused tea or capsules provide a stronger option for achieving a restful night's sleep. Incorporating hops into her regimen ensures she has a natural, effective method to support deep and uninterrupted sleep cycles, aligning with her preference for sustainable and natural health practices.

By using these herbs thoughtfully, individuals can develop an effective, natural strategy for improving sleep quality and achieving relaxation. For Emma, these herbs offer a holistic and adaptable approach that integrates seamlessly into her wellness routine, supporting her in maintaining restful sleep and overall health.

Remedies for Sleep Support and Restorative Rest

Valerian Root Sleep Aid Tea

INGREDIENTS

- 1 teaspoon dried valerian root
- 1 cup boiling water

PREPARATION

1. Steep valerian root in boiling water for 10-15 minutes.
2. Strain and drink 30 minutes before bedtime.

Benefits: Valerian root is well-known for its sedative effects, helping to promote deep, restful sleep. It works by calming the nervous system, making it effective for reducing insomnia and anxiety. Regular consumption of this tea can lead to better sleep quality and relaxation.

Passionflower Restful Sleep Tincture

INGREDIENTS

- 1/4 cup dried passionflower
- 1/2 cup alcohol (vodka or glycerin for non-alcoholic option)

PREPARATION

1. Place the dried passionflower in a jar and cover with alcohol or glycerin.
2. Seal the jar and let it sit for 4-6 weeks, shaking occasionally.
3. Strain and store the tincture in a dark bottle. Take 1-2 droppers before bed.

Benefits: Passionflower helps increase levels of GABA in the brain, promoting relaxation and reducing anxiety. This tincture is perfect for those who struggle with restlessness, racing thoughts, or difficulty falling asleep.

Hops and Lavender Sleep Pillow Sachet

INGREDIENTS

- 1 tablespoon dried hops flowers
- 1 tablespoon dried lavender buds
- Small fabric sachet

PREPARATION

1. Mix the dried hops and lavender buds together.
2. Fill the fabric sachet with the mixture.
3. Place the sachet inside your pillowcase before bed.

Benefits: Hops and lavender are both calming herbs that promote relaxation and better sleep. The gentle fragrance of this sachet soothes the senses, reducing stress and anxiety, and creating a calming sleep environment. It's especially helpful for those who have trouble unwinding before bed.

Lemon Balm Evening Calming Elixir

INGREDIENTS

- 1 teaspoon dried lemon balm leaves
- 1 teaspoon honey
- 1 cup hot water

PREPARATION

1. Steep lemon balm leaves in hot water for 10 minutes.
2. Strain, then add honey and stir.
3. Drink warm 30 minutes before bedtime.

Benefits: Lemon balm is a gentle sedative that helps ease stress, anxiety, and mild insomnia. This calming elixir helps to relax both the mind and body, preparing you for a peaceful night's sleep. It's also beneficial for reducing digestive discomfort that can disrupt sleep.

California Poppy Nighttime Relaxation Capsules

INGREDIENTS

- 1 tablespoon dried California poppy powder
- Capsule shells

PREPARATION

1. Fill capsule shells with California poppy powder.
2. Take 1-2 capsules 30 minutes before bed.

Benefits: California poppy is a mild sedative that helps promote relaxation and reduce anxiety. It is particularly useful for those who suffer from difficulty falling asleep or staying asleep. Regular use can help regulate sleep patterns and improve sleep quality.

Chamomile and Skullcap Sleep-Inducing Infusion

INGREDIENTS

- 1 teaspoon dried chamomile flowers
- 1 teaspoon dried skullcap leaves
- 1 cup boiling water

PREPARATION

1. Steep chamomile and skullcap in boiling water for 10 minutes.
2. Strain and drink 30 minutes before bed.

Benefits: Chamomile is widely known for its calming properties, while skullcap helps to quiet the mind and relax the nervous system. This combination is perfect for inducing sleep, especially for those experiencing stress-related insomnia. Regular consumption helps improve sleep quality.

Ashwagandha Stress Relief Sleep Tonic

INGREDIENTS

- 1 teaspoon dried ashwagandha root powder
- 1 cup warm milk (or dairy alternative)
- 1 teaspoon honey

PREPARATION

1. Mix ashwagandha root powder into warm milk.
2. Add honey and stir well.
3. Drink 30 minutes before bedtime.

Benefits: Ashwagandha is an adaptogen that helps the body manage stress, making it easier to fall asleep. This tonic helps to calm the mind and body, reducing anxiety and promoting restorative sleep. It's particularly beneficial for people who experience sleep disturbances due to stress or worry.

Magnolia Bark Tranquility Drops

INGREDIENTS

- 1/4 cup magnolia bark
- 1/2 cup alcohol (vodka or glycerin for non-alcoholic option)

PREPARATION

1. Place magnolia bark in a jar and cover with alcohol or glycerin.
2. Seal the jar and let it sit for 4-6 weeks, shaking occasionally.
3. Strain and store in a dark bottle. Take 1-2 droppers 30 minutes before bed.

Benefits: Magnolia bark has sedative properties that promote relaxation and reduce cortisol levels, helping you to fall asleep faster and stay asleep longer. It is an excellent remedy for people with insomnia or anxiety-related sleep disturbances.

Catnip and Honey Sleepy Time Tea

INGREDIENTS

- 1 teaspoon dried catnip leaves
- 1 teaspoon honey
- 1 cup boiling water

PREPARATION

1. Steep catnip leaves in boiling water for 10 minutes.
2. Strain and add honey before drinking.

Benefits: Catnip has gentle sedative properties that help relax the mind and body, making it easier to fall asleep. The honey adds sweetness and helps calm the digestive system, making this tea a perfect bedtime drink for a restful night's sleep.

Linden Flower Bedtime Relaxation Tea

INGREDIENTS

- 1 teaspoon dried linden flowers
- 1 cup boiling water

PREPARATION

1. Steep linden flowers in boiling water for 10 minutes.
2. Strain and drink 30 minutes before bed.

Benefits: Linden flowers have calming properties that help to reduce tension and anxiety, promoting a state of relaxation before sleep. This tea is especially useful for people who experience stress-induced insomnia or restlessness. Regular consumption helps improve overall sleep quality.

Lavender and Lemon Verbena Sleep Balm

INGREDIENTS

- 1 tablespoon dried lavender flowers
- 1 tablespoon dried lemon verbena leaves
- 1/4 cup coconut oil

PREPARATION

1. Infuse lavender and lemon verbena in melted coconut oil using a double boiler for 30 minutes.
2. Strain and pour into a jar, allowing it to cool.
3. Apply the balm to your temples and wrists before bed.

Benefits: Lavender and lemon verbena are both calming herbs that promote relaxation and ease anxiety. This sleep balm helps to calm the nervous system and reduce stress, making it easier to fall asleep. It's especially helpful for people with anxiety or racing thoughts at bedtime.

Blue Vervain Night Calm Capsules

INGREDIENTS

- 1 tablespoon dried blue vervain powder
- Capsule shells

PREPARATION

1. Fill capsule shells with blue vervain powder.
2. Take 1-2 capsules 30 minutes before bed.

Benefits: Blue vervain is known for its calming effects on the nervous system, making it an excellent remedy for reducing stress and promoting restful sleep. It helps alleviate anxiety and tension, which can interfere with falling asleep or staying asleep.

Holy Basil (Tulsi) and Mint Evening Tea

INGREDIENTS

- 1 teaspoon dried holy basil (tulsi) leaves
- 1 teaspoon dried mint leaves
- 1 cup boiling water

PREPARATION

1. Steep holy basil and mint leaves in boiling water for 10 minutes.
2. Strain and drink 30 minutes before bed.

Benefits: Holy basil is an adaptogen that helps reduce stress and anxiety, while mint has a calming effect on the digestive system. This combination promotes relaxation and helps prepare the body and mind for a peaceful night's sleep.

Sweet Marjoram Aromatherapy Oil

INGREDIENTS

- 1 tablespoon sweet almond oil
- 5 drops sweet marjoram essential oil

PREPARATION

1. Mix sweet almond oil with sweet marjoram essential oil.

2. Apply to pulse points or use in a diffuser before bed.

Benefits: Sweet marjoram has calming and sedative properties that help reduce anxiety and promote restful sleep. The soothing aroma helps to create a peaceful environment, making it easier to relax and unwind before bedtime. It is especially beneficial for those who have difficulty falling asleep due to stress or worry.

Reishi Mushroom Sleep Support Decoction

INGREDIENTS

- 1 teaspoon dried reishi mushroom powder
- 1 cup water

PREPARATION

1. Simmer reishi mushroom powder in water for 15 minutes.
2. Strain and drink 30 minutes before bed.

Benefits: Reishi mushroom is an adaptogen that helps balance the body's stress response and supports restorative sleep. It promotes relaxation and enhances sleep quality by calming the nervous system. Regular consumption helps improve overall sleep patterns.

St. John's Wort Relaxation Elixir

INGREDIENTS

- 1 teaspoon dried St. John's wort leaves
- 1 cup boiling water
- 1 teaspoon honey

PREPARATION

1. Steep St. John's wort leaves in boiling water for 10 minutes.
2. Strain and add honey before drinking.

Benefits: St. John's wort is known for its mood-boosting and calming effects, making it an excellent remedy for reducing anxiety and promoting relaxation. This elixir helps calm the mind and body, making it easier to fall asleep and stay asleep through the night.

Ziziphus (Jujube) Sleep Aid Capsules

INGREDIENTS

- 1 tablespoon dried ziziphus powder
- Capsule shells

PREPARATION

1. Fill capsule shells with ziziphus powder.
2. Take 1-2 capsules 30 minutes before bed.

Benefits: Ziziphus is a traditional herb used in Chinese medicine for its sedative and sleep-inducing properties. It helps calm the mind and promote deep, restful sleep, making it an excellent remedy for insomnia or sleep disturbances.

Poppy Seed Night Rest Syrup

INGREDIENTS

- 1 tablespoon poppy seeds
- 1/4 cup honey
- 1/4 cup water

PREPARATION

1. Simmer poppy seeds in water for 10 minutes, then strain.
2. Mix the strained liquid with honey until fully dissolved.
3. Take 1-2 teaspoons of the syrup before bedtime.

Benefits: Poppy seeds have natural sedative properties that help induce sleep and relaxation. This syrup calms the nervous system and promotes a restful night's sleep, making it especially useful for people with insomnia or restlessness.

Licorice Root Sleep Harmony Tea

INGREDIENTS

- 1 teaspoon dried licorice root
- 1 cup boiling water

PREPARATION

1. Steep licorice root in boiling water for 10 minutes.
2. Strain and drink 30 minutes before bed.

Benefits: Licorice root is known for its soothing effects on the digestive and respiratory systems, both of which can affect sleep quality. It also helps reduce stress and promotes relaxation, creating a calming effect that encourages deep, restorative sleep.

Wild Lettuce Relaxing Drops

INGREDIENTS

- 1 teaspoon wild lettuce extract
- 1/4 cup water

PREPARATION

1. Mix wild lettuce extract with water.
2. Take 1-2 droppers of the mixture before bed.

Benefits: Wild lettuce has natural sedative and calming properties that help ease anxiety and reduce restlessness, making it easier to fall asleep. This remedy is especially beneficial for those who experience sleep disturbances due to chronic pain or muscle tension.

Fennel and Orange Blossom Sleep-Enhancing Tea

INGREDIENTS

- 1 teaspoon fennel seeds
- 1 teaspoon dried orange blossom petals
- 1 cup boiling water

PREPARATION

1. Steep fennel seeds and orange blossom petals in boiling water for 10 minutes.
2. Strain and drink 30 minutes before bedtime.

Benefits: Fennel helps relax the digestive system, while orange blossom promotes a sense of calm and relaxation. This tea is ideal for people who have trouble falling asleep due to digestive discomfort or stress. It creates a peaceful environment that supports restful sleep.

Rose Petal and Lavender Bedtime Bath Salts

INGREDIENTS

- 1/2 cup Epsom salts
- 1 tablespoon dried rose petals
- 1 tablespoon dried lavender buds

PREPARATION

1. Mix Epsom salts with rose petals and lavender buds.
2. Add the mixture to a warm bath and soak for 20-30 minutes before bed.

Benefits: This soothing bath blend combines the relaxing effects of lavender and rose petals with the muscle-relaxing properties of Epsom salts. It helps ease muscle tension, reduce stress, and create a calm, peaceful environment for restful sleep.

Lemon Balm and Rosemary Sleep Lotion

INGREDIENTS

- 1 tablespoon dried lemon balm leaves
- 1 tablespoon dried rosemary leaves
- 1/4 cup coconut oil

PREPARATION

1. Infuse lemon balm and rosemary in melted coconut oil using a double boiler for 30 minutes.
2. Strain and pour into a jar, allowing it to cool.
3. Apply the lotion to your hands and feet before bed.

Benefits: Lemon balm promotes relaxation, while rosemary helps improve circulation. This sleep lotion is perfect for easing tension and calming the body before bed, allowing for deeper and more restful sleep.

Hop Flower Evening Tea Blend

INGREDIENTS

- 1 teaspoon dried hop flowers
- 1 teaspoon dried chamomile flowers
- 1 cup boiling water

PREPARATION

1. Steep hop flowers and chamomile in boiling water for 10 minutes.
2. Strain and drink 30 minutes before bed.

Benefits: Hop flowers have natural sedative properties, making them perfect for promoting sleep. Combined with chamomile, this tea blend helps to relax the body and mind, reducing anxiety and preparing you for a peaceful night's sleep.

Anise Seed Digestive and Sleep Tea

INGREDIENTS

- 1 teaspoon anise seeds
- 1 cup boiling water

PREPARATION

1. Steep anise seeds in boiling water for 10 minutes.
2. Strain and drink 30 minutes before bed.

Benefits: Anise seeds help soothe digestive discomfort, which can often interfere with sleep. This tea is particularly beneficial for those who experience bloating or indigestion at night. It calms the stomach and promotes relaxation, making it easier to fall asleep.

Angelica Root Nighttime Infusion

INGREDIENTS

- 1 teaspoon dried angelica root
- 1 cup boiling water

PREPARATION

1. Steep angelica root in boiling water for 10 minutes.
2. Strain and drink 30 minutes before bed.

Benefits: Angelica root has calming properties that help reduce stress and promote relaxation. This infusion is particularly useful for people who experience difficulty falling asleep due to anxiety or nervous tension. It supports a calm and peaceful night's rest.

Wood Betony Relaxing Tincture

INGREDIENTS

- 1/4 cup dried wood betony leaves
- 1/2 cup alcohol (vodka or glycerin for non-alcoholic option)

PREPARATION

1. Place wood betony leaves in a jar and cover with alcohol or glycerin.
2. Seal the jar and let it sit for 4-6 weeks, shaking occasionally.
3. Strain and take 1-2 droppers before bed.

Benefits: Wood betony is an herb known for its ability to calm the nervous system and promote relaxation. This tincture helps to reduce anxiety, ease stress, and support deep, restful sleep. It's especially useful for people with insomnia or racing thoughts.

Hawthorn Berry Sleep Support Capsules

INGREDIENTS

- 1 tablespoon dried hawthorn berry powder
- Capsule shells

PREPARATION

1. Fill capsule shells with hawthorn berry powder.
2. Take 1-2 capsules 30 minutes before bed.

Benefits: Hawthorn berries are known for their calming effects on the heart and circulatory system, which can improve sleep quality. These capsules help reduce anxiety, lower blood pressure, and promote a sense of calm, making them ideal for supporting restful sleep.

Mugwort Dream-Enhancing Infusion

INGREDIENTS

- 1 teaspoon dried mugwort leaves
- 1 cup boiling water

PREPARATION

1. Steep mugwort leaves in boiling water for 10 minutes.
2. Strain and drink 30 minutes before bed.

Benefits: Mugwort is an herb traditionally used to enhance dreams and promote deep sleep. This infusion helps to stimulate vivid dreams and improve dream recall, while also promoting relaxation and reducing restlessness during the night.

Pine Needle Night Rest Steam

INGREDIENTS

- 1/4 cup fresh pine needles
- 1 bowl hot water

PREPARATION

1. Add fresh pine needles to a bowl of hot water.
2. Lean over the bowl, cover your head with a towel, and inhale the steam for 10-15 minutes.

Benefits: Pine needles have calming and respiratory-clearing properties. This steam treatment helps open airways, making it easier to breathe during sleep, while the calming scent promotes relaxation and restful sleep. It's especially helpful for those who suffer from congestion or respiratory issues at night.

Chamomile and Ginger Sleep Warming Drink

INGREDIENTS

- 1 teaspoon dried chamomile flowers
- 1/2 teaspoon grated ginger
- 1 cup boiling water

PREPARATION

1. Steep chamomile flowers and grated ginger in boiling water for 10 minutes.
2. Strain and drink warm 30 minutes before bed.

Benefits: Chamomile calms the nervous system, while ginger provides warmth and supports digestion. This warming drink helps relax the body and mind, promoting a peaceful night's sleep. It's particularly useful for those who experience cold extremities or digestive discomfort at night.

Skullcap and Honey Bedtime Tea

INGREDIENTS

- 1 teaspoon dried skullcap leaves
- 1 teaspoon honey
- 1 cup boiling water

PREPARATION

1. Steep skullcap leaves in boiling water for 10 minutes.
2. Strain and stir in honey before drinking.

Benefits: Skullcap is a calming herb that helps to quiet the mind and reduce anxiety, while honey adds a soothing sweetness that promotes relaxation. This bedtime tea is perfect for winding down after a stressful day and preparing for a restful night's sleep.

Baikal Skullcap Sleep Support Capsules

INGREDIENTS

- 1 tablespoon dried Baikal skullcap root powder
- Capsule shells

PREPARATION

1. Fill capsule shells with Baikal skullcap root powder.
2. Take 1-2 capsules 30 minutes before bed.

Benefits: Baikal skullcap is a traditional Chinese herb used for its sedative and calming properties. These capsules help to reduce anxiety, promote relaxation, and support deep, restorative sleep. They are particularly beneficial for people who struggle with insomnia or stress-related sleep disturbances.

Sweet Violet Restorative Night Tea

INGREDIENTS

- 1 teaspoon dried sweet violet leaves
- 1 cup boiling water

PREPARATION

1. Steep sweet violet leaves in boiling water for 10 minutes.
2. Strain and drink 30 minutes before bed.

Benefits: Sweet violet leaves have gentle sedative properties that promote relaxation and ease tension. This restorative tea helps to calm the mind and body, making it easier to fall asleep and stay asleep throughout the night. Regular consumption supports better sleep quality and overall well-being.

BOOK 10

Herbal Nutrition and Superfoods

Nutrient-Rich Herbs for Daily Use

EVERYDAY HERBS FOR NUTRIENT-RICH LIVING

Herbs are not just flavor enhancers; they are powerful sources of vitamins, minerals, and antioxidants that can significantly boost daily nutrition. Integrating nutrient-rich herbs into everyday meals is an effective way to support overall health, enhance energy levels, and promote wellness. For individuals like Emma, who seek natural ways to optimize their nutrition, these herbs provide accessible, versatile solutions that align with holistic health practices. Below, we explore some of the most nutrient-rich herbs for daily use, each offering specific benefits that contribute to a well-rounded and healthy diet.

Nettle: A Multivitamin in Plant Form

Nettle, often referred to as "nature's multivitamin," is packed with a wide array of nutrients, including vitamins A, C, K, and several B vitamins, as well as minerals like calcium, magnesium, and iron. This makes it an excellent herb for supporting bone health, energy levels, and immune function. Nettle is particularly beneficial for individuals who may experience fatigue or need a boost in their daily nutrient intake.

Nettle can be used in various ways: as an infusion (tea), added to soups, or sautéed like spinach. For Emma, incorporating nettle tea into her morning routine provides a simple and effective way to start the day with a nutrient boost. It's an ideal herb for those looking to naturally enhance their intake of essential vitamins and minerals while supporting overall vitality.

Dandelion: A Rich Source of Minerals

Dandelion is another powerhouse herb rich in essential nutrients like potassium, calcium, iron, and vitamins A, C, and E. Traditionally used for detoxification, dandelion supports liver health and digestion while also providing nutrients that contribute to bone strength and immune function. It is especially beneficial for maintaining hydration and electrolyte balance due to its high potassium content.

Dandelion leaves can be used in salads, added to green smoothies, or brewed as a tea. For someone like Emma, who values versatile and easy-to-use options, dandelion tea offers a convenient way to access its benefits throughout the day. Using fresh dandelion leaves in meals is also a great way to boost nutritional intake while adding a slight, pleasant bitterness that enhances digestion.

Parsley: More Than a Garnish

Often underestimated, parsley is a nutrient-rich herb that provides significant health benefits beyond its role as a garnish. It is high in vitamins A, C, and K, which are important for eye health, immune support, and blood clotting, respectively. Additionally, parsley is rich in flavonoids like apigenin, which have anti-inflammatory and antioxidant properties that support overall well-being.

Parsley can be incorporated into numerous dishes, such

as salads, soups, and sauces, making it an easy addition to daily meals. For Emma, adding fresh parsley to her meals ensures she gains the benefits of this nutrient-dense herb effortlessly, helping her maintain a balanced diet that aligns with her holistic health goals.

Basil: An Antioxidant Powerhouse

Basil is a well-loved herb not only for its flavor but also for its nutritional content. It contains vitamins A, C, and K, along with minerals such as calcium, magnesium, and iron. Basil is particularly rich in antioxidants, including beta-carotene and lutein, which help protect the body from oxidative stress and support vision and skin health.

Fresh basil leaves are a versatile ingredient that can be added to salads, pasta dishes, or blended into pesto. For Emma, who seeks to maximize her nutritional intake through simple and delicious means, using fresh basil in her cooking not only enhances the flavor of her meals but also ensures she benefits from its antioxidant properties, promoting both internal and external health.

Cilantro: Detoxifying and Nutritious

Cilantro is an herb well-known for its detoxifying properties, particularly in its ability to support heavy metal detoxification. Rich in vitamins A, C, and K, cilantro also provides important minerals like potassium and magnesium, supporting cardiovascular health and overall vitality. It is especially beneficial for individuals who may be exposed to environmental toxins, as its compounds bind to heavy metals, aiding in their removal from the body.

Cilantro can be used fresh in salads, salsas, and as a garnish for various dishes. For Emma, who appreciates herbs that serve dual functions—enhancing both flavor and health—cilantro is an excellent addition to her daily meals, offering a refreshing taste while supporting her body's natural detox processes.

Oregano: Immune Support in Every Leaf

Oregano is a potent herb rich in antioxidants like thymol and carvacrol, which have antibacterial, antiviral, and anti-inflammatory properties. It is also a good source of vitamin K, which is essential for bone health. Consuming oregano regularly can support the immune system and promote overall health, making it a valuable herb for individuals seeking to enhance their wellness naturally.

Oregano can be used fresh or dried, making it easy to incorporate into dishes such as soups, sauces, and salads. For Emma, who might prefer convenient options that integrate seamlessly into her cooking, oregano provides both flavor and health benefits, ensuring her meals are both delicious and nutritious.

Rosemary: Enhancing Cognitive Function

Rosemary is an herb traditionally used to support memory and cognitive function, thanks to its antioxidant and anti-inflammatory properties. It contains compounds like rosmarinic acid, which protects the brain from oxidative stress and supports overall brain health. Additionally, rosemary provides vitamins A, C, and B6, contributing to immune support and energy metabolism.

Adding fresh rosemary to roasted vegetables, meats, or soups allows individuals like Emma to access its cognitive and nutritional benefits effortlessly. Incorporating rosemary into meals not only enhances flavor but also offers a natural way to boost brain function, aligning with her goal of maintaining overall wellness through simple, natural methods.

These nutrient-rich herbs provide an accessible and effective way to boost daily nutrition while supporting a wide range of health benefits. For Emma, integrating these herbs into her routine offers a balanced approach to holistic wellness, ensuring her dietary needs are met naturally and sustainably.

Integrating Superfoods into a Balanced Diet

INCORPORATING SUPERFOODS INTO EVERYDAY NUTRITION

Superfoods are nutrient-dense foods that provide an array of health benefits beyond basic nutrition. Integrating these powerhouse foods into a balanced diet is an effective way to enhance overall wellness, boost energy levels, and support long-term health. For individuals like Emma, who prioritize natural solutions for optimal health, superfoods offer a convenient and versatile approach to elevate daily meals. Understanding how to include these foods in a balanced and sustainable manner ensures that they can become a regular and enjoyable part of the diet.

The Role of Superfoods in a Balanced Diet

Superfoods are rich in essential nutrients such as vitamins, minerals, antioxidants, and healthy fats. They work synergistically with other foods to boost immunity, improve digestion, and support heart and brain health. Incorporating superfoods like **chia seeds**, **spirulina**, and **goji berries** can turn simple meals into nutrient-packed options that support the body's needs.

For Emma, who may have a busy schedule, integrating superfoods into her meals must be both practical and efficient. Using superfoods in easy-to-prepare dishes like smoothies, salads, and snacks ensures she gets their benefits without spending too much time in the kitchen. Whether sprinkled over yogurt or blended into morning smoothies, superfoods can be seamlessly added to daily routines.

Simple Ways to Add Superfoods to Meals

Integrating superfoods doesn't require complex recipes or significant changes to daily habits. In fact, many superfoods are easy to incorporate into existing meals, enhancing their nutritional profile without much effort. Below are some accessible ways to add nutrient-dense superfoods into a balanced diet:

1. **Smoothie Boosters**

Smoothies are an excellent way to include superfoods in a daily diet. Ingredients like **spirulina**, **acai**, and **chia seeds** can be blended into smoothies to create nutrient-rich drinks that support energy and immune function. Spirulina, for example, is high in protein and B vitamins, making it ideal for those who need an energy boost. For Emma, preparing a smoothie each morning with added superfoods offers a quick and efficient way to start her day on a nutritious note.

2. **Salad Toppers**

Adding superfoods like **hemp seeds**, **goji berries**, and **quinoa** to salads is another simple method to boost nutrition. Hemp seeds provide essential fatty acids, while goji berries add antioxidants and vitamins that support overall health. Quinoa, a protein-rich grain, can turn a basic salad into a filling, balanced meal. For Emma, who might seek variety in her meals, using these superfoods as salad toppers ensures she gains diverse nutrients in an enjoyable way.

3. **Nutritious Snacks**

Superfoods can also be integrated into snacks, making

them a convenient option for busy lifestyles. **Almonds**, **walnuts**, and **dark chocolate** are all considered superfoods due to their high levels of antioxidants and healthy fats. Mixing these into a trail mix or simply consuming them as on-the-go snacks offers Emma a way to stay energized throughout her day without compromising her health goals.

Cooking with Superfoods

Cooking with superfoods can enhance the flavor and nutritional content of everyday meals. Superfoods like **turmeric**, **garlic**, and **kale** are versatile ingredients that can be added to various dishes, transforming them into nutrient-rich options that support overall wellness.

Turmeric, known for its anti-inflammatory properties, can be added to soups, stews, or golden milk. Its active compound, curcumin, supports joint health and boosts immunity, making it particularly beneficial for those seeking holistic wellness. For Emma, using turmeric in her cooking not only enhances flavor but also ensures she receives its therapeutic benefits regularly.

Garlic is another powerful superfood that promotes heart health and provides antibacterial properties. Incorporating fresh garlic into stir-fries, roasted vegetables, or pasta dishes is an easy way to boost flavor and nutrition simultaneously. Emma can benefit from garlic's immune-supporting properties while enhancing the taste of her meals.

Kale, a nutrient-dense leafy green, is rich in vitamins A, C, and K, as well as antioxidants. Adding kale to smoothies, salads, or sautéed dishes increases the intake of essential nutrients that support skin health, vision, and overall immunity. For Emma, who might enjoy quick, nutritious meals, using kale is a versatile way to maximize nutrient intake without much preparation.

Balancing Superfoods with Other Nutrients

While superfoods offer numerous health benefits, they should be integrated as part of a balanced diet that includes a variety of other nutrient-rich foods. It's important to ensure that superfoods complement whole grains, lean proteins, fruits, and vegetables to create well-rounded meals that provide all essential nutrients.

For example, combining **quinoa** with vegetables like **broccoli** or **sweet potatoes** offers a balance of protein, fiber, and vitamins, creating a complete and satisfying meal. Similarly, adding **avocado** to salads or wraps provides healthy fats that enhance the absorption of fat-soluble vitamins, supporting skin health and brain function.

Creating Balanced Meals with Superfoods

A balanced meal plan incorporating superfoods can be as simple as structuring meals around key food groups while using superfoods to enhance their nutritional value. Below is an example meal plan for Emma to illustrate how superfoods can be integrated throughout the day:

Meal	Ingredients	Superfoods Included
Breakfast	Smoothie with spinach, banana, almond milk	Chia seeds, spirulina
Lunch	Quinoa salad with chickpeas, kale, and avocado	Hemp seeds, goji berries
Dinner	Grilled salmon with turmeric-spiced vegetables	Garlic, turmeric, broccoli

This approach ensures Emma receives a balanced mix of nutrients, supporting her holistic health goals and providing energy throughout her busy day.

Integrating superfoods into a balanced diet is not only practical but also essential for optimizing health. For individuals like Emma, these strategies offer versatile and effective ways to boost nutrition, ensuring that meals remain both delicious and nutrient-dense.

Remedies for Herbal Nutrition and Energy Boost

Spirulina and Lemon Energy Smoothie

INGREDIENTS

- 1 teaspoon spirulina powder
- 1 cup coconut water
- 1/2 banana
- 1 tablespoon fresh lemon juice
- 1/4 cup spinach leaves

PREPARATION

1. Place all ingredients in a blender.
2. Blend until smooth.
3. Drink immediately for an energy boost.

Benefits: Spirulina is a nutrient-dense superfood packed with protein, vitamins, and minerals. Combined with the electrolytes in coconut water and the vitamin C in lemon, this smoothie provides a refreshing energy boost while promoting overall health and vitality.

Nettle Leaf Iron Boost Tea

INGREDIENTS

- 1 teaspoon dried nettle leaves
- 1 cup boiling water

PREPARATION

1. Steep nettle leaves in boiling water for 10 minutes.
2. Strain and drink warm.

Benefits: Nettle leaf is a rich source of iron and other essential minerals, making it a powerful remedy for boosting iron levels naturally. It helps combat fatigue and supports overall energy production, making it ideal for people with low iron or anemia.

Moringa Leaf Nutrient-Rich Capsules

INGREDIENTS

- 1 tablespoon dried moringa leaf powder
- Capsule shells

PREPARATION

1. Fill capsule shells with moringa leaf powder.

2. Take 1-2 capsules daily.

Benefits: Moringa is often called the "miracle tree" due to its high nutrient content. It provides essential vitamins, minerals, and antioxidants that support overall health, boost energy, and enhance immune function. Regular consumption can improve vitality and well-being.

Alfalfa Sprout Detox Salad

INGREDIENTS

- 1 cup fresh alfalfa sprouts
- 1/2 cucumber, sliced
- 1/4 cup shredded carrots
- 1 tablespoon lemon juice
- 1 tablespoon olive oil

PREPARATION

1. Combine alfalfa sprouts, cucumber, and carrots in a bowl.
2. Drizzle with lemon juice and olive oil.
3. Toss well and serve.

Benefits: Alfalfa sprouts are rich in vitamins, minerals, and enzymes that support detoxification. This salad helps cleanse the liver and digestive system, while providing a nutrient-rich boost for energy and vitality.

Maca Root Energy Elixir

INGREDIENTS

- 1 teaspoon maca root powder
- 1 cup almond milk
- 1 teaspoon honey

PREPARATION

1. Mix maca root powder with warm almond milk.
2. Stir in honey and drink.

Benefits: Maca root is an adaptogen that supports energy, stamina, and hormonal balance. This elixir helps increase vitality and reduces fatigue, making it a perfect drink for boosting energy levels naturally without stimulants.

Ashwagandha Adaptogenic Superfood Latte

INGREDIENTS

- 1 teaspoon ashwagandha powder
- 1 cup warm oat milk
- 1 teaspoon maple syrup
- 1/4 teaspoon cinnamon

PREPARATION

1. Mix ashwagandha powder with warm oat milk.
2. Add maple syrup and cinnamon, then stir well.
3. Drink once a day for best results.

Benefits: Ashwagandha is a powerful adaptogen that helps the body manage stress and boosts energy. This superfood latte supports adrenal health and provides sustained energy throughout the day while calming the mind and reducing anxiety.

Wheatgrass Green Juice

INGREDIENTS

- 1 ounce wheatgrass juice
- 1/2 cucumber
- 1/2 apple
- 1/4 lemon, peeled

PREPARATION

1. Juice the wheatgrass, cucumber, apple, and lemon together.
2. Drink immediately for a green energy boost.

Benefits: Wheatgrass is one of the most potent sources of chlorophyll, vitamins, and minerals. This green juice helps detoxify the body, boost energy, and support overall health. It's perfect for a morning energy boost or midday pick-me-up.

Chlorella Detox Tonic

INGREDIENTS

- 1 teaspoon chlorella powder
- 1 cup water
- 1 tablespoon fresh lemon juice

PREPARATION

1. Mix chlorella powder with water and lemon juice.
2. Drink on an empty stomach for best detox results.

Benefits: Chlorella is a powerful detoxifying agent that binds to heavy metals and toxins in the body, helping to flush them out. This tonic supports liver function, boosts immune health, and enhances energy levels by clearing out harmful substances.

Goji Berry Immune-Boosting Snack Mix

INGREDIENTS

- 1/4 cup dried goji berries
- 1/4 cup raw almonds
- 1/4 cup pumpkin seeds
- 1 tablespoon cacao nibs

PREPARATION

1. Combine all ingredients in a bowl.
2. Store in an airtight container and enjoy as a snack.

Benefits: Goji berries are rich in antioxidants and vitamins that support the immune system and improve energy levels. This snack mix provides a quick and nutritious boost, ideal for busy days when you need sustained energy and immune support.

Acai Berry Antioxidant Smoothie Bowl

INGREDIENTS

- 1/2 cup frozen acai berry pulp
- 1/2 banana
- 1/4 cup almond milk
- Toppings: sliced fruit, granola, chia seeds

PREPARATION

1. Blend acai berry pulp, banana, and almond milk until smooth.
2. Pour into a bowl and add your choice of toppings.
3. Enjoy immediately for an antioxidant boost.

Benefits: Acai berries are packed with antioxidants that fight free radicals and support overall health. This smoothie bowl is rich in vitamins and minerals, making it perfect for boosting energy, enhancing skin health, and supporting the immune system.

Dandelion Greens Vitamin Salad

INGREDIENTS

- 1 cup fresh dandelion greens
- 1/2 avocado, sliced
- 1 tablespoon olive oil
- 1 teaspoon lemon juice

PREPARATION

1. Toss dandelion greens and avocado in a bowl.
2. Drizzle with olive oil and lemon juice, then toss again.
3. Serve immediately.

Benefits: Dandelion greens are high in vitamins A, C, and K, and support liver health and detoxification. This salad provides a nutrient-dense meal that helps boost energy, improve digestion, and enhance skin health.

Baobab Citrus Hydration Drink

INGREDIENTS

- 1 teaspoon baobab powder
- 1 cup coconut water
- Juice of 1/2 lemon

PREPARATION

1. Mix baobab powder, coconut water, and lemon juice in a glass.
2. Stir well and drink for hydration.

Benefits: Baobab is rich in vitamin C and antioxidants, while coconut water provides natural electrolytes. This drink helps hydrate the body, boosts immune health, and supports energy levels, making it ideal for recovery after physical activity or as a refreshing energy boost.

Bee Pollen Protein Boost Shake

INGREDIENTS

- 1 teaspoon bee pollen
- 1 cup almond milk
- 1/2 banana
- 1 tablespoon almond butter

PREPARATION

1. Blend all ingredients until smooth.
2. Drink immediately for a protein boost.

Benefits: Bee pollen is a complete protein source and is packed with essential nutrients. This protein shake helps build muscle, improve energy, and boost immunity. It's perfect for post-workout recovery or as a meal replacement for sustained energy.

Camu Camu Vitamin C Immune Tea

INGREDIENTS

- 1 teaspoon camu camu powder
- 1 cup warm water
- 1 teaspoon honey

PREPARATION

1. Mix camu camu powder with warm water.
2. Stir in honey and drink.

Benefits: Camu camu is one of the richest natural sources of vitamin C, making this tea a potent immune booster. Regular consumption helps improve immunity, fight infections, and increase overall energy levels. It's especially beneficial during cold and flu season.

Holy Basil (Tulsi) Metabolic Support Capsules

INGREDIENTS

- 1 tablespoon dried holy basil (tulsi) powder
- Capsule shells

PREPARATION

1. Fill capsule shells with holy basil powder.
2. Take 1-2 capsules daily.

Benefits: Holy basil, or tulsi, is an adaptogen that helps support metabolism and reduce stress. Regular use of these capsules boosts energy, promotes a healthy metabolic rate, and supports overall wellness by balancing hormones and reducing inflammation.

Fenugreek Seed Protein-Rich Sprouts

INGREDIENTS

- 2 tablespoons fenugreek seeds
- Water for soaking

PREPARATION

1. Soak fenugreek seeds in water for 6-8 hours.
2. Rinse and drain the seeds, then place them in a sprouting jar or tray.
3. Rinse the seeds twice daily for 3-4 days until they sprout.
4. Enjoy the sprouts in salads or as a snack.

Benefits: Fenugreek sprouts are a rich source of plant-based protein and essential nutrients. They help support muscle growth, improve digestion, and provide sustained energy, making them an excellent addition to any diet.

Astragalus Root Immune-Enhancing Broth

INGREDIENTS

- 1 tablespoon dried astragalus root
- 4 cups water

PREPARATION

1. Simmer astragalus root in water for 30 minutes.
2. Strain the broth and drink warm or use as a base for soups.

Benefits: Astragalus is a powerful adaptogen that supports immune function and increases energy. This immune-enhancing broth helps protect the body from infections, boosts stamina, and supports recovery from illness. It's ideal for daily consumption during flu season.

Reishi Mushroom Energy and Vitality Decoction

INGREDIENTS

- 1 teaspoon dried reishi mushroom powder
- 2 cups water

PREPARATION

1. Simmer reishi mushroom powder in water for 20-30 minutes.
2. Strain and drink warm.

Benefits: Reishi mushrooms are known for their ability to boost energy, support the immune system, and promote longevity. This decoction helps increase vitality, reduce fatigue, and enhance overall well-being by balancing the body's stress response.

Ginseng Root Energizing Tea

INGREDIENTS

- 1 teaspoon dried ginseng root
- 1 cup boiling water

PREPARATION

1. Steep ginseng root in boiling water for 10-15 minutes.
2. Strain and drink.

Benefits: Ginseng is a natural stimulant that helps boost energy levels, improve mental clarity, and enhance physical endurance. This tea is ideal for anyone looking for a natural way to increase energy without the jitters of caffeine. Regular consumption supports overall vitality.

Red Clover Blossom Mineral Tonic

INGREDIENTS

- 1 teaspoon dried red clover blossoms
- 1 cup boiling water

PREPARATION

1. Steep red clover blossoms in boiling water for 10 minutes.
2. Strain and drink warm.

Benefits: Red clover is rich in minerals like calcium, magnesium, and potassium, making this tonic excellent for supporting bone health, detoxification, and overall well-being. It helps balance hormones, improve circulation, and promote clear skin.

Oatstraw Calcium Boost Infusion

INGREDIENTS

- 1 tablespoon dried oatstraw
- 1 cup boiling water

PREPARATION

1. Steep oatstraw in boiling water for 20 minutes.
2. Strain and drink warm.

Benefits: Oatstraw is a natural source of calcium and other minerals that support bone health and promote relaxation. This infusion helps strengthen bones, improve mood, and enhance energy levels by providing essential nutrients.

Burdock Root Detox Soup

INGREDIENTS

- 1 tablespoon dried burdock root
- 4 cups vegetable broth
- 1 carrot, chopped
- 1 celery stalk, chopped

PREPARATION

1. Simmer burdock root, carrot, and celery in vegetable broth for 30 minutes.
2. Strain if desired and serve warm.

Benefits: Burdock root is a powerful detoxifying herb that helps cleanse the liver and improve digestion. This detox soup supports the body's natural detox processes, boosts energy, and provides essential nutrients for overall health.

Shatavari Rejuvenating Herbal Drink

INGREDIENTS

- 1 teaspoon shatavari powder
- 1 cup warm almond milk
- 1 teaspoon honey

PREPARATION

1. Mix shatavari powder into warm almond milk.
2. Stir in honey and drink.

Benefits: Shatavari is a rejuvenating herb that supports hormonal balance, enhances vitality, and improves energy levels. This drink helps nourish the body, reduce stress, and promote overall well-being, especially for women's health.

Elderberry and Hibiscus Immune Support Elixir

INGREDIENTS

- 1 tablespoon dried elderberries
- 1 teaspoon dried hibiscus flowers
- 1 cup water

PREPARATION

1. Simmer elderberries and hibiscus flowers in water for 10 minutes.
2. Strain and drink warm.

Benefits: Elderberries are packed with antioxidants and are known for their immune-boosting properties, while hibiscus is rich in vitamin C. This elixir helps fight infections, boost immune health, and support overall vitality. It's especially beneficial during cold and flu season.

Chia Seed and Mint Hydration Water

INGREDIENTS

- 1 tablespoon chia seeds
- 1 teaspoon fresh mint leaves
- 1 cup water

PREPARATION

1. Add chia seeds and mint leaves to water.
2. Stir well and let sit for 10 minutes, stirring occasionally to prevent clumping.
3. Drink for hydration.

Benefits: Chia seeds are rich in omega-3 fatty acids, fiber, and protein, making this drink highly nourishing and hydrating. Mint adds a refreshing taste and helps soothe digestion. This hydration water is perfect for boosting energy and staying hydrated throughout the day.

Ginger and Turmeric Anti-Inflammatory Shot

INGREDIENTS

- 1 teaspoon grated fresh ginger
- 1 teaspoon grated fresh turmeric
- Juice of 1/2 lemon

PREPARATION

1. Mix ginger, turmeric, and lemon juice together in a small glass.
2. Drink immediately.

Benefits: Ginger and turmeric are both potent anti-inflammatory herbs that help reduce pain, fight inflammation, and boost immunity. This shot provides a quick energy boost while promoting overall wellness and reducing inflammation in the body.

Cat's Claw Immune-Boost Capsules

INGREDIENTS

- 1 tablespoon dried cat's claw powder
- Capsule shells

PREPARATION

1. Fill capsule shells with cat's claw powder.
2. Take 1-2 capsules daily.

Benefits: Cat's claw is a powerful immune-boosting herb that helps protect the body from infections and inflammation. These capsules support immune health, improve energy, and help the body recover from illness more quickly.

Schisandra Berry Energy Tonic

INGREDIENTS

- 1 teaspoon dried schisandra berries
- 1 cup water

PREPARATION

Simmer schisandra berries

1. in water for 10 minutes.
2. Strain and drink warm.

Benefits: Schisandra berries are adaptogens that help improve energy, stamina, and mental clarity. This tonic supports endurance, reduces stress, and enhances overall vitality, making it ideal for people with demanding schedules or those who need an energy boost.

Matcha Green Tea Energizer

INGREDIENTS

- 1 teaspoon matcha green tea powder
- 1 cup hot water

PREPARATION

1. Mix matcha green tea powder with hot water.
2. Stir well and drink immediately for an energy boost.

Benefits: Matcha is rich in antioxidants and provides a steady, sustained energy boost without the crash associated with caffeine. It also helps improve mental clarity and focus, making it an excellent drink for boosting productivity and enhancing physical performance.

Lemon Balm and Honey Nutrient Infusion

INGREDIENTS

- 1 teaspoon dried lemon balm leaves
- 1 teaspoon honey
- 1 cup boiling water

PREPARATION

1. Steep lemon balm leaves in boiling water for 10 minutes.
2. Strain and stir in honey before drinking.

Benefits: Lemon balm helps calm the mind, reduces anxiety, and supports digestion. This nutrient infusion is rich in antioxidants and helps soothe the nervous system while boosting immunity. Honey adds additional soothing and antibacterial properties, making this a perfect drink for overall well-being.

Hemp Seed Protein Power Bars

INGREDIENTS

- 1/2 cup hemp seeds
- 1/4 cup almond butter
- 1/4 cup rolled oats
- 1 tablespoon honey

PREPARATION

1. Mix hemp seeds, almond butter, rolled oats, and honey in a bowl.
2. Press the mixture into a lined baking dish.
3. Refrigerate for 1 hour, then cut into bars.
4. Store in an airtight container.

Benefits: Hemp seeds are a complete source of plant-based protein and contain essential fatty acids. These power bars are perfect for a protein boost, providing sustained energy and supporting muscle recovery. They are ideal for post-workout snacks or as a healthy, nutritious treat.

Blueberry and Nettle Antioxidant Smoothie

INGREDIENTS

- 1/2 cup fresh or frozen blueberries
- 1 teaspoon dried nettle leaf powder
- 1/2 cup almond milk
- 1 teaspoon honey

PREPARATION

1. Blend blueberries, nettle leaf powder, almond milk, and honey until smooth.
2. Drink immediately for a nutrient boost.

Benefits: Blueberries are rich in antioxidants that help fight free radicals, while nettle provides a wealth of vitamins and minerals, including iron and calcium. This smoothie supports immune health, boosts energy, and promotes healthy skin. It's a great way to start the day or as a mid-day refreshment.

Licorice Root Digestive Support Chews

INGREDIENTS

- 1 tablespoon dried licorice root powder
- 1/4 cup honey

PREPARATION

1. Mix licorice root powder with honey until a thick paste forms.
2. Roll the paste into small balls or chews.
3. Refrigerate for 1 hour to firm up before consuming.

Benefits: Licorice root is well-known for its digestive soothing properties, helping to relieve indigestion, heartburn, and stomach discomfort. These chews are a convenient and natural way to support digestion, reduce inflammation, and boost energy levels.

Rose Hip Vitamin C-Rich Tea

INGREDIENTS

- 1 tablespoon dried rose hips
- 1 cup boiling water

PREPARATION

1. Steep rose hips in boiling water for 10-15 minutes.
2. Strain and drink warm.

Benefits: Rose hips are one of the best natural sources of vitamin C, which supports immune function, skin health, and overall vitality. This tea is a refreshing and nourishing way to boost your intake of antioxidants, protect against illness, and promote radiant skin.

BOOK 11

Cardiovascular Health

Herbs for Heart Health and Circulation

NATURAL HERBS FOR ENHANCING HEART HEALTH AND CIRCULATION

Maintaining heart health and promoting proper circulation are essential for overall wellness. Herbs offer a natural and effective way to support cardiovascular function, improve blood flow, and reduce the risk of heart disease. For individuals like Emma, who prefer natural approaches, integrating heart-healthy herbs into their daily routines can provide numerous benefits without the side effects often associated with synthetic medications. Below, we explore several powerful herbs that promote heart health and enhance circulation, each contributing uniquely to cardiovascular wellness.

Hawthorn: The Ultimate Heart Tonic

Hawthorn is one of the most widely recognized herbs for cardiovascular health. It has been used for centuries in traditional medicine to strengthen the heart and improve blood circulation. Hawthorn berries, leaves, and flowers are rich in flavonoids, powerful antioxidants that protect the heart by reducing oxidative stress and inflammation. These compounds also help dilate blood vessels, improving blood flow and lowering blood pressure.

Hawthorn works as a heart tonic by enhancing the contraction of the heart muscle, supporting its ability to pump blood efficiently. This makes it especially beneficial for individuals experiencing heart fatigue or arrhythmias. For Emma, incorporating hawthorn as a tea or tincture offers a gentle yet effective way to support her heart health, especially if she is proactive about maintaining a balanced cardiovascular system. Regular use of hawthorn not only strengthens the heart but also improves overall circulation, ensuring her body remains well-oxygenated and energized.

Garlic: The Natural Cholesterol Buster

Garlic is another potent herb known for its cardiovascular benefits, particularly in reducing cholesterol levels and improving circulation. Allicin, the active compound in garlic, has been shown to lower LDL (bad) cholesterol and triglycerides while increasing HDL (good) cholesterol. Additionally, garlic helps prevent the buildup of plaque in the arteries, reducing the risk of atherosclerosis and heart disease.

Garlic also acts as a natural blood thinner, promoting smooth blood flow and preventing clots. For Emma, incorporating fresh garlic into her meals is a simple and effective way to gain these cardiovascular benefits. Whether added to soups, salads, or used as a seasoning for roasted vegetables, garlic offers an accessible approach to enhancing heart health. Its versatility in cooking makes it an easy addition to Emma's diet, ensuring consistent support for her cardiovascular system.

Cayenne Pepper: Enhancing Blood Circulation

Cayenne pepper is well-known for its ability to stimulate blood flow and improve circulation. The active compound **capsaicin** helps dilate blood vessels, allowing for better blood flow and reducing pressure on the heart.

Cayenne also supports the metabolism, ensuring that the body utilizes energy efficiently, which is crucial for overall cardiovascular function.

By adding a small amount of cayenne pepper to meals or using it in tea, Emma can boost circulation and enjoy the herb's warming, invigorating effects. Cayenne is particularly useful for those who experience cold hands and feet, as it helps improve peripheral circulation. For Emma, who may prefer easy and practical solutions, incorporating cayenne pepper into her cooking provides a natural way to promote blood flow and maintain cardiovascular health.

Ginkgo Biloba: Supporting Vascular Health

Ginkgo biloba is an ancient herb traditionally used to improve circulation and support vascular health. It works by dilating blood vessels and enhancing blood flow, particularly to the brain and extremities. This makes ginkgo not only beneficial for heart health but also for cognitive function and overall vitality. The herb's antioxidant properties further protect blood vessels from damage, ensuring long-term cardiovascular wellness.

Ginkgo can be taken as a tea, tincture, or capsule, offering flexibility in how it is consumed. For Emma, who might seek ways to enhance both her heart health and mental clarity, ginkgo provides dual benefits. Regular use of ginkgo ensures that blood circulates effectively, delivering oxygen and nutrients throughout the body while also supporting cognitive function.

Ginger: Anti-Inflammatory and Circulation Enhancer

Ginger is a versatile herb known for its anti-inflammatory and circulation-enhancing properties. It contains **gingerol**, an active compound that supports blood vessel health and reduces inflammation in the cardiovascular system. Ginger helps prevent blood clot formation, promoting smooth blood flow and reducing the risk of heart-related conditions like hypertension and stroke.

Ginger tea is a simple way to integrate this herb into a daily routine, offering Emma an accessible and warming remedy that supports both her heart and digestive health. Fresh ginger can also be added to meals, smoothies, or juices, providing a consistent way to enjoy its benefits. For Emma, who values practical and efficient solutions, using ginger in her daily meals or as a tea ensures she receives the herb's cardiovascular support while also enjoying its refreshing and zesty flavor.

Turmeric: Protecting the Heart with Antioxidants

Turmeric, with its active compound **curcumin**, is a powerful herb for protecting heart health. Curcumin is a potent anti-inflammatory and antioxidant that reduces arterial inflammation and protects the cardiovascular system from oxidative damage. Turmeric also helps maintain healthy cholesterol levels and supports smooth blood flow, making it beneficial for those seeking comprehensive heart support.

Adding turmeric to meals, such as soups, stews, or even smoothies, is an easy way for Emma to incorporate this superfood into her diet. Turmeric can also be consumed as a tea or used in golden milk for additional benefits. For Emma, using turmeric regularly not only supports heart health but also provides anti-inflammatory effects that benefit her overall well-being, ensuring a balanced approach to holistic health.

Motherwort: Calming the Heart

Motherwort is an herb specifically known for its calming effects on the heart. Traditionally used to manage heart palpitations and anxiety, motherwort is an excellent choice for individuals who may experience stress-related cardiovascular issues. The herb helps to reduce high blood pressure by calming the nervous system and improving circulation.

For Emma, using motherwort as a tea or tincture can provide a natural way to manage stress and support her heart's function. Regular use of motherwort helps maintain a calm and steady heart rate, aligning with her preference for nurturing remedies that promote balance and well-being.

By incorporating these herbs into her lifestyle, Emma can naturally support her heart health and circulation, ensuring her cardiovascular system remains strong and resilient. Each herb offers unique benefits that align with holistic wellness, providing practical and effective solutions for long-term heart health.

Managing Blood Pressure and Cholesterol Naturally

NATURAL STRATEGIES FOR BALANCING BLOOD PRESSURE AND CHOLESTEROL

Maintaining balanced blood pressure and healthy cholesterol levels are crucial for cardiovascular health. Many individuals turn to pharmaceuticals to manage these conditions, but herbs offer a natural and effective alternative that supports the body without the side effects associated with medications. For those like Emma, who seek holistic and sustainable solutions, understanding how to use these herbs provides a powerful way to manage these common issues naturally. Below, we explore a range of herbs known for their effectiveness in supporting heart health through blood pressure regulation and cholesterol management.

Hawthorn: Supporting Blood Vessel Health

Hawthorn is one of the most effective herbs for managing blood pressure naturally. It helps dilate blood vessels, improving circulation and reducing the pressure within arteries. The flavonoids and procyanidins found in hawthorn not only support blood flow but also protect against the hardening of arteries, which can lead to hypertension and heart disease.

Hawthorn's ability to improve the elasticity of blood vessels makes it particularly beneficial for those dealing with high blood pressure. For Emma, incorporating hawthorn as a tea or tincture can be a simple and effective way to support her cardiovascular health. Its mild flavor and ease of use make it accessible, ensuring she can maintain her routine without significant changes to her daily habits.

Garlic: Nature's Cholesterol Reducer

Garlic is well-known for its cholesterol-lowering properties. Allicin, the active compound in garlic, has been shown to reduce LDL (bad) cholesterol levels while supporting the production of HDL (good) cholesterol. Regular consumption of garlic not only helps balance cholesterol levels but also prevents the formation of arterial plaque, reducing the risk of atherosclerosis.

Garlic also possesses mild blood-thinning properties, promoting smooth blood flow and lowering blood pressure. For Emma, using fresh garlic in her cooking offers a practical way to reap these cardiovascular benefits. Whether added to soups, stir-fries, or salads, garlic's versatility ensures it can be included in various dishes, making it a consistent part of her natural wellness strategy.

Hibiscus: The Blood Pressure Regulator

Hibiscus tea is another powerful tool for managing blood pressure. Studies have shown that hibiscus can effectively lower systolic and diastolic blood pressure levels due to its diuretic properties and its ability to relax blood vessels. This makes it a valuable herb for those who seek to manage hypertension naturally.

Hibiscus tea is not only effective but also refreshing and easy to prepare. For Emma, drinking a cup of hibiscus tea daily provides a flavorful and natural way to regulate her blood pressure. Its vibrant color and tangy taste make it a pleasant addition to her routine, offering health benefits while also promoting relaxation.

Turmeric: Combating Inflammation and Cholesterol

Turmeric, with its active compound curcumin, is a powerful anti-inflammatory herb that supports heart health by reducing inflammation within blood vessels. It helps prevent the oxidation of cholesterol, a process that contributes to plaque buildup and arterial damage. Turmeric's ability to maintain cholesterol levels and improve blood vessel function makes it a valuable ally in cardiovascular health.

Adding turmeric to meals, such as soups, stews, or even smoothies, offers Emma a practical way to include this herb in her daily routine. Turmeric supplements are also available for those who prefer a concentrated form. By using turmeric regularly, Emma can not only manage her cholesterol levels but also support overall heart health through its anti-inflammatory effects.

Olive Leaf: A Natural Blood Pressure Solution

Olive leaf extract is another effective herb for managing blood pressure naturally. The compound **oleuropein** in olive leaves has been shown to dilate blood vessels and improve circulation, which helps lower blood pressure. Additionally, olive leaf extract supports heart health by reducing LDL cholesterol levels and preventing oxidative damage to blood vessels.

For Emma, who may prefer convenient options, olive leaf extract capsules offer an easy way to incorporate this herb into her daily regimen. Alternatively, olive leaf tea provides a simple and effective method to gain the same benefits. Regular use of olive leaf ensures that Emma maintains balanced blood pressure levels while supporting her overall cardiovascular wellness.

Fenugreek: Balancing Cholesterol Levels

Fenugreek seeds are rich in soluble fiber, which helps reduce cholesterol levels by binding to cholesterol molecules and preventing their absorption in the digestive tract. Fenugreek also supports liver function, promoting the breakdown of excess cholesterol and triglycerides. By balancing cholesterol levels, fenugreek plays a critical role in reducing the risk of heart disease and supporting vascular health.

Fenugreek can be used in various ways, such as in teas, capsules, or added to meals as a spice. For Emma, fenugreek tea offers an accessible way to benefit from its cholesterol-lowering properties. Adding fenugreek seeds to meals, like curries or salads, also provides a simple way to integrate this herb into her diet naturally.

Cinnamon: Improving Blood Sugar and Cholesterol

Cinnamon is not only a delicious spice but also a powerful herb for managing cholesterol and blood pressure. It helps lower blood sugar levels, which in turn supports balanced blood pressure, as high blood sugar is often linked to hypertension. Cinnamon also aids in reducing LDL cholesterol and triglyceride levels, further promoting cardiovascular health.

Adding cinnamon to breakfast dishes like oatmeal, smoothies, or yogurt is a practical way for Emma to enjoy its benefits. Cinnamon tea is another effective option, providing a warm and comforting way to support heart health. By incorporating cinnamon regularly, Emma can manage both her cholesterol levels and blood pressure naturally.

Dandelion: A Diuretic for Blood Pressure Management

Dandelion is a natural diuretic that supports blood pressure management by helping the body eliminate excess fluids and sodium. By reducing fluid retention, dandelion lowers the pressure on blood vessels, making it an effective herb for those with hypertension. It also provides potassium, a vital mineral that supports cardiovascular health and maintains electrolyte balance.

Dandelion tea is an easy way to consume this herb and can be integrated into Emma's routine as a simple, daily beverage. The gentle diuretic effect of dandelion not only aids in regulating blood pressure but also promotes detoxification, aligning with Emma's preference for natural, holistic solutions.

These herbs provide effective and natural ways to manage blood pressure and cholesterol levels, offering a comprehensive approach to cardiovascular health. For Emma, integrating these herbs into her daily routine supports her heart health goals, ensuring her wellness strategy is both balanced and sustainable.

Remedies for Cardiovascular Wellness

Hawthorn Berry Heart Tonic Tea

INGREDIENTS

- 1 teaspoon dried hawthorn berries
- 1 cup boiling water

PREPARATION

1. Steep the hawthorn berries in boiling water for 10-15 minutes.
2. Strain and drink warm.

Benefits: Hawthorn berries are well-known for their heart-strengthening properties. They improve blood circulation, reduce blood pressure, and enhance the strength of the heart muscles, making this tea ideal for overall cardiovascular health. Regular consumption may help reduce the risk of heart-related issues.

Motherwort Heart Health Tincture

INGREDIENTS

- 1/4 cup dried motherwort leaves
- 1/2 cup alcohol (vodka or glycerin for non-alcoholic option)

PREPARATION

1. Place the dried motherwort leaves in a jar and cover with alcohol or glycerin.
2. Seal and let it sit for 4-6 weeks, shaking occasionally.
3. Strain and take 1-2 droppers daily for heart health.

Benefits: Motherwort is a calming herb that supports heart health by regulating heart rhythms, reducing palpitations, and calming anxiety. This tincture helps balance the nervous system, making it particularly useful for stress-related heart conditions.

Garlic and Lemon Blood Pressure Elixir

INGREDIENTS

- 3 cloves garlic, minced
- Juice of 1 lemon
- 1 cup water

PREPARATION

1. Mix the minced garlic and lemon juice with water.
2. Drink the mixture once daily in the morning.

Benefits: Garlic is known for its ability to lower blood pressure by improving blood circulation and reducing cholesterol levels. Lemon adds antioxidants and helps to cleanse the arteries, making this elixir effective for maintaining healthy blood pressure.

Hibiscus Cholesterol-Lowering Infusion

INGREDIENTS

- 1 tablespoon dried hibiscus petals
- 1 cup boiling water

PREPARATION

1. Steep the hibiscus petals in boiling water for 10 minutes.
2. Strain and drink once daily.

Benefits: Hibiscus is a powerful herb for reducing cholesterol and improving cardiovascular health. Its antioxidants help lower LDL (bad cholesterol) levels and promote better circulation, making this infusion beneficial for maintaining a healthy heart.

Cayenne Pepper Circulation Boost Capsules

INGREDIENTS

- 1 tablespoon cayenne pepper powder
- Capsule shells

PREPARATION

1. Fill the capsule shells with cayenne pepper powder.
2. Take 1-2 capsules daily.

Benefits: Cayenne pepper boosts circulation, reduces blood pressure, and helps prevent blood clots by thinning the blood. These capsules are a natural way to improve circulation and support overall heart health, especially for those with poor blood flow.

Linden Flower Heart Calming Tea

INGREDIENTS

- 1 teaspoon dried linden flowers
- 1 cup boiling water

PREPARATION

1. Steep the linden flowers in boiling water for 10 minutes.
2. Strain and drink before bed.

Benefits: Linden flowers have gentle sedative and calming properties that help reduce stress and lower blood pressure. This tea is perfect for calming the heart and supporting cardiovascular health, particularly for people dealing with stress-related heart issues.

Ginkgo Biloba Circulatory Support Capsules

INGREDIENTS

- 1 tablespoon dried ginkgo biloba leaf powder
- Capsule shells

PREPARATION

1. Fill capsule shells with ginkgo biloba powder.
2. Take 1-2 capsules daily for circulatory support.

Benefits: Ginkgo biloba improves circulation by increasing blood flow to the extremities and brain, making it an excellent remedy for cardiovascular health. Regular use can enhance cognitive function, reduce the risk of blood clots, and improve overall blood flow.

Yarrow Blood Pressure Regulation Tea

INGREDIENTS

- 1 teaspoon dried yarrow leaves
- 1 cup boiling water

PREPARATION

1. Steep the yarrow leaves in boiling water for 10 minutes.
2. Strain and drink once daily.

Benefits: Yarrow helps regulate blood pressure by improving circulation and reducing inflammation. This tea supports overall heart health by helping to balance blood pressure naturally, making it a great addition to a cardiovascular wellness routine.

Dandelion Leaf Heart Health Salad

INGREDIENTS

- 1 cup fresh dandelion leaves
- 1/2 cucumber, sliced
- 1 tablespoon olive oil
- 1 teaspoon lemon juice

PREPARATION

1. Toss dandelion leaves and cucumber in a bowl.
2. Drizzle with olive oil and lemon juice.
3. Serve fresh as a heart-healthy salad.

Benefits: Dandelion leaves are rich in potassium and other heart-healthy nutrients. They help reduce blood pressure, support healthy cholesterol levels, and promote overall cardiovascular health. This salad is a delicious and nutritious way to boost heart function.

Arjuna Bark Cardiovascular Support Capsules

INGREDIENTS

- 1 tablespoon dried arjuna bark powder
- Capsule shells

PREPARATION

1. Fill capsule shells with arjuna bark powder.
2. Take 1-2 capsules daily for cardiovascular support.

Benefits: Arjuna bark is a traditional Ayurvedic remedy for strengthening the heart and improving cardiovascular function. It helps regulate blood pressure, reduce cholesterol, and improve overall heart health. Regular use can enhance cardiac strength and resilience.

Turmeric and Black Pepper Heart Tonic

INGREDIENTS

- 1 teaspoon turmeric powder
- 1/4 teaspoon black pepper
- 1 cup warm water

PREPARATION

1. Mix turmeric and black pepper in warm water.
2. Drink once daily for heart health.

Benefits: Turmeric contains curcumin, which has powerful anti-inflammatory and antioxidant properties that support heart health. Black pepper enhances the absorption of curcumin, making this tonic highly effective for reducing inflammation, improving circulation, and protecting the heart from oxidative stress.

Celery Seed Blood Pressure Drops

INGREDIENTS

- 1 tablespoon dried celery seeds
- 1/4 cup alcohol (vodka or glycerin for non-alcoholic option)

PREPARATION

1. Infuse celery seeds in alcohol or glycerin for 4-6 weeks.
2. Strain and take 1-2 droppers daily.

Benefits: Celery seeds are known for their ability to lower blood pressure and reduce inflammation. This tincture helps improve circulation, lower blood pressure naturally, and support overall heart health. It's an excellent remedy for hypertension.

Blueberry and Ginger Heart-Healthy Smoothie

INGREDIENTS

- 1/2 cup fresh or frozen blueberries
- 1/2 teaspoon grated ginger
- 1/2 cup almond milk
- 1 teaspoon honey

PREPARATION

1. Blend all ingredients together until smooth.
2. Drink immediately for heart health benefits.

Benefits: Blueberries are packed with antioxidants that protect the heart and improve circulation, while ginger helps reduce inflammation. This smoothie supports cardiovascular health by providing vital nutrients and promoting healthy blood pressure and cholesterol levels.

Olive Leaf Cholesterol Management Extract

INGREDIENTS

- 1 tablespoon dried olive leaves
- 1/4 cup alcohol (vodka or glycerin for non-alcoholic option)

PREPARATION

1. Infuse the dried olive leaves in alcohol or glycerin for 4-6 weeks.
2. Strain and take 1-2 droppers daily.

Benefits: Olive leaves contain compounds that help lower cholesterol and improve heart function. This extract supports healthy cholesterol levels, reduces inflammation, and promotes overall cardiovascular wellness. Regular use helps protect the arteries and improve circulation.

Ginger and Hawthorn Circulation Boosting Decoction

INGREDIENTS

- 1 tablespoon dried hawthorn berries
- 1 teaspoon grated fresh ginger
- 2 cups water
- Instructions: (#p#)
- Simmer hawthorn berries and ginger in water for 15 minutes.
- Strain and drink warm.
- Benefits: This combination of hawthorn and ginger helps improve circulation, reduce blood pressure, and strengthen the heart. Hawthorn supports heart function, while ginger reduces inflammation and enhances blood flow. This decoction is perfect for boosting cardiovascular health.
- Beetroot and Apple Cider Vinegar Heart Health Tonic
- Ingredients
- 1/4 cup beetroot juice
- 1 tablespoon apple cider vinegar
- 1 cup water

PREPARATION

1. Mix beetroot juice and apple cider vinegar with water.
2. Drink once daily.

Benefits: Beetroot is known for its ability to improve blood flow and lower blood pressure, while apple cider vinegar supports cholesterol management. This tonic helps enhance cardiovascular health, reduce hypertension, and improve overall circulation.

Valerian and Lemon Balm Relaxing Heart Tea

INGREDIENTS

- 1 teaspoon dried valerian root
- 1 teaspoon dried lemon balm leaves
- 1 cup boiling water

PREPARATION

1. Steep valerian root and lemon balm in boiling water for 10 minutes.
2. Strain and drink before bedtime for heart relaxation.

Benefits: Valerian and lemon balm are calming herbs that help reduce stress and anxiety, which can benefit heart health. This tea helps lower blood pressure, calm the nervous system, and support overall cardiovascular function, especially for stress-related heart conditions.

Rosemary and Thyme Blood Flow Capsules

INGREDIENTS

- 1 tablespoon dried rosemary leaves
- 1 tablespoon dried thyme leaves
- Capsule shells

PREPARATION

1. Grind rosemary and thyme leaves into a fine powder.
2. Fill capsule shells with the powder.
3. Take 1-2 capsules daily to improve blood flow.

Benefits: Rosemary and thyme are natural circulatory stimulants that help improve blood flow and reduce inflammation in the blood vessels. These herbs also support healthy cholesterol levels and enhance overall cardiovascular wellness.

Bilberry Eye and Heart Health Capsules

INGREDIENTS

- 1 tablespoon dried bilberry powder
- Capsule shells

PREPARATION

1. Fill capsule shells with bilberry powder.
2. Take 1-2 capsules daily for eye and heart health.

Benefits: Bilberries are rich in antioxidants that support both eye and heart health by improving blood flow to these areas. They help reduce blood pressure, strengthen blood vessels, and protect against oxidative damage, supporting cardiovascular and visual wellness.

Reishi Mushroom Heart Support Tea

INGREDIENTS

- 1 teaspoon dried reishi mushroom powder
- 1 cup boiling water

PREPARATION

1. Steep reishi mushroom powder in boiling water for 15 minutes.
2. Strain and drink warm.

Benefits: Reishi mushrooms are adaptogens that support heart health by reducing stress, inflammation, and blood pressure. Regular consumption of this tea helps protect the cardiovascular system, enhance blood flow, and improve overall heart function.

Ginger and Cinnamon Cholesterol Control Drink

INGREDIENTS

- 1 teaspoon grated ginger
- 1/2 teaspoon cinnamon powder
- 1 cup warm water

PREPARATION

1. Mix ginger and cinnamon in warm water.
2. Drink once daily to support cholesterol management.

Benefits: Ginger and cinnamon both have anti-inflammatory and cholesterol-lowering properties. This drink helps reduce LDL (bad cholesterol) levels and improve heart health by supporting healthy circulation and reducing plaque buildup in the arteries.

Horse Chestnut Vein Support Tincture

INGREDIENTS

- 1 tablespoon dried horse chestnut seeds
- 1/4 cup alcohol (vodka or glycerin for non-alcoholic option)

PREPARATION

1. Place horse chestnut seeds in a jar and cover with alcohol or glycerin.
2. Seal and let it infuse for 4-6 weeks, shaking occasionally.

3. Strain and take 1-2 droppers daily to support vein health.

Benefits: Horse chestnut is widely used for improving vein health and reducing varicose veins. This tincture helps strengthen veins, improve blood circulation, and reduce swelling in the legs, making it an effective remedy for vein and cardiovascular health.

Clove and Honey Heart Warming Elixir

INGREDIENTS

- 1 teaspoon clove powder
- 1 tablespoon honey
- 1 cup warm water

PREPARATION

1. Mix clove powder and honey in warm water.
2. Stir well and drink once daily for heart support.

Benefits: Cloves have warming and anti-inflammatory properties that support circulation and reduce cholesterol. Honey adds heart-protecting antioxidants, making this elixir a comforting and effective remedy for cardiovascular health, particularly for improving blood flow.

Green Tea and Hibiscus Blood Pressure Tea

INGREDIENTS

- 1 teaspoon green tea leaves
- 1 teaspoon dried hibiscus petals
- 1 cup boiling water

PREPARATION

1. Steep green tea and hibiscus petals in boiling water for 10 minutes.
2. Strain and drink once daily for blood pressure control.

Benefits: Green tea is rich in antioxidants that support heart health, while hibiscus helps lower blood pressure. This tea combination improves circulation, reduces inflammation, and helps maintain healthy blood pressure levels, making it ideal for daily cardiovascular support.

Garlic and Olive Oil Heart-Healthy Capsules

INGREDIENTS

- 1 tablespoon garlic powder
- 1 tablespoon olive oil
- Capsule shells

PREPARATION

1. Mix garlic powder with olive oil to form a paste.
2. Fill capsule shells with the mixture.
3. Take 1-2 capsules daily for heart health.

Benefits: Garlic is a well-known remedy for lowering cholesterol and improving heart health. Olive oil adds heart-healthy fats that support circulation and reduce inflammation. These capsules are perfect for maintaining healthy blood pressure and cholesterol levels.

Ashwagandha Stress and Heart Support Capsules

INGREDIENTS

- 1 tablespoon dried ashwagandha root powder
- Capsule shells

PREPARATION

1. Fill capsule shells with ashwagandha root powder.
2. Take 1-2 capsules daily to reduce stress and support heart health.

Benefits: Ashwagandha is an adaptogen that helps the body manage stress, which in turn supports cardiovascular health. These capsules help reduce cortisol levels, lower blood pressure, and protect the heart from stress-related damage, making them beneficial for both mental and physical health.

Passionflower Heart Calming Infusion

INGREDIENTS

- 1 teaspoon dried passionflower
- 1 cup boiling water

PREPARATION

1. Steep passionflower in boiling water for 10 minutes.
2. Strain and drink before bed to calm the heart.

Benefits: Passionflower is a calming herb that helps reduce stress, anxiety, and heart palpitations. This infusion is particularly beneficial for people who experience anxiety-related heart issues, as it promotes relaxation and supports overall cardiovascular wellness.

Grapeseed Extract Antioxidant Capsules

INGREDIENTS

- 1 tablespoon grapeseed extract powder
- Capsule shells

PREPARATION

1. Fill capsule shells with grapeseed extract powder.
2. Take 1-2 capsules daily for antioxidant support.

Benefits: Grapeseed extract is rich in antioxidants that protect the cardiovascular system from oxidative damage. Regular consumption helps reduce inflammation, lower cholesterol, and improve circulation, supporting overall heart health and longevity.

Black Garlic Circulation Support Syrup

INGREDIENTS

- 2 cloves black garlic
- 1 tablespoon honey
- 1 cup water

PREPARATION

1. Simmer black garlic in water for 15 minutes.
2. Strain and stir in honey.
3. Drink once daily for circulation support.

Benefits: Black garlic is rich in antioxidants and has powerful circulation-boosting properties. Combined with honey, this syrup helps improve blood flow, reduce cholesterol, and support overall heart health, making it an effective remedy for cardiovascular wellness.

Flaxseed Omega-3 Heart Health Smoothie

INGREDIENTS

- 1 tablespoon ground flaxseeds
- 1/2 banana
- 1/2 cup almond milk
- 1 teaspoon honey

PREPARATION

1. Blend all ingredients together until smooth.
2. Drink immediately for heart health.

Benefits: Flaxseeds are rich in omega-3 fatty acids, which support heart health by reducing inflammation, lowering cholesterol, and improving circulation. This smoothie provides a nutrient-dense boost to protect and strengthen the cardiovascular system.

Burdock Root Blood Purifier Tonic

INGREDIENTS

- 1 tablespoon dried burdock root
- 2 cups water

PREPARATION

1. Simmer burdock root in water for 20 minutes.
2. Strain and drink once daily.

Benefits: Burdock root is known for its blood-purifying properties, which help remove toxins and improve circulation. This tonic supports cardiovascular health by cleansing the blood, improving artery health, and promoting better blood flow throughout the body.

Marjoram Blood Pressure Support Tea

INGREDIENTS

- 1 teaspoon dried marjoram leaves
- 1 cup boiling water

PREPARATION

Steep marjoram leaves in boiling water

1. for 10 minutes.
2. Strain and drink once daily for blood pressure support.

Benefits: Marjoram helps relax blood vessels, reduce inflammation, and support healthy blood pressure levels. This tea is a gentle yet effective remedy for maintaining healthy blood pressure and supporting overall cardiovascular wellness.

Lemon Balm and Ginger Heart Support Elixir

INGREDIENTS

- 1 teaspoon dried lemon balm leaves
- 1/2 teaspoon grated ginger
- 1 cup boiling water

PREPARATION

1. Steep lemon balm and ginger in boiling water for 10 minutes.
2. Strain and drink once daily for heart support.

Benefits: Lemon balm calms the nervous system, while ginger boosts circulation and reduces inflammation. This elixir helps soothe stress-related heart issues, improve blood flow, and support overall heart health. It's particularly beneficial for those dealing with high stress levels.

Mistletoe Cardiovascular Balance Capsules

INGREDIENTS

- 1 tablespoon dried mistletoe powder
- Capsule shells

PREPARATION

1. Fill capsule shells with mistletoe powder.
2. Take 1-2 capsules daily to balance cardiovascular function.

Benefits: Mistletoe has been traditionally used to support cardiovascular health by lowering blood pressure and improving circulation. These capsules help balance the cardiovascular system, reduce hypertension, and protect the heart from stress and inflammation.

BOOK 12

Herbal Remedies for Children

Safe and Gentle Herbs for Kids

GENTLE HERBAL SOLUTIONS FOR CHILDREN'S WELLBEING

When it comes to children's health, choosing safe and gentle herbs is essential. Children's bodies are more sensitive and respond differently compared to adults, requiring mild yet effective remedies that promote wellness without side effects. For parents like Emma, who prioritize natural and holistic approaches for their children, understanding the right herbs for everyday use can empower them to manage minor health concerns safely and naturally. Below, we explore several herbs that are both gentle and effective for children, focusing on their benefits and ways to incorporate them into daily routines.

Chamomile: The Ultimate Calming Herb

Chamomile is one of the most trusted and widely used herbs for children. Its mild sedative properties make it ideal for calming anxiety, soothing digestive upsets, and promoting restful sleep. Chamomile's anti-inflammatory and antispasmodic effects are also beneficial for easing colic and teething pain, making it a versatile remedy for young children.

Chamomile tea is a simple way to administer this herb. For infants, a few cooled drops can be given via a dropper, while older children can enjoy a small cup of mild tea. For Emma, who seeks convenient and natural options, having chamomile tea on hand provides an easy solution for calming her child during restless nights or minor stomach upsets. Chamomile's gentle nature ensures that it can be used regularly without concerns about safety.

Fennel: Soothing Digestive Aid

Fennel is another child-friendly herb, particularly effective for digestive issues such as gas, bloating, and colic. It has been traditionally used to relieve stomach discomfort and promote digestion. Fennel seeds contain compounds that relax the muscles of the digestive tract, making it suitable for infants and children who experience tummy troubles.

Fennel tea can be made by steeping crushed fennel seeds in hot water, and a few drops can be given to infants. For older children, a diluted tea is safe and effective. Emma can use fennel tea as a go-to remedy for her child's digestive issues, ensuring relief with a gentle, natural approach. Its mild flavor is generally well-accepted by children, making it a practical addition to her herbal toolkit.

Lavender: Calming and Skin-Soothing

Lavender is a gentle herb known for its calming properties, making it suitable for children who struggle with restlessness, anxiety, or sleep disturbances. Its soothing aroma helps relax the nervous system, creating a sense of calm and comfort. Additionally, lavender's anti-inflammatory and antiseptic properties make it useful for minor skin irritations, such as insect bites or rashes.

Lavender essential oil can be diluted and applied to the skin or added to bathwater to create a calming effect before bedtime. For Emma, using lavender oil in her child's bath or as a bedtime spray provides an easy way to create a peaceful environment, promoting restful sleep. The versatility of lavender allows her to use it for both calming and skin-soothing purposes, ensuring her child feels comfortable and relaxed.

Calendula: The Skin Healer

Calendula, also known as marigold, is a gentle herb perfect for children's skin issues. It has anti-inflammatory and antibacterial properties, making it effective for treating diaper rash, eczema, and minor cuts or scrapes. Calendula is safe for young skin and can be used daily to promote healing and soothe irritation.

Calendula can be applied as an infused oil, cream, or salve. For Emma, having a calendula salve available provides a quick and effective remedy for her child's minor skin concerns, ensuring comfort and relief. The mild nature of calendula means it can be used without worry, offering parents a reliable, gentle solution for their child's skincare needs.

Lemon Balm: Easing Tension and Discomfort

Lemon balm is a mild herb known for its calming effects, making it suitable for children experiencing stress, restlessness, or digestive discomfort. It has antiviral properties, which can help manage cold sores and other viral infections in children. Lemon balm tea is mild and has a pleasant, lemony flavor that is generally well-received by children.

For Emma, offering lemon balm tea to her child can provide a simple way to relieve mild tension or digestive upset. A few drops of cooled tea can be administered to infants, while older children can enjoy it as a warm, soothing beverage. The gentle nature of lemon balm ensures that it supports her child's well-being without the risk of overstimulation or adverse effects.

Ginger: A Gentle Remedy for Nausea

Ginger is another safe herb for children when used in small amounts. It is effective for relieving nausea, motion sickness, and mild digestive discomfort. The anti-inflammatory properties of ginger also make it a valuable herb for supporting the immune system, particularly during colds or flu.

For older children, a mild ginger tea made from fresh ginger slices can be given in small sips to ease nausea. For Emma, using ginger as a remedy for travel sickness or during minor stomach upsets offers a quick and natural solution. Ginger's warming and soothing effects make it a versatile herb for children's health, as long as it is administered in appropriately small doses.

Peppermint: Supporting Digestion and Comfort

Peppermint is known for its cooling and soothing effects, particularly on the digestive system. It can help relieve stomach cramps, gas, and bloating, making it suitable for children who experience digestive discomfort. The menthol in peppermint also has mild analgesic properties, which can help soothe headaches or muscle aches.

Peppermint tea is a safe option for children when given in diluted forms. Emma can prepare a mild tea for her child, offering a refreshing and effective way to ease tummy troubles or discomfort. Its familiar taste is often enjoyable for children, making it a practical herb to use when needed.

These herbs provide a gentle and effective approach to managing children's minor health concerns naturally. For Emma, integrating these safe herbal remedies into her child's routine offers peace of mind, ensuring that her child receives the benefits of holistic care without compromising safety.

Boosting Immunity and Managing Common Illnesses

STRENGTHENING IMMUNITY AND ADDRESSING COMMON ILLNESSES IN CHILDREN

Children are naturally exposed to various pathogens as they grow, and developing a strong immune system is essential for their overall health. For parents like Emma, who seek natural ways to boost their children's immunity and manage common illnesses effectively, herbs provide safe and effective solutions. Herbs can be integrated into daily routines to support children's immune systems, helping them build resilience and recover from common ailments. Below, we explore some of the best herbs for boosting immunity and managing illnesses like colds, flu, and digestive upsets in children.

Echinacea: A Powerful Immune Booster

Echinacea is one of the most well-known herbs for enhancing the immune system, making it a valuable tool for children who frequently encounter germs, especially during cold and flu season. It works by stimulating the production of white blood cells, which are essential for fighting infections. Echinacea also has anti-inflammatory and antiviral properties, helping to reduce the severity and duration of colds and other respiratory infections.

Echinacea can be given to children as a tea, tincture, or in a syrup form mixed with honey for a palatable flavor. For Emma, offering echinacea at the first sign of illness provides a proactive approach to boosting her child's immune response. Using it during the early stages of a cold or flu can significantly shorten the duration of the illness, ensuring her child recovers faster and stays active.

Elderberry: Supporting Respiratory Health

Elderberry is another essential herb for immune support, particularly for respiratory health. Rich in antioxidants and vitamins A, B, and C, elderberry strengthens the immune system and helps prevent respiratory infections. Its antiviral properties make it effective against the common cold and influenza, reducing the duration and intensity of symptoms.

Elderberry syrup is a popular and child-friendly way to administer this herb. The sweet flavor makes it enjoyable for children, and Emma can incorporate it into her child's daily routine as a preventative measure or during the onset of cold symptoms. By using elderberry syrup, Emma ensures her child's respiratory health is supported naturally, minimizing the reliance on over-the-counter medications.

Astragalus: Building Long-Term Immunity

Astragalus is a less commonly known herb but is highly effective for boosting immunity, particularly in children who may be prone to frequent illnesses. It is an adaptogen, meaning it helps the body adapt to stress and boosts the immune system's capacity over time. Astragalus is particularly beneficial for strengthening the body's defenses against viruses and bacteria, making it an excellent addition to a child's long-term wellness plan.

Astragalus can be used as a tea or added to soups and broths, making it easy to incorporate into meals. For Emma, adding astragalus root to homemade soups provides her child with immune support in a comforting and natural way. This method not only makes the herb palatable but also ensures that its immune-boosting properties are consumed regularly, promoting long-term resilience against illnesses.

Ginger: Natural Remedy for Digestive Upsets

Ginger is a versatile herb that not only boosts immunity but also helps manage digestive issues, which are common among children. It has anti-inflammatory and antibacterial properties, making it effective for soothing stomachaches, nausea, and indigestion. Ginger also helps to warm the body and promote circulation, supporting overall immune function during cold weather or illness.

Ginger tea, made by steeping fresh ginger slices, can be given in small sips to children experiencing digestive discomfort or early signs of a cold. Emma can also add a bit of honey to enhance the flavor, making it more enjoyable for her child. The soothing and warming properties of ginger provide a gentle, natural way to support her child's health, ensuring comfort and relief from common digestive and respiratory complaints.

Lemon Balm: Calming and Immune-Enhancing

Lemon balm is a mild herb known for its calming properties and immune-boosting effects. It is particularly effective for children who experience stress or anxiety, which can weaken the immune system. Lemon balm also has antiviral properties, making it suitable for preventing and managing illnesses like cold sores and mild viral infections.

Lemon balm tea is an easy way to administer this herb to children. For Emma, offering lemon balm tea during stressful periods or when her child shows signs of illness provides a comforting and effective way to boost immunity while calming the nervous system. The pleasant, lemony flavor of the tea makes it an appealing option for children, ensuring they receive its benefits consistently.

Thyme: Protecting Against Respiratory Infections

Thyme is a powerful herb for respiratory health, with antiseptic and antibacterial properties that make it effective against coughs, bronchitis, and sore throats. It supports the immune system by helping to clear congestion and soothe irritated airways, making it a valuable herb during cold and flu season.

Thyme tea or a thyme-infused steam inhalation can be used to relieve respiratory symptoms in children. For Emma, preparing a thyme tea or using it as a steam treatment when her child experiences cough or congestion provides a simple and effective way to manage these symptoms naturally. Thyme's ability to support respiratory health without the side effects of synthetic cough medicines ensures that her child remains comfortable and protected.

Licorice Root: Soothing Colds and Coughs

Licorice root is a gentle herb that offers both immune-boosting and anti-inflammatory effects, making it ideal for managing coughs and sore throats in children. It soothes mucous membranes and acts as a natural expectorant, helping to clear phlegm and ease breathing.

Licorice root tea can be sweetened with honey and given to children to alleviate cold symptoms. For Emma, this herb provides a natural and child-friendly way to manage her child's respiratory symptoms, ensuring her child receives relief from discomfort in a safe and gentle manner.

These herbs provide effective strategies for boosting children's immunity and managing common illnesses naturally. By integrating these herbs into her child's routine, Emma can feel confident in providing natural support that aligns with her preference for holistic wellness solutions.

Child-Friendly Remedies for Parents

Chamomile Calming Tea for Kids

INGREDIENTS

- 1 teaspoon dried chamomile flowers
- 1 cup boiling water

PREPARATION

1. Steep chamomile flowers in boiling water for 5-10 minutes.
2. Strain and allow the tea to cool before serving.

Benefits: Chamomile has gentle calming properties, making it ideal for soothing fussy or anxious children. It helps to relax the muscles and the mind, promoting restful sleep and easing digestive discomfort. This tea is safe and mild for children of all ages.

Elderberry Immune Boosting Syrup

INGREDIENTS

- 1/2 cup dried elderberries
- 2 cups water
- 1/4 cup honey (omit for children under 1 year)

PREPARATION

1. Simmer elderberries in water for 20 minutes.
2. Strain the mixture and stir in honey.
3. Store in the fridge and give 1-2 teaspoons daily.

Benefits: Elderberries are rich in antioxidants and vitamins, especially vitamin C, which helps strengthen the immune system. This syrup is excellent for preventing colds and flu and can also reduce the severity and duration of symptoms if illness occurs.

Lemon Balm Digestive Relief Drops

INGREDIENTS

- 1 teaspoon dried lemon balm leaves
- 1/2 cup water

PREPARATION

1. Steep lemon balm leaves in boiling water for 10 minutes.
2. Strain and allow to cool.
3. Give 1-2 droppers to children for digestive relief.

Benefits: Lemon balm is a gentle herb that helps soothe upset stomachs, gas, and indigestion in children. These drops are perfect for relieving digestive discomfort without the use of harsh medications. They also promote relaxation and calmness.

Marshmallow Root Cough Soothing Syrup

INGREDIENTS

- 1 tablespoon dried marshmallow root
- 1 cup water
- 1/4 cup honey (omit for children under 1 year)

PREPARATION

1. Simmer marshmallow root in water for 15 minutes.
2. Strain and stir in honey.
3. Give 1 teaspoon as needed to soothe coughs.

Benefits: Marshmallow root has mucilage properties that coat and soothe irritated throats, making it effective for easing coughs and respiratory discomfort. This syrup is gentle enough for children and can be used to provide relief from dry, scratchy throats.

Catnip and Fennel Colic Relief Tea

INGREDIENTS

- 1 teaspoon dried catnip leaves
- 1/2 teaspoon fennel seeds
- 1 cup boiling water

PREPARATION

1. Steep catnip leaves and fennel seeds in boiling water for 10 minutes.
2. Strain and cool before giving to the child.
3. Give 1-2 teaspoons for colic relief.

Benefits: Catnip is calming and helps relax the digestive system, while fennel relieves gas and bloating. This combination is especially effective for soothing colic in infants and easing digestive discomfort in children.

Calendula Diaper Rash Cream

INGREDIENTS

- 1 tablespoon dried calendula flowers
- 1/4 cup coconut oil

PREPARATION

1. Infuse calendula flowers in melted coconut oil using a double boiler for 30 minutes.
2. Strain and pour into a jar.
3. Apply to diaper rash as needed.

Benefits: Calendula is a gentle anti-inflammatory herb that helps soothe and heal irritated skin. This cream is perfect for treating diaper rash, as it promotes healing and provides a protective barrier against further irritation. The coconut oil adds moisturizing and antibacterial properties.

Echinacea Immune Support Gummies

INGREDIENTS

- 1/2 cup echinacea tea
- 1 tablespoon gelatin
- 1 tablespoon honey (optional)

PREPARATION

1. Brew echinacea tea and allow it to cool slightly.
2. Dissolve gelatin in the tea, stirring well.
3. Pour into silicone molds and refrigerate until set.
4. Give 1-2 gummies daily for immune support.

Benefits: Echinacea is a well-known immune booster that helps protect children from infections. These gummies are a fun and effective way to strengthen the immune system and prevent colds, flu, and other common childhood illnesses.

Slippery Elm Throat Lozenge

INGREDIENTS

- 1 tablespoon slippery elm powder
- 1 tablespoon honey

PREPARATION

1. Mix slippery elm powder and honey to form a thick paste.
2. Roll the paste into small balls and refrigerate until firm.
3. Give 1 lozenge as needed for throat relief.

Benefits: Slippery elm is soothing to the throat and helps ease irritation caused by coughing. These lozenges coat the throat and provide relief from dryness, scratchiness, and soreness, making them an ideal natural remedy for children with sore throats.

Ginger Tummy Comfort Tea

INGREDIENTS

- 1/2 teaspoon grated fresh ginger
- 1 cup boiling water

PREPARATION

1. Steep ginger in boiling water for 10 minutes.
2. Strain and allow the tea to cool before serving.

Benefits: Ginger is known for its ability to soothe upset stomachs, reduce nausea, and relieve gas. This tea is gentle enough for children and can help provide relief from indigestion, motion sickness, and general tummy discomfort.

Lavender and Aloe Skin Soothing Gel

INGREDIENTS

- 1 tablespoon aloe vera gel
- 5 drops lavender essential oil

PREPARATION

1. Mix aloe vera gel with lavender essential oil.
2. Apply to irritated or sunburned skin as needed.

Benefits: Lavender has soothing and anti-inflammatory properties, while aloe vera is cooling and hydrating. This gel provides relief for irritated skin, sunburns, and minor cuts or scrapes, making it a versatile remedy for children's skin issues.

Licorice Root Cough Ease Tincture

INGREDIENTS

- 1 tablespoon dried licorice root
- 1/4 cup water

PREPARATION

1. Simmer licorice root in water for 15 minutes.
2. Strain and allow to cool before giving 1-2 droppers for cough relief.

Benefits: Licorice root has expectorant properties that help ease coughs by loosening mucus and soothing the throat. This tincture provides gentle, effective relief for children with persistent coughs or respiratory irritation.

Nettle Infusion for Iron Support

INGREDIENTS

- 1 teaspoon dried nettle leaves
- 1 cup boiling water

PREPARATION

1. Steep nettle leaves in boiling water for 10 minutes.
2. Strain and allow to cool before giving to the child.

Benefits: Nettle is rich in iron and other essential minerals, making this infusion a great way to support healthy iron levels in children. It helps prevent anemia and boosts energy levels in a natural, gentle way.

Dill Seed Baby Gripe Water

INGREDIENTS

- 1 teaspoon dill seeds
- 1 cup water

PREPARATION

1. Simmer dill seeds in water for 10 minutes.
2. Strain and allow to cool before giving 1-2 teaspoons to the baby.

Benefits: Dill seed is effective in relieving colic, gas, and indigestion in babies. This gripe water provides gentle digestive support and can help calm fussy babies by soothing their stomachs and reducing discomfort.

Orange Peel and Peppermint Tummy Tonic

INGREDIENTS

- 1 teaspoon dried orange peel
- 1/2 teaspoon dried peppermint leaves
- 1 cup boiling water

PREPARATION

1. Steep orange peel and peppermint leaves in boiling water for 10 minutes.

Strain and allow to cool

2. before giving 1-2 teaspoons to children.

Benefits: Orange peel and peppermint are both excellent for relieving digestive discomfort. This tummy tonic helps ease gas, bloating, and indigestion, making it a soothing remedy for children with upset stomachs.

Rose Hip Vitamin C Syrup

INGREDIENTS

- 1/4 cup dried rose hips
- 1 cup water
- 1/4 cup honey (omit for children under 1 year)

PREPARATION

1. Simmer rose hips in water for 10 minutes.
2. Strain and stir in honey.
3. Give 1-2 teaspoons daily for vitamin C support.

Benefits: Rose hips are high in vitamin C, which supports the immune system and promotes overall health. This syrup is an easy and delicious way to ensure children receive their daily dose of vitamin C, especially during cold and flu season.

Blueberry and Lemon Immune-Boosting Smoothie

INGREDIENTS

- 1/2 cup fresh or frozen blueberries
- 1/4 cup plain yogurt
- 1 tablespoon lemon juice

PREPARATION

1. Blend all ingredients until smooth.
2. Serve immediately for an immune boost.

Benefits: Blueberries are packed with antioxidants, and lemon adds vitamin C, making this smoothie a powerful immune booster for kids. The yogurt provides probiotics, which support gut health and strengthen the immune system. It's a tasty way to promote wellness.

Chamomile and Lemon Balm Sleepy Time Lotion

INGREDIENTS

- 1 tablespoon dried chamomile flowers
- 1 tablespoon dried lemon balm leaves
- 1/4 cup coconut oil

PREPARATION

1. Infuse chamomile flowers and lemon balm leaves in melted coconut oil for 30 minutes.
2. Strain and pour into a jar.
3. Massage into the child's skin before bed.

Benefits: Chamomile and lemon balm are calming herbs that help relax the mind and body. This sleepy time lotion soothes the skin while promoting restful sleep, making it an excellent remedy for fussy or restless children.

Ginger and Honey Warm Elixir

INGREDIENTS

- 1/2 teaspoon grated fresh ginger
- 1 teaspoon honey (omit for children under 1 year)
- 1/2 cup warm water

PREPARATION

1. Mix the grated ginger and honey in warm water.
2. Stir well and give 1-2 teaspoons to children for soothing.

Benefits: Ginger helps to settle the stomach and soothe nausea, while honey coats the throat and eases discomfort. This elixir is gentle enough for children and can be used to treat both stomach upset and mild colds.

Plantain Leaf Boo-Boo Balm

INGREDIENTS

- 1 tablespoon dried plantain leaves
- 1/4 cup coconut oil

PREPARATION

1. Infuse dried plantain leaves in melted coconut oil for 30 minutes using a double boiler.
2. Strain and pour into a small jar.
3. Apply to cuts, scrapes, and minor wounds as needed.

Benefits: Plantain has natural wound-healing and anti-inflammatory properties. This balm provides relief from cuts, scrapes, and insect bites, promoting faster healing and soothing the skin. It's a safe and effective remedy for minor skin irritations in children.

Peppermint and Marshmallow Digestive Aid

INGREDIENTS

- 1 teaspoon dried peppermint leaves
- 1 teaspoon dried marshmallow root
- 1 cup boiling water

PREPARATION

1. Steep peppermint leaves and marshmallow root in boiling water for 10 minutes.
2. Strain and allow to cool before serving.

Benefits: Peppermint helps ease indigestion and gas, while marshmallow root soothes the digestive tract. This digestive aid is a gentle and effective remedy for children experiencing tummy troubles, including bloating and discomfort.

Hibiscus Hydration Tea

INGREDIENTS

- 1 tablespoon dried hibiscus petals
- 1 cup boiling water

PREPARATION

1. Steep hibiscus petals in boiling water for 10 minutes.
2. Strain and cool before serving to children.

Benefits: Hibiscus is rich in antioxidants and provides gentle hydration for children. This tea is a healthy alternative to sugary drinks, helping to replenish fluids and keep children hydrated, especially during hot weather or after physical activity.

Oatstraw Calcium Support Infusion

INGREDIENTS

- 1 tablespoon dried oatstraw
- 1 cup boiling water

PREPARATION

1. Steep oatstraw in boiling water for 20-30 minutes.
2. Strain and cool before serving.

Benefits: Oatstraw is an excellent source of calcium and other essential minerals. This infusion helps support strong bones and teeth, making it a great way to provide children with the nutrients they need for healthy growth and development.

Thyme and Elderflower Fever Reducer

INGREDIENTS

- 1 teaspoon dried thyme
- 1 teaspoon dried elderflower
- 1 cup boiling water

PREPARATION

1. Steep thyme and elderflower in boiling water for 10 minutes.
2. Strain and allow the tea to cool before giving 1-2 teaspoons to children.

Benefits: Thyme has antimicrobial properties, while elderflower helps reduce fever and boost the immune system. This tea provides natural relief from fevers in children and can be used alongside other treatments to help lower body temperature.

Rose Petal Emotional Support Drops

INGREDIENTS

- 1 tablespoon dried rose petals
- 1/2 cup water

PREPARATION

1. Steep rose petals in boiling water for 10 minutes.
2. Strain and allow the tea to cool.
3. Give 1-2 droppers to children to help calm their emotions.

Benefits: Rose petals are known for their calming and uplifting effects on emotions. These drops help children manage feelings of anxiety, sadness, or irritability, making them a gentle remedy for emotional support.

Chickweed Itch Relief Cream

INGREDIENTS

- 1 tablespoon dried chickweed
- 1/4 cup coconut oil

PREPARATION

1. Infuse chickweed in melted coconut oil using a double boiler for 30 minutes.
2. Strain and pour into a jar.
3. Apply to itchy skin as needed.

Benefits: Chickweed is known for its ability to relieve itching and soothe irritated skin. This cream is effective for treating rashes, bug bites, and other skin irritations in children, providing quick relief and promoting healing.

Sage and Honey Sore Throat Spray

INGREDIENTS

- 1 teaspoon dried sage leaves
- 1/4 cup water
- 1 tablespoon honey (omit for children under 1 year)

PREPARATION

1. Steep sage leaves in boiling water for 10 minutes.
2. Strain and mix with honey.
3. Pour into a spray bottle and spritz onto the throat as needed.

Benefits: Sage has antibacterial and anti-inflammatory properties, making it effective for soothing sore throats. The honey adds a protective coating and further helps relieve throat irritation. This spray is a natural way to ease throat pain in children.

Fennel Seed Digestive Drops

INGREDIENTS

- 1 teaspoon fennel seeds
- 1/2 cup water

PREPARATION

1. Simmer fennel seeds in water for 10 minutes.
2. Strain and cool before giving 1-2 droppers for digestive support.

Benefits: Fennel seeds are known for their ability to relieve gas, bloating, and indigestion. These digestive drops are gentle and effective for easing tummy troubles in children, providing quick relief from discomfort.

Linden Flower Comforting Tea

INGREDIENTS

- 1 teaspoon dried linden flowers
- 1 cup boiling water

PREPARATION

1. Steep linden flowers in boiling water for 10 minutes.
2. Strain and allow to cool before serving to children.

Benefits: Linden flowers have calming properties that help ease anxiety and promote relaxation. This tea is perfect for comforting children who are feeling upset, anxious, or restless, providing gentle emotional and physical support.

Violet Leaf Rash Soothing Balm

INGREDIENTS

- 1 tablespoon dried violet leaves
- 1/4 cup coconut oil

PREPARATION

1. Infuse violet leaves in melted coconut oil for 30 minutes.
2. Strain and pour into a jar.
3. Apply to rashes or irritated skin as needed.

Benefits: Violet leaves are known for their ability to soothe skin irritations and reduce inflammation. This balm is effective for treating rashes, eczema, and other skin issues in children, promoting healing and providing relief from itching and discomfort.

Grape Seed Antioxidant Snack Mix

INGREDIENTS

- 1/4 cup dried grape seeds
- 1/4 cup almonds
- 1/4 cup dried cranberries

PREPARATION

1. Combine all ingredients in a bowl.
2. Store in an airtight container and serve as a snack.

Benefits: Grape seeds are rich in antioxidants that help protect the body from free radical damage. This snack mix provides a healthy, antioxidant-rich boost for children, supporting their overall health and immune function in a delicious and easy-to-eat way.

Lemon Verbena Calming Bath Oil

INGREDIENTS

- 1 tablespoon dried lemon verbena leaves
- 1/4 cup olive oil

PREPARATION

1. Infuse lemon verbena leaves in olive oil using a double boiler for 30 minutes.
2. Strain and pour into a bottle.
3. Add 1-2 tablespoons to a warm bath for a calming effect.

Benefits: Lemon verbena is known for its relaxing and calming properties. This bath oil helps soothe the nerves and promote relaxation, making it an ideal remedy for calming children before bedtime or after a long, stressful day.

Parsley and Dandelion Iron Boost Tea

INGREDIENTS

- 1 teaspoon dried parsley
- 1 teaspoon dried dandelion leaves
- 1 cup boiling water

PREPARATION

1. Steep parsley and dandelion leaves in boiling water for 10 minutes.
2. Strain and allow to cool before serving.

Benefits: Parsley and dandelion are both rich in iron and other essential nutrients. This tea provides a natural way to boost iron levels in children, supporting healthy blood production and energy levels, especially for those prone to low iron.

Chamomile and Ginger Teething Relief Gel

INGREDIENTS

- 1 teaspoon dried chamomile flowers
- 1/2 teaspoon grated ginger
- 1/4 cup water

PREPARATION

1. Simmer chamomile and ginger in water for 10 minutes.
2. Strain and allow to cool.
3. Apply the gel to the gums for teething relief.

Benefits: Chamomile and ginger help soothe inflammation and reduce discomfort associated with teething. This gentle gel provides natural pain relief for teething babies, helping to calm them and ease the pain in their gums.

BOOK 13

Herbal Support for Aging and Longevity

Herbs for Cognitive Health and Memory

NATURAL HERBS TO ENHANCE COGNITIVE FUNCTION AND MEMORY

As individuals age, maintaining cognitive health and memory becomes increasingly important. Herbs offer a natural, effective way to support brain function, improve focus, and enhance memory retention. For those like Emma, who seek holistic and sustainable solutions to promote cognitive wellness, understanding which herbs to incorporate can make a significant difference in their daily routines. Below, we explore several herbs that are known for their cognitive benefits, detailing how they work and how they can be used to boost brain health and memory naturally.

Ginkgo Biloba: The Memory Enhancer

Ginkgo biloba is one of the oldest and most researched herbs for cognitive health. It has been used for centuries in traditional medicine to improve memory and mental clarity. Ginkgo works by increasing blood flow to the brain, delivering oxygen and nutrients essential for cognitive function. Its antioxidant properties also protect brain cells from damage caused by free radicals, which can accelerate cognitive decline.

Ginkgo biloba is particularly effective for older individuals experiencing mild memory issues or those seeking to maintain sharp mental function as they age. It can be taken as a supplement, tea, or tincture. For Emma, who may prefer convenient and consistent solutions, ginkgo biloba capsules offer a practical way to integrate this herb into her daily regimen. Regular use supports long-term memory retention and mental acuity, aligning with her goals of sustaining cognitive health naturally.

Bacopa Monnieri: Promoting Mental Clarity

Bacopa monnieri, also known as Brahmi, is an herb traditionally used in Ayurvedic medicine to enhance cognitive function and memory. It works by supporting neurotransmitter activity in the brain, which improves communication between neurons and enhances cognitive processes. Bacopa also acts as an adaptogen, reducing stress and anxiety—factors that can impair memory and focus over time.

Research has shown that bacopa monnieri not only enhances memory retention but also improves learning and information processing speed. For Emma, who values holistic solutions for maintaining cognitive health, bacopa can be taken as a supplement or consumed as an infusion. Incorporating bacopa into her daily routine provides a sustainable way to promote mental clarity and focus, ensuring she continues to feel sharp and alert as she ages.

Rosemary: The Herb of Remembrance

Rosemary is a well-known culinary herb that also offers significant benefits for cognitive health. The compounds in rosemary, particularly **carnosic acid**, protect the brain from oxidative damage and reduce inflammation. Rosemary has been shown to enhance memory and concentration, making it an ideal herb for those looking to boost cognitive performance naturally.

Incorporating rosemary into meals is an easy and practical way for Emma to enjoy its cognitive benefits. Fresh rosemary can be added to roasted vegetables, meats, or soups, providing both flavor and health support. Alternatively, using rosemary essential oil in a diffuser or applying it topically can also help improve focus and memory retention. Emma can include rosemary in her daily habits without making significant lifestyle changes, ensuring consistent support for her brain health.

Gotu Kola: Supporting Cognitive Longevity

Gotu kola, another herb rooted in traditional Ayurvedic and Chinese medicine, is renowned for its cognitive-enhancing properties. It helps improve circulation, especially to the brain, ensuring that neurons receive adequate oxygen and nutrients. Gotu kola is also known for its ability to reduce mental fatigue and enhance memory, making it beneficial for those experiencing age-related cognitive decline.

Gotu kola can be consumed as a tea, tincture, or capsule. For Emma, who may seek versatile and easy-to-use options, gotu kola tea provides a relaxing and effective way to support cognitive health. Regular use not only enhances mental clarity but also supports long-term brain function, helping Emma maintain sharpness and focus throughout the aging process.

Ashwagandha: Combating Cognitive Decline

Ashwagandha is an adaptogenic herb that offers numerous benefits for cognitive health. It works by reducing stress and inflammation, both of which can impair brain function over time. Ashwagandha supports the production of acetylcholine, a neurotransmitter crucial for learning and memory retention. It also helps combat oxidative stress, protecting the brain from age-related damage.

Ashwagandha is effective for older adults looking to maintain mental sharpness and reduce the impact of stress on cognitive performance. For Emma, incorporating ashwagandha capsules into her daily routine offers a simple way to support cognitive longevity. This herb not only enhances brain function but also promotes overall wellness, aligning with her holistic approach to health.

Sage: A Boost for Memory and Concentration

Sage is another herb that has been traditionally used to enhance memory and concentration. Compounds in sage, such as rosmarinic acid, provide antioxidant and anti-inflammatory effects that protect the brain from damage. Studies have shown that sage improves cognitive performance, particularly in memory and attention, making it valuable for those seeking to sustain sharp mental function.

Sage can be consumed as a tea or used as a culinary herb in daily cooking. For Emma, adding sage to her meals—whether in soups, dressings, or herbal teas—offers a flavorful and natural way to enhance cognitive health. Regular use ensures she benefits from its brain-boosting properties while also enjoying its distinct taste.

These herbs provide a natural and effective approach to supporting cognitive health and memory, particularly as individuals age. By integrating these herbs into her routine, Emma can enjoy enhanced mental clarity and long-term cognitive support, ensuring she maintains a sharp and vibrant mind well into her later years.

Strengthening Bones and Joints with Natural Solutions

NATURAL HERBS FOR STRENGTHENING BONES AND SUPPORTING JOINT HEALTH

Maintaining strong bones and flexible joints is essential for healthy aging, as these factors greatly influence mobility, independence, and overall quality of life. Herbs and natural remedies provide effective ways to support bone density, reduce inflammation, and improve joint function, offering a holistic approach to longevity. For individuals like Emma, who prefer natural and sustainable solutions, understanding the herbs that promote bone and joint health is crucial for developing a wellness routine that supports aging gracefully. Below, we explore various herbs known for their ability to strengthen bones and joints, detailing their benefits and practical applications.

Horsetail: A Rich Source of Silica

Horsetail is an ancient herb renowned for its high silica content, which is essential for bone strength and health. Silica aids in the formation of collagen, a vital component of bones, joints, and connective tissues. By increasing collagen production, horsetail supports bone density and helps repair and maintain cartilage, making it an effective herb for those experiencing age-related bone loss or joint stiffness.

Horsetail can be consumed as a tea or tincture, providing a gentle and natural way to boost silica levels. For Emma, integrating horsetail tea into her daily routine offers a simple and effective way to strengthen her bones and support joint health. Its mineral-rich composition ensures that she receives consistent support, promoting flexibility and mobility as she ages.

Nettle: Calcium-Rich and Anti-Inflammatory

Nettle is another powerful herb that supports bone health, thanks to its high calcium, magnesium, and vitamin K content. These nutrients are critical for maintaining bone density and preventing osteoporosis. In addition to its rich mineral profile, nettle also possesses anti-inflammatory properties, which help alleviate joint pain and stiffness.

For Emma, nettle tea is a practical way to consume this herb regularly. The tea provides a soothing, nutrient-rich beverage that not only supports bone health but also reduces inflammation in the joints. Additionally, fresh nettle leaves can be added to soups or salads, offering a versatile approach to incorporating this herb into her diet and ensuring she benefits from its full spectrum of nutrients.

Turmeric: Reducing Inflammation and Supporting Joint Flexibility

Turmeric, with its active compound curcumin, is widely known for its anti-inflammatory properties, making it invaluable for joint health. Chronic inflammation is a major contributor to joint pain and stiffness, particularly as individuals age. Curcumin helps reduce this inflammation, alleviating pain and improving mobility. Turmeric also supports the maintenance of bone health by protecting against oxidative stress, which can weaken bones over time.

Turmeric can be incorporated into daily meals, such as soups, curries, or even smoothies, providing Emma with a versatile and flavorful way to enhance her diet. Additionally, turmeric supplements are available for those seeking a more concentrated dose. Using turmeric regularly helps Emma manage joint pain naturally, ensuring her joints remain flexible and her bones strong as she ages.

Red Clover: Supporting Bone Density

Red clover is a herb rich in phytoestrogens, which mimic the effects of estrogen in the body. Estrogen plays a critical role in maintaining bone density, especially in women as they age and go through menopause. The decline in estrogen levels can lead to bone loss and osteoporosis. Red clover helps counteract this effect, making it a valuable ally for women aiming to strengthen their bones naturally.

Red clover can be consumed as a tea or taken in capsule form. For Emma, drinking red clover tea provides a gentle and enjoyable way to support her bone health. Incorporating this herb into her daily regimen ensures that she proactively addresses the risk of bone density loss, aligning with her holistic approach to health and aging.

Devil's Claw: Easing Joint Pain

Devil's claw is a herb traditionally used for its anti-inflammatory and analgesic properties, making it an effective remedy for joint pain and stiffness. It is particularly beneficial for individuals with arthritis or those who experience chronic joint discomfort. The active compounds in devil's claw, known as harpagosides, help reduce inflammation in the joints, promoting flexibility and ease of movement.

Devil's claw is commonly available as a capsule or tincture, providing Emma with an easy way to include it in her routine. Using devil's claw ensures that her joint health is supported naturally, without relying on synthetic pain relief medications. This herb's ability to alleviate pain and inflammation makes it a valuable addition for those seeking long-term joint support.

Alfalfa: Boosting Mineral Absorption

Alfalfa is another herb rich in essential nutrients for bone health, including calcium, magnesium, and phosphorus. These minerals are vital for maintaining bone density and strength. Alfalfa also supports the absorption of these minerals, enhancing their effectiveness and promoting overall skeletal health.

Alfalfa can be consumed as a tea or added to salads as fresh sprouts. For Emma, alfalfa tea provides an accessible way to increase her mineral intake, ensuring her bones receive the nutrients needed for optimal strength. Regular consumption of alfalfa supports not only her bone health but also her overall vitality, making it a holistic solution for aging gracefully.

Boswellia: Enhancing Joint Flexibility

Boswellia, also known as frankincense, is a herb traditionally used to improve joint health due to its anti-inflammatory properties. It is particularly effective in managing arthritis symptoms and improving joint flexibility by reducing inflammation and protecting the cartilage. For individuals experiencing joint stiffness or discomfort, boswellia provides a natural alternative to conventional anti-inflammatory medications.

Boswellia can be taken as a capsule or tincture, making it easy for Emma to incorporate into her wellness routine. Its long-term use helps ensure that her joints remain flexible and pain-free, supporting her active lifestyle and helping her maintain mobility as she ages.

These natural solutions offer effective ways to strengthen bones and support joint health through the aging process. For Emma, integrating these herbs into her routine ensures that she maintains her physical mobility and bone density, supporting her holistic wellness goals in a sustainable and natural manner.

Remedies for Healthy Aging and Vitality

Ginkgo Biloba Memory Tea

INGREDIENTS

- 1 teaspoon dried ginkgo biloba leaves
- 1 cup boiling water

PREPARATION

1. Steep ginkgo biloba leaves in boiling water for 10 minutes.
2. Strain and drink once daily.

Benefits: Ginkgo biloba is renowned for its ability to improve memory and cognitive function by increasing blood flow to the brain. Regular consumption of this tea supports healthy aging by enhancing focus, memory retention, and mental clarity. It may also help reduce symptoms of cognitive decline in the elderly.

Ashwagandha Energy Boost Capsules

INGREDIENTS

- 1 tablespoon dried ashwagandha root powder
- Capsule shells

PREPARATION

1. Fill capsule shells with ashwagandha root powder.
2. Take 1-2 capsules daily for an energy boost.

Benefits: Ashwagandha is an adaptogen known for its ability to reduce stress, boost energy levels, and improve stamina. These capsules help combat fatigue, enhance physical and mental endurance, and support overall vitality, making them a powerful remedy for aging individuals looking to maintain their energy and strength.

Bacopa Brain Function Tincture

INGREDIENTS

- 1 tablespoon dried bacopa herb
- 1/4 cup alcohol (vodka or glycerin for a non-alcoholic option)

PREPARATION

1. Infuse dried bacopa herb in alcohol or glycerin for 4-6 weeks, shaking occasionally.
2. Strain and take 1-2 droppers daily for brain support.

Benefits: Bacopa has long been used in Ayurvedic medicine to enhance brain function and memory. This tincture promotes cognitive clarity, improves concentration, and supports overall brain health, making it an ideal supplement for aging adults concerned about cognitive decline.

Eleuthero Anti-Fatigue Elixir

INGREDIENTS

- 1 teaspoon dried eleuthero root
- 1 cup water

PREPARATION

1. Simmer eleuthero root in water for 20 minutes.
2. Strain and drink once daily to reduce fatigue.

Benefits: Eleuthero is a powerful adaptogen that helps reduce fatigue, improve endurance, and increase mental and physical energy. This elixir is excellent for combating the effects of stress and aging, helping the body maintain vitality and resilience.

Hawthorn Berry Heart Tonic

INGREDIENTS

- 1 teaspoon dried hawthorn berries
- 1 cup boiling water

PREPARATION

1. Steep hawthorn berries in boiling water for 10-15 minutes.
2. Strain and drink once daily to support heart health.

Benefits: Hawthorn berries are well-known for their ability to strengthen the heart and improve circulation. This tonic helps maintain healthy blood pressure, reduces the risk of heart disease, and promotes overall cardiovascular health, making it an essential remedy for aging adults.

Turmeric and Ginger Anti-Inflammatory Paste

INGREDIENTS

- 1 teaspoon turmeric powder
- 1/2 teaspoon grated fresh ginger
- 1 tablespoon coconut oil

PREPARATION

1. Mix turmeric powder, grated ginger, and coconut oil into a paste.
2. Apply to sore joints or muscles to reduce inflammation.

Benefits: Turmeric and ginger are both potent anti-inflammatory agents that help reduce pain and swelling in the joints. This paste is especially beneficial for individuals suffering from arthritis or age-related joint pain, offering a natural remedy to manage discomfort.

Reishi Mushroom Longevity Decoction

INGREDIENTS

- 1 tablespoon dried reishi mushroom slices
- 2 cups water

PREPARATION

1. Simmer reishi mushroom slices in water for 30 minutes.
2. Strain and drink daily for longevity support.

Benefits: Reishi mushrooms are known for their adaptogenic properties and ability to promote longevity and vitality. This decoction helps balance the body's stress response, boosts immune function, and supports healthy aging by protecting against the effects of stress and illness.

Gotu Kola Cognitive Clarity Capsules

INGREDIENTS

- 1 tablespoon dried gotu kola powder
- Capsule shells

PREPARATION

1. Fill capsule shells with gotu kola powder.
2. Take 1-2 capsules daily for cognitive clarity.

Benefits: Gotu kola is a powerful herb that supports mental clarity, improves memory, and enhances focus. These capsules are particularly beneficial for aging individuals looking to maintain cognitive function and prevent cognitive decline.

Red Clover Hormone Balance Tea

INGREDIENTS

- 1 teaspoon dried red clover blossoms
- 1 cup boiling water

PREPARATION

1. Steep red clover blossoms in boiling water for 10 minutes.
2. Strain and drink once daily for hormone balance.

Benefits: Red clover contains phytoestrogens that help balance hormone levels in aging women. This tea is especially useful for women going through menopause, as it helps alleviate symptoms such as hot flashes, mood swings, and hormonal imbalances.

St. John's Wort Mood Lift Drops

INGREDIENTS

- 1 tablespoon dried St. John's wort leaves
- 1/4 cup alcohol (vodka or glycerin for non-alcoholic option)

PREPARATION

1. Infuse dried St. John's wort leaves in alcohol or glycerin for 4-6 weeks.
2. Strain and take 1-2 droppers daily for mood support.

Benefits: St. John's wort is a well-known herb for improving mood and reducing symptoms of depression. These drops help alleviate feelings of sadness, anxiety, and stress, making them particularly beneficial for individuals experiencing mood fluctuations as they age.

Horsetail Bone Strength Infusion

INGREDIENTS

- 1 tablespoon dried horsetail herb
- 1 cup boiling water

PREPARATION

1. Steep horsetail herb in boiling water for 20 minutes.
2. Strain and drink daily for bone strength support.

Benefits: Horsetail is rich in silica, a mineral that supports bone density and strength. This infusion helps maintain strong bones and joints, making it an excellent remedy for aging individuals concerned about osteoporosis or age-related bone loss.

Nettle Joint Support Tea

INGREDIENTS

- 1 teaspoon dried nettle leaves
- 1 cup boiling water

PREPARATION

1. Steep nettle leaves in boiling water for 10 minutes.
2. Strain and drink once daily for joint support.

Benefits: Nettle is rich in minerals and anti-inflammatory compounds that help support joint health. This tea is particularly useful for individuals dealing with joint pain, stiffness, or inflammation, as it helps reduce discomfort and improve mobility.

Bilberry Eye Health Capsules

INGREDIENTS

- 1 tablespoon dried bilberry powder
- Capsule shells

PREPARATION

1. Fill capsule shells with bilberry powder.
2. Take 1-2 capsules daily for eye health.

Benefits: Bilberries are rich in antioxidants that support eye health and improve vision. These capsules help protect the eyes from age-related conditions such as macular degeneration and cataracts, making them an essential remedy for aging individuals seeking to maintain good vision.

Ginseng Longevity Tonic

INGREDIENTS

- 1 teaspoon dried ginseng root
- 1 cup boiling water

PREPARATION

1. Steep ginseng root in boiling water for 15 minutes.
2. Strain and drink once daily for longevity support.

Benefits: Ginseng is a renowned adaptogen that boosts energy, enhances endurance, and promotes overall vitality. This tonic helps support longevity by improving mental and physical stamina, reducing fatigue, and enhancing the body's resilience to stress.

Rose Hip Antioxidant Powder

INGREDIENTS

- 1 tablespoon dried rose hip powder

PREPARATION

1. Mix rose hip powder into smoothies or sprinkle over food.
2. Consume daily for antioxidant support.

Benefits: Rose hips are one of the richest natural sources of vitamin C and antioxidants. Regular consumption of rose hip powder helps protect the body from oxidative stress, supports immune function, and promotes healthy skin, making it an essential remedy for healthy aging.

Schisandra Berry Vitality Elixir

INGREDIENTS

- 1 tablespoon dried schisandra berries
- 1 cup water

PREPARATION

1. Simmer schisandra berries in water for 20 minutes.
2. Strain and drink daily for vitality support.

Benefits: Schisandra is an adaptogen that improves stamina, endurance, and overall vitality. This elixir helps combat the effects of aging by boosting energy levels, enhancing mental clarity, and supporting the body's ability to handle physical and emotional stress.

Holy Basil (Tulsi) Stress Relief Tea

INGREDIENTS

- 1 teaspoon dried holy basil leaves
- 1 cup boiling water

PREPARATION

1. Steep holy basil leaves in boiling water for 10 minutes.
2. Strain and drink once daily to reduce stress.

Benefits: Holy basil is an adaptogen that helps the body manage stress and reduce cortisol levels. This tea promotes relaxation, calms the mind, and supports emotional well-being, making it an excellent remedy for aging individuals dealing with stress or anxiety.

Moringa Leaf Mineral Boost Capsules

INGREDIENTS

- 1 tablespoon dried moringa leaf powder
- Capsule shells

PREPARATION

1. Fill capsule shells with moringa leaf powder.
2. Take 1-2 capsules daily for a mineral boost.

Benefits: Moringa is packed with essential vitamins, minerals, and antioxidants that support overall health and vitality. These capsules help strengthen bones, boost immune function, and provide a natural source of energy, making them perfect for maintaining health during the aging process.

Elderflower Anti-Aging Skin Serum

INGREDIENTS

- 1 tablespoon dried elderflowers
- 1/4 cup almond oil

PREPARATION

1. Infuse dried elderflowers in almond oil using a double boiler for 30 minutes.
2. Strain and pour into a dropper bottle.
3. Apply a few drops to the skin daily for anti-aging support.

Benefits: Elderflower is known for its skin-rejuvenating properties, helping to reduce wrinkles, improve skin elasticity, and promote a youthful glow. This serum nourishes the skin with antioxidants and provides anti-inflammatory benefits, making it ideal for aging skin.

Saffron Memory Support Drops

INGREDIENTS

- 1/4 teaspoon saffron threads
- 1/4 cup alcohol (vodka or glycerin for non-alcoholic option)

PREPARATION

1. Infuse saffron threads in alcohol or glycerin for 4-6 weeks.
2. Strain and take 1-2 droppers daily for memory support.

Benefits: Saffron has been shown to improve cognitive function and enhance memory. These drops provide natural support for brain health and are particularly beneficial for aging individuals looking to preserve memory and mental clarity.

Astragalus Immune Strength Capsules

INGREDIENTS

- 1 tablespoon dried astragalus root powder
- Capsule shells

PREPARATION

1. Fill capsule shells with astragalus root powder.
2. Take 1-2 capsules daily to strengthen the immune system.

Benefits: Astragalus is a powerful immune-boosting herb that helps protect the body from infections and reduces the impact of stress on the immune system. These capsules support overall vitality, helping aging individuals maintain a strong and resilient immune system.

Fennel and Licorice Digestive Tea

INGREDIENTS

- 1/2 teaspoon fennel seeds
- 1/2 teaspoon dried licorice root
- 1 cup boiling water

PREPARATION

1. Steep fennel seeds and licorice root in boiling water for 10 minutes.
2. Strain and drink once daily for digestive support.

Benefits: Fennel and licorice are both soothing to the digestive system, helping to relieve bloating, indigestion, and other gastrointestinal discomforts. This tea supports healthy digestion and provides relief from age-related digestive issues.

Meadowsweet Joint Support Capsules

INGREDIENTS

- 1 tablespoon dried meadowsweet powder
- Capsule shells

PREPARATION

1. Fill capsule shells with meadowsweet powder.
2. Take 1-2 capsules daily to support joint health.

Benefits: Meadowsweet is known for its anti-inflammatory properties, making it an effective remedy for joint pain and stiffness. These capsules help reduce inflammation and support joint flexibility, providing relief from arthritis and other age-related joint issues.

Lemon Balm Restorative Sleep Tea

INGREDIENTS

- 1 teaspoon dried lemon balm leaves
- 1 cup boiling water

PREPARATION

1. Steep lemon balm leaves in boiling water for 10 minutes.
2. Strain and drink before bed for restful sleep.

Benefits: Lemon balm is a calming herb that promotes relaxation and reduces anxiety. This tea helps soothe the nervous system, making it easier to fall asleep and stay asleep, which is particularly beneficial for aging individuals struggling with insomnia or restless sleep.

Valerian Root Muscle Relaxant Capsules

INGREDIENTS

- 1 tablespoon dried valerian root powder
- Capsule shells

PREPARATION

1. Fill capsule shells with valerian root powder.
2. Take 1-2 capsules before bed to relax muscles.

Benefits: Valerian root is known for its muscle-relaxing properties, making it helpful for relieving tension and muscle cramps. These capsules are ideal for aging individuals experiencing muscle stiffness or nighttime muscle spasms, promoting relaxation and better sleep.

Blueberry Antioxidant Smoothie

INGREDIENTS

- 1/2 cup fresh or frozen blueberries
- 1/2 cup almond milk
- 1 tablespoon honey

PREPARATION

1. Blend blueberries, almond milk, and honey until smooth.
2. Drink immediately for antioxidant support.

Benefits: Blueberries are packed with antioxidants that protect the body from oxidative stress and support healthy aging. This smoothie is a delicious and easy way to boost your intake of antioxidants, improve brain health, and support heart health.

Burdock Root Blood Purifier Infusion

INGREDIENTS

- 1 tablespoon dried burdock root
- 2 cups boiling water

PREPARATION

1. Simmer burdock root in water for 15 minutes.
2. Strain and drink daily for blood purification.

Benefits: Burdock root is known for its detoxifying properties, helping to cleanse the blood and support liver health. This infusion promotes better circulation, clearer skin, and overall vitality, making it a great remedy for aging individuals looking to purify their system.

Yarrow Skin Regeneration Cream

INGREDIENTS

- 1 tablespoon dried yarrow flowers
- 1/4 cup coconut oil

PREPARATION

1. Infuse yarrow flowers in melted coconut oil using a double boiler for 30 minutes.
2. Strain and pour into a jar.
3. Apply to skin as needed for regeneration.

Benefits: Yarrow is known for its ability to promote skin regeneration and healing. This cream helps reduce the appearance of scars, wrinkles, and age spots, making it a great anti-aging remedy for maintaining youthful, healthy skin.

Dandelion and Milk Thistle Liver Support Tea

INGREDIENTS

- 1 teaspoon dried dandelion root
- 1 teaspoon dried milk thistle seeds
- 1 cup boiling water

PREPARATION

1. Steep dandelion root and milk thistle seeds in boiling water for 10 minutes.
2. Strain and drink daily to support liver health.

Benefits: Dandelion and milk thistle are both known for their liver-supporting properties, helping to detoxify the liver and improve its function. This tea helps cleanse the body, improve digestion, and promote overall vitality, making it an essential remedy for healthy aging.

Angelica Root Hormone Balance Drops

INGREDIENTS

- 1 tablespoon dried angelica root
- 1/4 cup alcohol (vodka or glycerin for non-alcoholic option)

PREPARATION

1. Infuse angelica root in alcohol or glycerin for 4-6 weeks.
2. Strain and take 1-2 droppers daily to support hormone balance.

Benefits: Angelica root helps balance hormones and alleviate symptoms related to hormonal changes, such as hot flashes and mood swings. These drops are particularly beneficial for aging women going through menopause, providing natural relief from discomfort.

Alfalfa Sprout Longevity Salad

INGREDIENTS

- 1 cup fresh alfalfa sprouts
- 1/2 cucumber, sliced
- 1 tablespoon olive oil
- 1 teaspoon lemon juice

PREPARATION

1. Toss alfalfa sprouts and cucumber together in a bowl.
2. Drizzle with olive oil and lemon juice, then serve fresh.

Benefits: Alfalfa sprouts are rich in vitamins and minerals that support overall health and longevity. This salad provides essential nutrients that promote healthy digestion, boost energy, and support the immune system, making it a perfect addition to a longevity-focused diet.

Pine Bark Extract Anti-Aging Capsules

INGREDIENTS

- 1 tablespoon pine bark extract powder
- Capsule shells

PREPARATION

1. Fill capsule shells with pine bark extract powder.
2. Take 1-2 capsules daily for anti-aging benefits.

Benefits: Pine bark extract is rich in antioxidants that protect the body from free radicals and oxidative stress. These capsules help reduce inflammation, improve skin health, and support overall vitality, making them a powerful remedy for healthy aging.

Sea Buckthorn Skin Nourishing Oil

INGREDIENTS

- 1 tablespoon sea buckthorn oil

PREPARATION

1. Apply sea buckthorn oil directly to the skin for nourishment.
2. Massage gently until absorbed.

Benefits: Sea buckthorn oil is packed with vitamins and fatty acids that nourish the skin and promote hydration. It helps reduce the appearance of wrinkles and fine lines, making it an excellent remedy for maintaining youthful, radiant skin. Regular use helps improve skin texture and elasticity.

BOOK 14

Herbal First Aid

Essential Herbs for Cuts, Burns, and Injuries

NATURAL REMEDIES FOR CUTS, BURNS, AND MINOR INJURIES

Herbs have been used for centuries as natural remedies for treating wounds, burns, and other minor injuries. They provide an effective and gentle approach to promoting healing, reducing pain, and preventing infection. For those like Emma, who prioritize a holistic lifestyle and wish to maintain a natural first aid kit, understanding these essential herbs offers an opportunity to manage minor injuries effectively without relying on synthetic products. Below, we explore several herbs known for their wound-healing, antibacterial, and anti-inflammatory properties, detailing how they work and how they can be applied safely.

Aloe Vera: The Soothing Healer

Aloe vera is one of the most commonly used herbs for burns and skin injuries due to its soothing and healing properties. The gel from the aloe leaf has anti-inflammatory, antibacterial, and antioxidant effects, which make it ideal for treating burns, sunburns, and cuts. Its cooling effect provides immediate relief, while its compounds promote skin regeneration and reduce the risk of infection.

To use aloe vera, the fresh gel can be applied directly to the affected area. For Emma, keeping an aloe vera plant at home offers a convenient and sustainable way to access this remedy whenever needed. Applying fresh aloe gel ensures her family receives immediate, natural care for burns or minor skin abrasions, supporting quick and effective healing.

Calendula: Promoting Wound Healing

Calendula, also known as marigold, is another powerful herb for managing cuts and wounds. It possesses antiseptic and anti-inflammatory properties that help prevent infection and reduce swelling. Calendula also stimulates collagen production, which is essential for tissue regeneration, making it particularly effective for healing cuts, scrapes, and abrasions.

Calendula can be applied as an infused oil, salve, or poultice directly onto the wound. For Emma, having a calendula salve in her natural first aid kit ensures she has a quick and effective remedy for her family's minor injuries. Applying calendula regularly to cuts or wounds promotes faster healing while minimizing scarring, making it a reliable and gentle option for skin care.

Lavender: Antiseptic and Anti-Inflammatory Benefits

Lavender is well-known for its soothing aroma, but it also has antiseptic and anti-inflammatory properties that make it effective for treating minor burns and cuts. Lavender essential oil can be applied to clean wounds to reduce pain and promote healing. Additionally, its antibacterial qualities help prevent infection, ensuring wounds remain clean as they heal.

Lavender oil can be diluted with a carrier oil like coconut

oil before application. For Emma, lavender oil provides a versatile option that supports wound care while also offering relaxation benefits. Whether used for burns or minor scrapes, lavender oil serves as a dual-purpose remedy in her natural first aid kit.

Plantain: Nature's Anti-Inflammatory Leaf

Plantain, often considered a common weed, is a potent herb for wound care. The leaves of plantain have anti-inflammatory, antibacterial, and astringent properties that make them effective for treating cuts, insect bites, and burns. Plantain works by drawing out impurities, reducing swelling, and forming a protective layer over wounds to aid in the healing process.

Fresh plantain leaves can be crushed and applied directly to wounds as a poultice. For Emma, using plantain is a practical way to harness a readily available remedy that grows abundantly in nature. Applying a plantain poultice ensures her family benefits from its immediate soothing and healing effects, making it an invaluable addition to her natural remedy collection.

Yarrow: Staunching Bleeding and Promoting Healing

Yarrow has long been used for its wound-healing abilities, especially in stopping bleeding. Its astringent and antibacterial properties make it effective for cleansing wounds and reducing inflammation. Yarrow also promotes the formation of new tissue, which aids in the healing process and prevents infection.

Yarrow can be applied as a poultice using fresh leaves, or it can be made into a salve. For Emma, yarrow provides a reliable solution for more serious cuts where bleeding needs to be controlled quickly. By applying a yarrow poultice, she can manage bleeding naturally, supporting the wound's healing and preventing infection.

Comfrey: Supporting Tissue Regeneration

Comfrey, also known as "knitbone," is an herb traditionally used to promote the healing of bones, tissues, and skin. Its main compound, allantoin, stimulates cell regeneration and supports the growth of new tissue. Comfrey is particularly beneficial for treating bruises, sprains, and cuts, as it accelerates the healing process.

Comfrey leaves can be used fresh as a poultice or in an infused oil or salve form. Emma can keep a comfrey salve on hand to apply to bruises, cuts, or other minor injuries, ensuring that her family benefits from this herb's rapid healing properties. The versatility of comfrey makes it a must-have in a natural first aid kit.

Tea Tree: Natural Antiseptic for Infection Prevention

Tea tree oil is a powerful natural antiseptic that is effective for cleansing wounds and preventing infection. Its antimicrobial properties make it suitable for treating minor cuts, scrapes, and burns. Tea tree oil also reduces inflammation, helping wounds heal faster without becoming infected.

To use tea tree oil, it should be diluted with a carrier oil to avoid irritation. For Emma, adding tea tree oil to her first aid kit provides a reliable, natural antiseptic solution for various skin injuries. By applying diluted tea tree oil, she can ensure that wounds remain clean and heal efficiently, maintaining her preference for gentle, plant-based care.

These herbs provide practical and effective solutions for treating cuts, burns, and injuries naturally. For Emma, integrating these remedies into her routine ensures that she can manage her family's minor injuries holistically, using the power of nature to promote quick and effective healing.

Managing Bites, Stings, and Allergic Reactions Naturally

NATURAL SOLUTIONS FOR BITES, STINGS, AND ALLERGIC REACTIONS

Bites, stings, and allergic reactions are common occurrences that can cause discomfort, swelling, and inflammation. Herbs provide effective and gentle solutions to manage these issues naturally, offering relief without the need for synthetic medications. For those like Emma, who prefer holistic approaches, understanding which herbs to use in these situations ensures that minor emergencies can be managed safely and efficiently. Below, we explore several herbs known for their anti-inflammatory, antihistamine, and soothing properties, detailing how they work and how they can be applied effectively.

Plantain: A Go-To for Bites and Stings

Plantain is a powerful herb for treating insect bites and stings, thanks to its anti-inflammatory and antihistamine properties. It has long been used as a natural remedy to reduce itching, swelling, and pain caused by bites from mosquitoes, bees, and other insects. The compounds in plantain work to draw out toxins and soothe irritation, making it an ideal first aid herb.

To use plantain, the fresh leaves can be crushed and applied directly to the affected area as a poultice. For Emma, who may find herself or her child dealing with an unexpected sting or bite, keeping fresh plantain leaves or dried plantain powder on hand provides a quick and effective remedy. The immediate application helps relieve discomfort and reduce swelling, ensuring that the bite or sting heals faster and with less irritation.

Lavender: Calming Allergic Reactions and Reducing Swelling

Lavender is well-known for its soothing and anti-inflammatory effects, making it effective for managing mild allergic reactions and insect stings. Lavender's essential oil, when applied to the skin, can help reduce redness, swelling, and itching. Its natural antihistamine properties make it a useful herb for dealing with mild allergic reactions such as skin irritation or hives.

Lavender essential oil should be diluted with a carrier oil before applying it to the skin. For Emma, who values versatility in her natural remedies, having a small bottle of diluted lavender oil in her first aid kit allows her to address minor skin reactions and insect bites quickly. The soothing aroma of lavender also provides a calming effect, which can be beneficial during stressful first aid situations.

Calendula: Soothing and Healing Skin Irritations

Calendula is a gentle herb that is effective for treating skin irritations caused by allergic reactions or insect stings. Its anti-inflammatory and antibacterial properties help soothe inflamed skin and prevent infection. Calendula is particularly beneficial for sensitive skin, making it an excellent choice for children or those prone to allergic responses.

Calendula can be applied as a cream, salve, or poultice directly to the affected area. For Emma, having a calendula salve on hand provides a safe and effective way to manage skin irritations naturally. Applying calendula ensures that the inflammation is reduced, and the skin is protected, allowing the affected area to heal quickly and with minimal discomfort.

Echinacea: Supporting Immune Response

Echinacea is often used to boost the immune system, but it also has benefits for managing insect bites and stings. It works by stimulating the immune system's response, which can help reduce inflammation and swelling in reaction to insect venom. Echinacea's antibacterial properties further support healing, ensuring that bites or stings do not become infected.

Echinacea tincture can be applied topically to bites or stings, or it can be taken internally to support the body's immune response. For Emma, using echinacea tincture as both a topical and internal remedy provides a holistic approach to managing bites, ensuring her body receives support from within and externally. This dual action approach helps her feel confident in addressing common outdoor mishaps.

Chamomile: Reducing Itching and Inflammation

Chamomile is a gentle herb that effectively reduces itching and inflammation caused by insect bites and mild allergic skin reactions. It has anti-inflammatory and antihistamine properties, which make it suitable for calming skin irritations. Chamomile is especially helpful for sensitive skin and can be used on both adults and children.

Chamomile can be applied as a cool compress using chamomile tea or as a diluted essential oil. For Emma, having chamomile tea bags available provides a quick solution when a compress is needed. Applying a cool chamomile compress to an affected area helps reduce swelling and soothes the skin, offering relief without harsh chemicals.

Basil: Natural Antihistamine for Immediate Relief

Basil is an effective herb for treating insect stings due to its natural antihistamine properties. It contains compounds that help reduce inflammation and swelling, making it particularly useful for bites that result in quick reactions like bee or wasp stings. Basil's antimicrobial properties also aid in preventing infection.

Crushed basil leaves can be applied directly to the site of the sting to provide immediate relief. For Emma, who may find herself or her child in need of quick first aid outdoors, using fresh basil leaves offers an accessible and natural option. The herb's ability to neutralize the effects of insect venom ensures that swelling and irritation are minimized swiftly.

Witch Hazel: Astringent for Soothing Bites

Witch hazel is a powerful astringent that is commonly used for treating insect bites and allergic reactions. It works by tightening the skin, reducing inflammation, and calming irritation. Witch hazel also helps cleanse the affected area, which prevents further irritation or infection.

Witch hazel can be applied with a cotton pad directly to bites, stings, or areas of skin irritation. For Emma, having witch hazel in her first aid kit offers a convenient and fast-acting solution for managing skin reactions. Its cooling effect provides instant relief, making it a practical and effective addition to her holistic approach to health and wellness.

These herbs provide safe and effective solutions for managing bites, stings, and allergic reactions naturally. By incorporating them into her first aid routine, Emma can address these common issues with confidence, ensuring that her approach aligns with her preference for natural, plant-based care.

Remedies for First Aid and Emergency Situations

Arnica Muscle Pain Balm

INGREDIENTS

- 1 tablespoon dried arnica flowers
- 1/4 cup coconut oil
- 1 tablespoon beeswax

PREPARATION

1. Infuse arnica flowers in melted coconut oil using a double boiler for 30 minutes.
2. Strain the mixture and stir in melted beeswax.
3. Pour into a jar and allow to cool before use.

Benefits: Arnica is known for its ability to relieve muscle pain, bruising, and inflammation. This balm helps reduce soreness and speeds up the healing of muscle injuries, making it a great addition to any first aid kit for sprains or strains.

Plantain Leaf Wound Healing Poultice

INGREDIENTS

- 1 tablespoon fresh plantain leaves
- 1 teaspoon water

PREPARATION

1. Crush fresh plantain leaves and mix with water to form a paste.
2. Apply the paste directly to wounds or insect bites.
3. Cover with a clean cloth and leave for 30 minutes before rinsing.

Benefits: Plantain has natural antibacterial and anti-inflammatory properties that promote wound healing and soothe irritated skin. It helps stop bleeding, reduces swelling, and accelerates the recovery of cuts, scrapes, and bites.

Calendula Antiseptic Wash

INGREDIENTS

- 1 tablespoon dried calendula flowers
- 1 cup boiling water

PREPARATION

1. Steep calendula flowers in boiling water for 15 minutes.
2. Strain and cool the liquid.
3. Use as an antiseptic wash for cuts, wounds, or skin infections.

Benefits: Calendula has powerful antibacterial and healing properties. This wash cleanses wounds, prevents infection, and speeds up the healing process, making it an essential remedy for minor cuts and abrasions.

Yarrow Bleeding Control Powder

INGREDIENTS

- 1 tablespoon dried yarrow powder

PREPARATION

1. Sprinkle dried yarrow powder directly onto a wound to control bleeding.
2. Cover with a clean bandage.

Benefits: Yarrow is well-known for its ability to stop bleeding quickly. It works as a natural styptic and promotes the clotting of blood, making it a highly effective remedy for first aid situations involving cuts or scrapes.

Comfrey Bone Healing Compress

INGREDIENTS

- 1 tablespoon dried comfrey leaves
- 1 cup boiling water

PREPARATION

1. Steep comfrey leaves in boiling water for 10 minutes.
2. Soak a clean cloth in the infusion and apply it as a compress to the affected area.
3. Leave for 20 minutes before removing.

Benefits: Comfrey contains allantoin, which promotes the healing of bones and tissues. This compress helps speed up the recovery of fractures, sprains, and bruises, making it a valuable addition to any first aid treatment for bone injuries.

Goldenseal Antimicrobial Tincture

INGREDIENTS

- 1 tablespoon dried goldenseal root
- 1/4 cup alcohol (vodka or glycerin for a non-alcoholic option)

PREPARATION

1. Infuse goldenseal root in alcohol or glycerin for 4-6 weeks, shaking occasionally.
2. Strain and store in a dark bottle.
3. Take 1-2 droppers daily for antimicrobial support.

Benefits: Goldenseal is a powerful antimicrobial herb that helps fight infections and support the immune system. This tincture can be used both internally and externally to help treat wounds, sore throats, and skin infections.

Aloe Vera Burn Relief Gel

INGREDIENTS

- 2 tablespoons fresh aloe vera gel

PREPARATION

1. Apply fresh aloe vera gel directly to burns or sunburned skin.
2. Reapply as needed to soothe and cool the area.

Benefits: Aloe vera is widely known for its soothing and healing properties, especially for burns. It helps reduce pain, cools the skin, and speeds up the healing of burns, making it a must-have in any first aid kit for treating minor burns or sunburns.

Echinacea Immune Support Capsules

INGREDIENTS

- 1 tablespoon dried echinacea root powder
- Capsule shells

PREPARATION

1. Fill capsule shells with echinacea root powder.
2. Take 1-2 capsules daily to boost immunity.

Benefits: Echinacea is known for its immune-boosting properties. These capsules help the body fight off infections, colds, and flu, providing a natural way to strengthen the immune system and promote faster recovery during illness.

Lavender Bite and Sting Relief Oil

INGREDIENTS

- 10 drops lavender essential oil
- 1 tablespoon coconut oil

PREPARATION

1. Mix lavender essential oil with coconut oil.
2. Apply the mixture directly to insect bites or stings to reduce itching and inflammation.

Benefits: Lavender oil is a natural anti-inflammatory and antimicrobial agent that helps relieve the pain and itching caused by insect bites or stings. It also promotes faster healing, making it an excellent remedy for outdoor emergencies.

Witch Hazel Bruise and Swelling Spray

INGREDIENTS

- 1/4 cup witch hazel extract
- 1/4 cup water

PREPARATION

1. Mix witch hazel extract with water in a spray bottle.
2. Spray directly onto bruises or swollen areas as needed.

Benefits: Witch hazel helps reduce swelling and inflammation, making it ideal for treating bruises and minor injuries. This spray provides instant relief and helps the body recover more quickly from trauma.

Chickweed Itch Relief Salve

INGREDIENTS

- 1 tablespoon dried chickweed
- 1/4 cup coconut oil
- 1 tablespoon beeswax

PREPARATION

1. Infuse chickweed in melted coconut oil for 30 minutes.
2. Strain and stir in melted beeswax.
3. Pour into a jar and cool before use.

Benefits: Chickweed is a natural remedy for itching and irritated skin. This salve helps soothe insect bites, rashes, and other skin irritations, providing fast relief and promoting healing.

Lemon Balm Cold Sore Cream

INGREDIENTS

- 1 tablespoon dried lemon balm leaves
- 1/4 cup coconut oil

PREPARATION

1. Infuse lemon balm leaves in melted coconut oil for 30 minutes.
2. Strain and pour into a jar.
3. Apply to cold sores as needed.

Benefits: Lemon balm has antiviral properties that help reduce the severity and duration of cold sores. This cream soothes irritation and promotes faster healing, making it a go-to remedy for treating cold sores naturally.

Marshmallow Root Throat Relief Syrup

INGREDIENTS

- 1 tablespoon dried marshmallow root
- 1 cup water
- 1/4 cup honey

PREPARATION

1. Simmer marshmallow root in water for 15 minutes.
2. Strain and stir in honey.
3. Take 1-2 teaspoons as needed for throat relief.

Benefits: Marshmallow root has mucilage properties that coat and soothe the throat. This syrup provides fast relief for sore throats and coughs, making it an essential first aid remedy for respiratory discomfort.

Peppermint Cooling Spray for Burns

INGREDIENTS

- 1 teaspoon peppermint essential oil
- 1/4 cup water

PREPARATION

1. Mix peppermint essential oil with water in a spray bottle.
2. Spray onto burns for immediate cooling relief.

Benefits: Peppermint oil has cooling and pain-relieving properties, making this spray perfect for soothing burns and reducing inflammation. It provides quick relief from the pain and discomfort of minor burns.

Feverfew Headache Balm

INGREDIENTS

- 1 tablespoon dried feverfew leaves (#ul#)
- 1/4 cup coconut oil

PREPARATION

1. Infuse feverfew leaves in melted coconut oil for 30 minutes.
2. Strain and pour into a jar.
3. Apply to the temples for headache relief.

Benefits: Feverfew is known for its ability to relieve headaches and migraines. This balm provides fast-acting relief from tension headaches by soothing inflammation and relaxing the muscles in the head and neck.

Chamomile Insect Bite Poultice

INGREDIENTS

- 1 tablespoon dried chamomile flowers
- 1 teaspoon water

PREPARATION

1. Crush dried chamomile flowers and mix with water to form a paste.
2. Apply directly to insect bites and leave on for 20 minutes.

Benefits: Chamomile has anti-inflammatory and soothing properties that reduce itching and irritation caused by insect bites. This poultice helps calm the skin and speeds up the healing process.

Ginger Motion Sickness Drops

INGREDIENTS

- 1 tablespoon grated fresh ginger
- 1/4 cup honey

PREPARATION

1. Simmer grated ginger in water for 10 minutes, then strain.
2. Mix the ginger tea with honey and let it cool.
3. Take 1-2 drops before or during travel to prevent motion sickness.

Benefits: Ginger is known for its ability to prevent nausea and motion sickness. These drops provide natural relief from travel-related nausea and help settle the stomach, making them ideal for trips or long journeys.

Arnica Muscle Pain Balm

INGREDIENTS

- 1 tablespoon dried arnica flowers
- 1/4 cup coconut oil
- 1 tablespoon beeswax

PREPARATION

1. Infuse arnica flowers in melted coconut oil using a double boiler for 30 minutes.
2. Strain the mixture and stir in melted beeswax.
3. Pour into a jar and allow to cool before use.

Benefits: Arnica is known for its ability to relieve muscle pain, bruising, and inflammation. This balm helps reduce soreness and speeds up the healing of muscle injuries, making it a great addition to any first aid kit for sprains or strains.

Plantain Leaf Wound Healing Poultice

INGREDIENTS

- 1 tablespoon fresh plantain leaves
- 1 teaspoon water

PREPARATION

1. Crush fresh plantain leaves and mix with water to form a paste.
2. Apply the paste directly to wounds or insect bites.
3. Cover with a clean cloth and leave for 30 minutes before rinsing.

Benefits: Plantain has natural antibacterial and anti-inflammatory properties that promote wound healing and soothe irritated skin. It helps stop bleeding, reduces swelling, and accelerates the recovery of cuts, scrapes, and bites.

Calendula Antiseptic Wash

INGREDIENTS

- 1 tablespoon dried calendula flowers
- 1 cup boiling water

PREPARATION

1. Steep calendula flowers in boiling water for 15 minutes.
2. Strain and cool the liquid.
3. Use as an antiseptic wash for cuts, wounds, or skin infections.

Benefits: Calendula has powerful antibacterial and healing properties. This wash cleanses wounds, prevents infection, and speeds up the healing process, making it an essential remedy for minor cuts and abrasions.

Yarrow Bleeding Control Powder

INGREDIENTS

- 1 tablespoon dried yarrow powder

PREPARATION

1. Sprinkle dried yarrow powder directly onto a wound to control bleeding.
2. Cover with a clean bandage.

Benefits: Yarrow is well-known for its ability to stop bleeding quickly. It works as a natural styptic and promotes the clotting of blood, making it a highly effective remedy for first aid situations involving cuts or scrapes.

Comfrey Bone Healing Compress

INGREDIENTS

- 1 tablespoon dried comfrey leaves
- 1 cup boiling water

PREPARATION

1. Steep comfrey leaves in boiling water for 10 minutes.
2. Soak a clean cloth in the infusion and apply it as a compress to the affected area.
3. Leave for 20 minutes before removing.

Benefits: Comfrey contains allantoin, which promotes the healing of bones and tissues. This compress helps speed up the recovery of fractures, sprains, and bruises, making it a valuable addition to any first aid treatment for bone injuries.

Goldenseal Antimicrobial Tincture

INGREDIENTS

- 1 tablespoon dried goldenseal root
- 1/4 cup alcohol (vodka or glycerin for a non-alcoholic option)

PREPARATION

1. Infuse goldenseal root in alcohol or glycerin for 4-6 weeks, shaking occasionally.
2. Strain and store in a dark bottle.
3. Take 1-2 droppers daily for antimicrobial support.

Benefits: Goldenseal is a powerful antimicrobial herb that helps fight infections and support the immune system. This tincture can be used both internally and externally to help treat wounds, sore throats, and skin infections.

Aloe Vera Burn Relief Gel

INGREDIENTS

- 2 tablespoons fresh aloe vera gel

PREPARATION

1. Apply fresh aloe vera gel directly to burns or sunburned skin.
2. Reapply as needed to soothe and cool the area.

Benefits: Aloe vera is widely known for its soothing and healing properties, especially for burns. It helps reduce pain, cools the skin, and speeds up the healing of burns, making it a must-have in any first aid kit for treating minor burns or sunburns.

Echinacea Immune Support Capsules

INGREDIENTS

- 1 tablespoon dried echinacea root powder
- Capsule shells

PREPARATION

1. Fill capsule shells with echinacea root powder.
2. Take 1-2 capsules daily to boost immunity.

Benefits: Echinacea is known for its immune-boosting properties. These capsules help the body fight off infections, colds, and flu, providing a natural way to strengthen the immune system and promote faster recovery during illness.

Lavender Bite and Sting Relief Oil

INGREDIENTS

- 10 drops lavender essential oil
- 1 tablespoon coconut oil

PREPARATION

1. Mix lavender essential oil with coconut oil.
2. Apply the mixture directly to insect bites or stings to reduce itching and inflammation.

Benefits: Lavender oil is a natural anti-inflammatory and antimicrobial agent that helps relieve the pain and itching caused by insect bites or stings. It also promotes faster healing, making it an excellent remedy for outdoor emergencies.

Witch Hazel Bruise and Swelling Spray

INGREDIENTS

- 1/4 cup witch hazel extract
- 1/4 cup water

PREPARATION

1. Mix witch hazel extract with water in a spray bottle.
2. Spray directly onto bruises or swollen areas as needed.

Benefits: Witch hazel helps reduce swelling and inflammation, making it ideal for treating bruises and minor injuries. This spray provides instant relief and helps the body recover more quickly from trauma.

Chickweed Itch Relief Salve

INGREDIENTS

- 1 tablespoon dried chickweed
- 1/4 cup coconut oil
- 1 tablespoon beeswax

PREPARATION

1. Infuse chickweed in melted coconut oil for 30 minutes.
2. Strain and stir in melted beeswax.
3. Pour into a jar and cool before use.

Benefits: Chickweed is a natural remedy for itching and irritated skin. This salve helps soothe insect bites, rashes, and other skin irritations, providing fast relief and promoting healing.

Lemon Balm Cold Sore Cream

INGREDIENTS

- 1 tablespoon dried lemon balm leaves
- 1/4 cup coconut oil

PREPARATION

1. Infuse lemon balm leaves in melted coconut oil for 30 minutes.
2. Strain and pour into a jar.
3. Apply to cold sores as needed.

Benefits: Lemon balm has antiviral properties that help reduce the severity and duration of cold sores. This cream soothes irritation and promotes faster healing, making it a go-to remedy for treating cold sores naturally.

Marshmallow Root Throat Relief Syrup

INGREDIENTS

- 1 tablespoon dried marshmallow root
- 1 cup water
- 1/4 cup honey

PREPARATION

1. Simmer marshmallow root in water for 15 minutes.
2. Strain and stir in honey.
3. Take 1-2 teaspoons as needed for throat relief.

Benefits: Marshmallow root has mucilage properties that coat and soothe the throat. This syrup provides fast relief for sore throats and coughs, making it an essential first aid remedy for respiratory discomfort.

Peppermint Cooling Spray for Burns

INGREDIENTS

- 1 teaspoon peppermint essential oil
- 1/4 cup water

PREPARATION

1. Mix peppermint essential oil with water in a spray bottle.
2. Spray onto burns for immediate cooling relief.

Benefits: Peppermint oil has cooling and pain-relieving properties, making this spray perfect for soothing burns and reducing inflammation. It provides quick relief from the pain and discomfort of minor burns.

Feverfew Headache Balm

INGREDIENTS

- 1 tablespoon dried feverfew leaves (#ul#)
- 1/4 cup coconut oil

PREPARATION

1. Infuse feverfew leaves in melted coconut oil for 30 minutes.
2. Strain and pour into a jar.
3. Apply to the temples for headache relief.

Benefits: Feverfew is known for its ability to relieve headaches and migraines. This balm provides fast-acting relief from tension headaches by soothing inflammation and relaxing the muscles in the head and neck.

Chamomile Insect Bite Poultice

INGREDIENTS

- 1 tablespoon dried chamomile flowers
- 1 teaspoon water

PREPARATION

1. Crush dried chamomile flowers and mix with water to form a paste.
2. Apply directly to insect bites and leave on for 20 minutes.

Benefits: Chamomile has anti-inflammatory and soothing properties that reduce itching and irritation caused by insect bites. This poultice helps calm the skin and speeds up the healing process.

Ginger Motion Sickness Drops

INGREDIENTS

- 1 tablespoon grated fresh ginger
- 1/4 cup honey

PREPARATION

1. Simmer grated ginger in water for 10 minutes, then strain.
2. Mix the ginger tea with honey and let it cool.
3. Take 1-2 drops before or during travel to prevent motion sickness.

Benefits: Ginger is known for its ability to prevent nausea and motion sickness. These drops provide natural relief from travel-related nausea and help settle the stomach, making them ideal for trips or long journeys.

Elderflower Fever Reducer Tincture

INGREDIENTS

- 1 tablespoon dried elderflowers
- 1/4 cup alcohol (vodka or glycerin for a non-alcoholic option)

PREPARATION

1. Infuse dried elderflowers in alcohol or glycerin for 4-6 weeks.
2. Strain and take 1-2 droppers daily to reduce fever.

Benefits: Elderflower is known for its ability to reduce fever and soothe inflammation. This tincture helps lower body temperature naturally and provides relief during feverish conditions, making it a useful addition to any first aid kit.

Oregano Oil Antimicrobial Spray

INGREDIENTS

- 10 drops oregano essential oil
- 1/4 cup water

PREPARATION

1. Mix oregano oil with water in a spray bottle.
2. Spray onto cuts or wounds for antimicrobial protection.

Benefits: Oregano oil has powerful antimicrobial properties, making it effective for preventing infection in minor cuts, scrapes, and wounds. This spray helps disinfect and protect the skin, promoting faster healing.

Sage Sore Throat Gargle

INGREDIENTS

- 1 teaspoon dried sage leaves
- 1/2 cup warm water

PREPARATION

1. Steep sage leaves in warm water for 10 minutes.
2. Strain and use the liquid as a gargle for sore throats.

Benefits: Sage has antibacterial and anti-inflammatory properties that help soothe sore throats. This gargle provides quick relief from throat irritation and helps reduce inflammation, making it an effective remedy for sore throats and hoarseness.

Horsetail Antifungal Foot Soak

INGREDIENTS

- 1 tablespoon dried horsetail
- 1 quart warm water

PREPARATION

1. Steep horsetail in warm water for 15 minutes.
2. Soak feet in the solution for 20 minutes to treat fungal infections.

Benefits: Horsetail has antifungal and antibacterial properties that help treat athlete's foot and other fungal infections. This foot soak relieves itching and discomfort while promoting the healing of fungal infections.

Thyme Respiratory Support Steam

INGREDIENTS

- 1 tablespoon dried thyme
- 1 quart boiling water

PREPARATION

1. Add dried thyme to boiling water.
2. Inhale the steam for 10 minutes to support respiratory health.

Benefits: Thyme is known for its antimicrobial and expectorant properties. This steam helps clear congestion, ease breathing, and support respiratory function during colds, coughs, or respiratory infections.

Cinnamon and Clove Toothache Oil

INGREDIENTS

- 1/2 teaspoon cinnamon powder
- 1/2 teaspoon clove powder
- 1 tablespoon coconut oil

PREPARATION

1. Mix cinnamon and clove powders with coconut oil.
2. Apply the mixture to the affected tooth for pain relief.

Benefits: Cinnamon and clove both have analgesic and antibacterial properties that help relieve toothache pain and reduce infection. This oil provides fast relief from dental pain and helps protect against further infection.

St. John's Wort Nerve Pain Balm

INGREDIENTS

- 1 tablespoon dried St. John's wort leaves
- 1/4 cup coconut oil
- 1 tablespoon beeswax

PREPARATION

1. Infuse St. John's wort leaves in melted coconut oil for 30 minutes.
2. Strain and stir in melted beeswax.
3. Apply the balm to areas of nerve pain as needed.

Benefits: St. John's wort is known for its ability to relieve nerve pain and reduce inflammation. This balm helps soothe conditions like sciatica or neuralgia by calming irritated nerves and reducing discomfort.

Burdock Poison Ivy Relief Wash

INGREDIENTS

- 1 tablespoon dried burdock root
- 1 cup boiling water

PREPARATION

1. Steep burdock root in boiling water for 15 minutes.
2. Strain and use the liquid as a wash for poison ivy rashes.

Benefits: Burdock root has anti-inflammatory and detoxifying properties that help soothe poison ivy rashes and other skin irritations. This wash helps reduce itching and inflammation, promoting faster healing of irritated skin.

Lemongrass Muscle Relaxing Bath Salts

INGREDIENTS

- 1 cup Epsom salts
- 10 drops lemongrass essential oil

PREPARATION

1. Mix Epsom salts with lemongrass essential oil.
2. Add to a warm bath and soak for 20 minutes to relieve muscle tension.

Benefits: Lemongrass oil and Epsom salts work together to relax tense muscles and reduce soreness. This bath soak is perfect for relieving muscle aches, cramps, or tension after physical activity.

Licorice Throat Coat Tea

INGREDIENTS

- 1 teaspoon dried licorice root
- 1 cup boiling water

PREPARATION

1. Steep licorice root in boiling water for 10 minutes.
2. Strain and drink warm for throat relief.

Benefits: Licorice root helps coat and soothe irritated throats, making it an effective remedy for sore throats, coughs, or hoarseness. It also has expectorant properties that help clear mucus from the respiratory tract.

Red Clover Antihistamine Capsules

INGREDIENTS

- 1 tablespoon dried red clover powder
- Capsule shells

PREPARATION

1. Fill capsule shells with red clover powder.
2. Take 1-2 capsules daily to reduce allergy symptoms.

Benefits: Red clover acts as a natural antihistamine, helping to reduce allergic reactions such as hay fever, hives, or skin rashes. These capsules provide relief from allergy symptoms while supporting overall immune health.

Dandelion Flower Skin Healing Ointment

INGREDIENTS

- 1 tablespoon dried dandelion flowers
- 1/4 cup coconut oil
- 1 tablespoon beeswax

PREPARATION

1. Infuse dandelion flowers in melted coconut oil for 30 minutes.
2. Strain and stir in melted beeswax.
3. Apply the ointment to cuts, scrapes, or dry skin.

Benefits: Dandelion flowers are known for their skin-healing properties. This ointment helps soothe and heal cuts, scrapes, burns, and dry patches by promoting skin regeneration and reducing inflammation.

Blue Flag Snake Bite Poultice

INGREDIENTS

- 1 tablespoon dried blue flag root powder
- 1 teaspoon water

PREPARATION

1. Mix blue flag root powder with water to create a paste.
2. Apply the paste directly to the snake bite area.
3. Cover with a clean bandage and leave for 30 minutes before rinsing.

Benefits: Blue flag root is traditionally used to treat venomous bites and stings. It helps draw out toxins, reduce inflammation, and promote healing in cases of snake bites and other poisonous wounds. It should always be used as a first-aid remedy before seeking medical attention.

Bay Leaf Digestive Relief Elixir

INGREDIENTS

- 3 dried bay leaves
- 1 cup water
- 1 teaspoon honey

PREPARATION

1. Simmer bay leaves in water for 10 minutes.
2. Strain and mix with honey.
3. Take 1-2 teaspoons as needed for digestive relief.

Benefits: Bay leaf has carminative properties that help reduce gas, bloating, and indigestion. This elixir soothes the digestive system and provides quick relief from discomfort caused by overeating or digestive issues.

Hyssop Cold and Flu Support Tea

INGREDIENTS

- 1 teaspoon dried hyssop leaves
- 1 cup boiling water

PREPARATION

1. Steep hyssop leaves in boiling water for 10 minutes.
2. Strain and drink warm to relieve cold and flu symptoms.

Benefits: Hyssop has antiviral and expectorant properties that help relieve cold and flu symptoms, such as cough, congestion, and sore throat. This tea supports the respiratory system and promotes faster recovery from colds and flu.

Rue Muscle Tension Relief Drops

INGREDIENTS

- 1 tablespoon dried rue leaves
- 1/4 cup alcohol (vodka or glycerin for a non-alcoholic option)

PREPARATION

1. Infuse rue leaves in alcohol or glycerin for 4-6 weeks.
2. Strain and take 1-2 droppers as needed to relieve muscle tension.

Benefits: Rue is known for its muscle-relaxing properties, making it effective for relieving tension, cramps, and muscle pain. These drops help soothe tight muscles and provide natural relief from muscle aches and discomfort.

BOOK 15

Emotional and Mental Well-Being

Herbs for Mood Enhancement and Emotional BalanceChapter Title

NATURAL HERBS FOR ENHANCING MOOD AND ACHIEVING EMOTIONAL BALANCE

Emotional well-being plays a crucial role in overall health, influencing not only how we feel but also how we navigate daily challenges and maintain relationships. For individuals like Emma, who seek natural ways to uplift their mood and achieve emotional balance, herbs offer a gentle yet effective solution. Herbs have been used for centuries to support the nervous system, enhance mood, and promote a sense of calm and stability. Below, we explore several herbs known for their mood-enhancing and emotionally balancing properties, detailing how they work and how they can be incorporated into a holistic approach to emotional wellness.

St. John's Wort: The Natural Antidepressant

St. John's Wort is one of the most widely recognized herbs for supporting mood and managing mild to moderate depression. It works by increasing serotonin, dopamine, and norepinephrine levels in the brain—neurotransmitters that play a key role in regulating mood. This makes it an effective remedy for individuals experiencing low mood, irritability, or feelings of sadness.

St. John's Wort is typically consumed as a capsule, tincture, or tea. For Emma, integrating this herb into her daily routine offers a natural and accessible way to maintain emotional balance, particularly during periods of stress or seasonal mood changes. However, it is important to note that St. John's Wort can interact with certain medications, so consulting a healthcare professional before use is essential. By incorporating this herb cautiously, Emma can safely benefit from its mood-enhancing effects, ensuring her emotional well-being is supported holistically.

Lemon Balm: Calming Anxiety and Lifting Spirits

Lemon balm is another valuable herb for mood enhancement and emotional balance. Known for its calming properties, it is particularly effective for reducing anxiety, restlessness, and mild depression. Lemon balm works by soothing the nervous system, promoting a sense of relaxation and ease. Its mild sedative effect also makes it beneficial for improving sleep quality, which is closely linked to emotional well-being.

Lemon balm can be consumed as a tea, tincture, or added to meals for a subtle lemony flavor. For Emma, sipping lemon balm tea in the evening offers a practical and enjoyable way to unwind and relieve stress naturally. Its gentle, uplifting effects make it suitable for regular use, helping her maintain a balanced mood and manage daily stressors without resorting to synthetic solutions.

Ashwagandha: The Adaptogen for Stress Management

Ashwagandha is an adaptogenic herb that supports emotional resilience by helping the body adapt to stress. It works by regulating cortisol levels, the hormone associated with stress, and promoting overall balance in the nervous system. Ashwagandha's ability to reduce anxiety and fatigue makes it a valuable herb for those seeking to stabilize their mood and enhance emotional well-being, especially during periods of high stress or burnout.

Ashwagandha is commonly taken in capsule or powder form and can be added to smoothies or beverages. For Emma, using ashwagandha daily provides her with a natural way to build emotional resilience and maintain a stable mood, even in challenging situations. The herb's adaptogenic properties ensure that her body and mind remain balanced, supporting her overall emotional wellness journey.

Lavender: Promoting Calm and Emotional Stability

Lavender is well-known for its calming and soothing effects, making it an ideal herb for promoting emotional balance. It helps reduce anxiety, lift low mood, and promote relaxation through its impact on the nervous system. Lavender's aroma has been shown to enhance mood and reduce stress levels, offering an immediate sense of calm when inhaled or applied topically.

Lavender can be used as an essential oil, added to baths, or infused in teas. For Emma, diffusing lavender oil in her living space or adding it to her bath routine provides a quick and effective way to create a calming environment that supports her emotional well-being. Its versatility allows her to use lavender in various forms, ensuring she benefits from its mood-enhancing properties throughout the day.

Passionflower: Easing Restlessness and Anxiety

Passionflower is a mild sedative herb that is effective for reducing anxiety, restlessness, and insomnia—all factors that can negatively impact mood. It works by increasing levels of gamma-aminobutyric acid (GABA) in the brain, which helps calm the nervous system and promote a state of relaxation. Passionflower's gentle nature makes it suitable for regular use, particularly for those who experience frequent episodes of anxiety or difficulty winding down at night.

Passionflower tea is a popular way to consume this herb, offering a soothing and natural solution for promoting emotional stability. For Emma, incorporating passionflower tea into her nighttime routine helps her manage stress and achieve a restful state, ensuring her mood remains balanced and her sleep quality supports her overall well-being.

Rhodiola: Enhancing Mood and Mental Clarity

Rhodiola is another adaptogenic herb that helps manage stress and uplift mood by balancing neurotransmitter levels and supporting overall brain function. It is particularly effective for reducing fatigue, improving mental clarity, and boosting energy levels, which all contribute to a positive emotional state. Rhodiola also helps regulate serotonin and dopamine levels, essential for maintaining a balanced mood and sense of well-being.

Rhodiola is often taken as a supplement or tincture. For Emma, who may experience occasional low energy or mental fatigue, using rhodiola provides a natural way to uplift her mood and maintain emotional balance throughout the day. Its energizing and mood-enhancing properties ensure that she feels emotionally equipped to handle daily challenges without feeling overwhelmed.

Valerian: Soothing the Mind and Body

Valerian is a well-known herb for its sedative properties, making it effective for managing stress, anxiety, and emotional agitation. It helps calm the nervous system, promoting relaxation and emotional stability. Valerian is particularly beneficial for individuals who struggle with restlessness or insomnia, as it supports restful sleep—an essential factor in maintaining a balanced mood.

Valerian can be taken as a tincture, capsule, or tea. For Emma, incorporating valerian into her nighttime regimen provides a way to relax both her mind and body, ensuring she wakes up feeling refreshed and emotionally balanced. Its gentle effects make it a safe and natural option for managing mood disturbances linked to stress and poor sleep.

These herbs provide a natural and effective approach to enhancing mood and maintaining emotional balance. By integrating them into her daily routine, Emma can support her emotional well-being in a sustainable and holistic manner, ensuring she stays resilient and balanced even during challenging times.

Supporting Mental Clarity and Focus

HERBS THAT ENHANCE FOCUS AND PROMOTE MENTAL CLARITY

Maintaining mental clarity and focus is essential in today's fast-paced world, where distractions are constant and stress levels can easily overwhelm. For individuals like Emma, who seek natural methods to enhance cognitive function and improve focus, herbs offer a powerful and holistic solution. Various herbs have been traditionally used to sharpen the mind, enhance concentration, and support memory, making them invaluable tools for those striving to stay mentally clear and focused. Below, we explore some of the most effective herbs for enhancing mental clarity and focus, detailing their benefits and how they can be incorporated into daily routines.

Ginkgo Biloba: Improving Blood Flow to the Brain

Ginkgo biloba is a well-researched herb known for its cognitive-enhancing properties. It works by increasing blood flow to the brain, thereby improving oxygen and nutrient delivery, which are crucial for optimal brain function. The active compounds in ginkgo, such as flavonoids and terpenoids, help protect brain cells from oxidative damage, enhancing memory and concentration.

Ginkgo biloba can be consumed in capsule or tincture form, making it a convenient option for daily use. For Emma, who may be managing a busy lifestyle while maintaining focus, ginkgo biloba supplements offer a practical way to support her cognitive needs. By integrating ginkgo biloba into her routine, she can benefit from improved concentration and enhanced mental clarity, which can help her manage daily tasks more effectively.

Rosemary: The Herb of Remembrance

Rosemary is traditionally associated with memory enhancement and mental sharpness. The herb contains compounds such as carnosic acid that protect the brain from free radical damage and stimulate blood flow, which enhances concentration and clarity. The aroma of rosemary alone has been shown to improve focus and cognitive performance, making it a powerful tool for mental clarity.

Rosemary can be used in various ways, such as in teas, essential oils, or even as a culinary herb. For Emma, diffusing rosemary essential oil while working or studying can create an environment that supports mental focus. Alternatively, adding fresh rosemary to meals provides a flavorful and health-boosting option, ensuring she gains cognitive benefits naturally throughout the day.

Bacopa Monnieri: Enhancing Memory and Learning

Bacopa monnieri, also known as Brahmi, is an herb traditionally used in Ayurvedic medicine for its cognitive-enhancing properties. Bacopa helps improve memory retention and learning abilities by promoting the growth of dendrites, which are crucial for neuron communication. Additionally, it helps reduce anxiety, which can often interfere with focus and concentration.

Bacopa is available in capsules, tinctures, or as a tea. For Emma, taking bacopa capsules daily offers a convenient way to boost her mental clarity without disrupting her routine. By supporting neuron communication and reducing stress, bacopa helps her maintain focus, allowing her to stay productive and mentally sharp.

Gotu Kola: Supporting Brain Function and Clarity

Gotu kola is another herb used in Ayurvedic and Chinese medicine for its ability to improve cognitive function. It supports mental clarity by enhancing circulation and reducing oxidative stress in the brain. Gotu kola also acts as an adaptogen, helping the body adapt to physical and mental stress, which often impairs concentration and focus.

Gotu kola can be taken as a tea or in capsule form. For Emma, incorporating gotu kola tea into her morning routine provides a gentle and effective way to start the day with mental clarity. The herb's ability to enhance brain function ensures that her mind remains sharp and focused, supporting her throughout her daily activities and work.

Peppermint: A Quick Boost for Focus

Peppermint is an invigorating herb that is commonly used for its energizing effects. The scent of peppermint has been shown to enhance alertness and concentration, making it a useful tool for those who need a quick mental boost. The essential oils in peppermint stimulate the brain, promoting clarity and focus while also alleviating fatigue.

Peppermint tea is an easy and enjoyable way for Emma to benefit from this herb's cognitive-enhancing effects. Alternatively, using peppermint essential oil in a diffuser or applying it to her temples offers a quick method for gaining mental clarity. This herb's refreshing properties provide an instant pick-me-up, ensuring she stays focused and alert during demanding tasks.

Sage: Improving Cognitive Performance

Sage is another herb recognized for its memory-enhancing and focus-improving abilities. It contains compounds such as rosmarinic acid and antioxidants that protect the brain and enhance neurotransmitter function. Sage has been shown to improve cognitive performance, particularly in tasks that require sustained attention and focus.

Sage can be consumed as a tea or used in cooking. For Emma, drinking sage tea offers a simple and effective way to sharpen her mind and enhance focus, especially during work or study sessions. Its cognitive benefits, coupled with its soothing properties, make it a valuable addition to her herbal routine, supporting her mental clarity and overall well-being.

Rhodiola Rosea: Boosting Mental Stamina

Rhodiola rosea is an adaptogenic herb that is effective for improving focus and mental stamina. It helps reduce fatigue and enhances concentration by balancing neurotransmitters such as dopamine and serotonin, which are critical for maintaining mental clarity. Rhodiola is particularly useful for those who experience stress-induced fatigue or mental burnout.

Rhodiola is often taken as a capsule or tincture. For Emma, using rhodiola daily provides a way to sustain her mental energy and focus, especially during long and demanding days. The herb's ability to enhance mental endurance ensures she can maintain clarity and productivity, even when faced with stressful or overwhelming situations.

These herbs offer effective and natural solutions for enhancing mental clarity and focus. By integrating them into her routine, Emma can support her cognitive function holistically, ensuring she stays sharp, focused, and mentally resilient in her everyday life.

Remedies for Emotional Wellness and Mental Resilience

Lemon Balm Stress Relief Tea

INGREDIENTS

- 1 teaspoon dried lemon balm leaves
- 1 cup boiling water

PREPARATION

1. Steep lemon balm leaves in boiling water for 10 minutes.
2. Strain and drink once daily for stress relief.

Benefits: Lemon balm is a gentle herb that helps calm the nervous system, reduce stress, and ease anxiety. Regular consumption promotes emotional balance and relaxation, making it perfect for managing everyday stress and tension.

Skullcap Nerve Calming Drops

INGREDIENTS

- 1 tablespoon dried skullcap leaves
- 1/4 cup alcohol (vodka or glycerin for a non-alcoholic option)

PREPARATION

1. Infuse dried skullcap leaves in alcohol or glycerin for 4-6 weeks, shaking occasionally.
2. Strain and take 1-2 droppers daily for nerve calming support.

Benefits: Skullcap is known for its calming effects on the nervous system. These drops help reduce nervous tension, ease anxiety, and promote a sense of calm, making them ideal for those dealing with stress or restlessness.

Passionflower Mood Stabilizer Tincture

INGREDIENTS

- 1 tablespoon dried passionflower leaves
- 1/4 cup alcohol (vodka or glycerin for a non-alcoholic option)

PREPARATION

1. Infuse passionflower leaves in alcohol or glycerin for 4-6 weeks.
2. Strain and take 1-2 droppers daily to support mood stability.

Benefits: Passionflower is an excellent herb for stabilizing mood and alleviating symptoms of anxiety and depression. This tincture helps promote emotional well-being by calming the mind and soothing nervous tension.

Blue Vervain Anxiety Support Capsules

INGREDIENTS

- 1 tablespoon dried blue vervain powder
- Capsule shells

PREPARATION

1. Fill capsule shells with blue vervain powder.
2. Take 1-2 capsules daily for anxiety support.

Benefits: Blue vervain has natural anti-anxiety properties that help soothe the nervous system and reduce symptoms of stress and worry. These capsules provide gentle and effective support for those dealing with anxious feelings or mild depression.

Valerian Root Relaxation Oil

INGREDIENTS

- 1 tablespoon dried valerian root
- 1/4 cup carrier oil (such as coconut oil)

PREPARATION

1. Infuse valerian root in carrier oil using a double boiler for 30 minutes.
2. Strain and pour into a jar.
3. Massage onto the skin before bedtime to promote relaxation.

Benefits: Valerian root is widely known for its sedative properties, helping to relieve tension and promote deep relaxation. This oil helps soothe the nervous system and is ideal for calming the body before sleep or during stressful moments.

Rose Petal Uplifting Elixir

INGREDIENTS

- 1 tablespoon dried rose petals
- 1/4 cup honey
- 1/2 cup water

PREPARATION

1. Simmer rose petals in water for 10 minutes.
2. Strain and stir in honey.
3. Take 1-2 teaspoons daily to uplift mood.

Benefits: Rose petals have uplifting properties that can help lift the spirits and combat feelings of sadness or grief. This elixir provides emotional comfort and helps promote feelings of joy and well-being.

Chamomile and Lavender Sleepy Time Infusion

INGREDIENTS

- 1 teaspoon dried chamomile flowers
- 1/2 teaspoon dried lavender flowers
- 1 cup boiling water

PREPARATION

1. Steep chamomile and lavender flowers in boiling water for 10 minutes.
2. Strain and drink before bed to promote restful sleep.

Benefits: Chamomile and lavender are both known for their calming and sleep-promoting properties. This infusion helps reduce stress, relax the mind, and encourage deep, restful sleep, making it ideal for those struggling with insomnia or anxiety.

Motherwort Emotional Support Drops

INGREDIENTS

- 1 tablespoon dried motherwort leaves
- 1/4 cup alcohol (vodka or glycerin for a non-alcoholic option)

PREPARATION

1. Infuse motherwort leaves in alcohol or glycerin for 4-6 weeks.
2. Strain and take 1-2 droppers daily for emotional support.

Benefits: Motherwort is traditionally used to calm the heart and soothe emotional turmoil. These drops help ease feelings of anxiety, grief, and stress, providing natural emotional support and promoting inner peace.

Ashwagandha Mood Balance Capsules

INGREDIENTS

- 1 tablespoon dried ashwagandha root powder
- Capsule shells

PREPARATION

1. Fill capsule shells with ashwagandha root powder.
2. Take 1-2 capsules daily to support mood balance.

Benefits: Ashwagandha is an adaptogen known for its ability to balance mood, reduce stress, and promote mental clarity. These capsules help maintain emotional equilibrium and are particularly beneficial for those dealing with anxiety, depression, or chronic stress.

Holy Basil (Tulsi) Adaptogenic Tea

INGREDIENTS

- 1 teaspoon dried holy basil (tulsi) leaves
- 1 cup boiling water

PREPARATION

1. Steep holy basil leaves in boiling water for 10 minutes.
2. Strain and drink daily for adaptogenic support.

Benefits: Holy basil is a powerful adaptogen that helps the body manage stress, balance emotions, and promote mental clarity. This tea helps soothe the mind and body, making it an excellent remedy for maintaining emotional and mental resilience.

California Poppy Nerve Soothing Tincture

INGREDIENTS

- 1 tablespoon dried California poppy leaves
- 1/4 cup alcohol (vodka or glycerin for a non-alcoholic option)

PREPARATION

1. Infuse California poppy leaves in alcohol or glycerin for 4-6 weeks.
2. Strain and take 1-2 droppers daily for nerve support.

Benefits: California poppy is known for its sedative and calming effects, helping to ease nervous tension and promote relaxation. This tincture provides gentle relief from anxiety and helps soothe the nervous system, promoting a sense of calm.

Kava Kava Anxiety Relief Capsules

INGREDIENTS

- 1 tablespoon dried kava kava root powder
- Capsule shells

PREPARATION

1. Fill capsule shells with kava kava root powder.
2. Take 1-2 capsules daily to reduce anxiety.

Benefits: Kava kava is well-known for its ability to relieve anxiety, stress, and tension. These capsules provide natural anxiety relief, promoting relaxation without causing drowsiness, making them ideal for managing everyday stress.

Rhodiola Energy and Mood Boost Drops

INGREDIENTS

- 1 tablespoon dried rhodiola root
- 1/4 cup alcohol (vodka or glycerin for a non-alcoholic option)

PREPARATION

1. Infuse rhodiola root in alcohol or glycerin for 4-6 weeks.
2. Strain and take 1-2 droppers daily for energy and mood support.

Benefits: Rhodiola is an adaptogen that helps improve energy levels, reduce fatigue, and balance mood. These drops provide a natural boost for both physical and mental energy, making them ideal for combating stress and promoting emotional well-being.

Linden Flower Emotional Calming Tea

INGREDIENTS

- 1 teaspoon dried linden flowers
- 1 cup boiling water

PREPARATION

1. Steep linden flowers in boiling water for 10 minutes.
2. Strain and drink as needed for emotional calm.

Benefits: Linden flowers are known for their calming and sedative effects. This tea helps ease anxiety, calm emotional distress, and promote a sense of peace and well-being, making it a great remedy for stress-related emotional im balances.

Wild Oat Flower Remedy for Stress

INGREDIENTS

- 1 tablespoon dried wild oat flowers
- 1/4 cup alcohol (vodka or glycerin for a non-alcoholic option)

PREPARATION

1. Infuse wild oat flowers in alcohol or glycerin for 4-6 weeks.
2. Strain and take 1-2 droppers daily for stress relief.

Benefits: Wild oat flowers are known for their ability to relieve stress and anxiety. This remedy provides gentle emotional support for those dealing with feelings of overwhelm or emotional fatigue, helping to restore emotional balance.

Magnolia Bark Relaxation Capsules

INGREDIENTS

- 1 tablespoon dried magnolia bark powder
- Capsule shells

PREPARATION

1. Fill capsule shells with magnolia bark powder.
2. Take 1-2 capsules daily for relaxation.

Benefits: Magnolia bark is a natural sedative that helps promote relaxation and reduce feelings of anxiety and stress. These capsules provide gentle relaxation support, making them an effective remedy for calming the mind and body during stressful times.

Ziziphus Sleep and Calm Elixir

INGREDIENTS

- 1 tablespoon dried ziziphus seeds
- 1 cup boiling water

PREPARATION

1. Simmer ziziphus seeds in boiling water for 15 minutes.
2. Strain and drink before bed to promote calm and sleep.

Benefits: Ziziphus is known for its calming and sleep-promoting properties. This elixir helps soothe the mind and body, making it easier to fall asleep and stay asleep. It's particularly beneficial for individuals dealing with insomnia or anxiety-related sleep issues.

Hops and Lemon Verbena Bedtime Tea

INGREDIENTS

- 1 teaspoon dried hops flowers
- 1 teaspoon dried lemon verbena leaves
- 1 cup boiling water

PREPARATION

1. Steep hops flowers and lemon verbena leaves in boiling water for 10 minutes.
2. Strain and drink 30 minutes before bedtime.

Benefits: Hops and lemon verbena work together to calm the nervous system and promote restful sleep. This tea is perfect for those struggling with insomnia, helping to ease anxiety and encourage deep, undisturbed sleep.

Violet Leaf Emotional Balance Cream

INGREDIENTS

- 1 tablespoon dried violet leaves
- 1/4 cup coconut oil
- 1 tablespoon beeswax

PREPARATION

1. Infuse violet leaves in melted coconut oil for 30 minutes.
2. Strain and stir in melted beeswax.
3. Apply to the skin as needed to promote emotional balance.

Benefits: Violet leaves are known for their calming and grounding properties. This cream helps soothe emotional distress and brings a sense of calm, making it an excellent remedy for those dealing with emotional imbalance or anxiety.

Rosehip Stress Relief Bath Salts

INGREDIENTS

- 1 cup Epsom salts
- 1 tablespoon dried rosehip powder
- 10 drops lavender essential oil

PREPARATION

1. Mix Epsom salts, rosehip powder, and lavender essential oil.
2. Add the mixture to a warm bath and soak for 20 minutes.

Benefits: Rosehip is rich in antioxidants that help relieve stress, while lavender and Epsom salts relax the muscles and mind. This bath blend is perfect for unwinding after a long, stressful day, promoting emotional balance and relaxation.

Gotu Kola Memory and Mood Capsules

INGREDIENTS

- 1 tablespoon dried gotu kola powder
- Capsule shells

PREPARATION

1. Fill capsule shells with gotu kola powder.
2. Take 1-2 capsules daily for memory and mood support.

Benefits: Gotu kola is an adaptogen that helps improve cognitive function and enhance mood. These capsules support mental clarity and emotional balance, making them ideal for boosting both memory and mood in times of stress or mental fatigue.

Peppermint and Rosemary Mental Clarity Tincture

INGREDIENTS

- 1 teaspoon dried peppermint leaves
- 1 teaspoon dried rosemary leaves
- 1/4 cup alcohol (vodka or glycerin for a non-alcoholic option)

PREPARATION

1. Infuse peppermint and rosemary leaves in alcohol or glycerin for 4-6 weeks.
2. Strain and take 1-2 droppers as needed for mental clarity.

Benefits: Peppermint and rosemary are known for their ability to sharpen mental focus and enhance cognitive function. This tincture helps clear mental fog, improve concentration, and boost overall mental clarity, making it ideal for moments of mental exhaustion.

Lavender and Sage Aromatherapy Mist

INGREDIENTS

- 10 drops lavender essential oil
- 5 drops sage essential oil
- 1/4 cup water

PREPARATION

1. Mix lavender and sage essential oils with water in a spray bottle.
2. Spray around the room or onto linens to promote relaxation.

Benefits: Lavender and sage help calm the mind and reduce stress, making this aromatherapy mist perfect for creating a peaceful environment. It helps ease anxiety and promote emotional balance, especially during times of tension.

Lemon Verbena Uplifting Syrup

INGREDIENTS

- 1 tablespoon dried lemon verbena leaves
- 1/4 cup honey
- 1 cup water

PREPARATION

1. Simmer lemon verbena leaves in water for 10 minutes.
2. Strain and stir in honey.
3. Take 1-2 teaspoons as needed to uplift mood.

Benefits: Lemon verbena has uplifting properties that help improve mood and combat feelings of sadness or lethargy. This syrup provides a natural boost to the spirits, helping to promote joy and emotional well-being.

Chrysanthemum Calm Mind Tea

INGREDIENTS

- 1 teaspoon dried chrysanthemum flowers
- 1 cup boiling water

PREPARATION

1. Steep chrysanthemum flowers in boiling water for 10 minutes.
2. Strain and drink as needed to calm the mind.

Benefits: Chrysanthemum is known for its calming and cooling properties. This tea helps soothe the mind and body, making it an ideal remedy for relieving tension, stress, and emotional overwhelm.

Mimosa Bark Emotional Comfort Tincture

INGREDIENTS

- 1 tablespoon dried mimosa bark
- 1/4 cup alcohol (vodka or glycerin for a non-alcoholic option)

PREPARATION

1. Infuse mimosa bark in alcohol or glycerin for 4-6 weeks.
2. Strain and take 1-2 droppers daily for emotional comfort.

Benefits: Mimosa bark is often referred to as the "tree of happiness" for its ability to uplift the spirit and provide emotional comfort. This tincture helps soothe feelings of sadness, grief, or emotional distress, promoting a sense of calm and happiness.

Lemon Balm and Rose Tea Blend

INGREDIENTS

- 1 teaspoon dried lemon balm leaves
- 1 teaspoon dried rose petals
- 1 cup boiling water

PREPARATION

1. Steep lemon balm and rose petals in boiling water for 10 minutes.
2. Strain and drink to promote emotional balance.

Benefits: Lemon balm and rose combine to create a soothing and uplifting tea that helps balance emotions and reduce anxiety. This tea is perfect for calming the mind and promoting a sense of emotional well-being.

Fennel Seed Digestive Comfort Elixir

INGREDIENTS

- 1 teaspoon fennel seeds
- 1/2 cup water
- 1 teaspoon honey

PREPARATION

1. Simmer fennel seeds in water for 10 minutes.
2. Strain and stir in honey.
3. Take 1-2 teaspoons for digestive relief and emotional comfort.

Benefits: Fennel seed helps soothe digestive discomfort, and its calming effects extend to the emotions as well. This elixir supports both physical and emotional well-being, making it useful during times of stress or digestive upset.

Yarrow Nerve Strengthening Capsules

INGREDIENTS

- 1 tablespoon dried yarrow powder
- Capsule shells

PREPARATION

1. Fill capsule shells with yarrow powder.
2. Take 1-2 capsules daily for nerve support.

Benefits: Yarrow strengthens the nervous system, making it beneficial for those who feel emotionally fragile or easily overwhelmed. These capsules support nerve health and resilience, helping to calm anxiety and promote emotional stability.

Angelica Root Emotional Resilience Drops

INGREDIENTS

- 1 tablespoon dried angelica root
- 1/4 cup alcohol (vodka or glycerin for a non-alcoholic option)

PREPARATION

1. Infuse angelica root in alcohol or glycerin for 4-6 weeks.

2. Strain and take 1-2 droppers daily for emotional resilience.

Benefits: Angelica root helps promote emotional resilience and calm, making it an effective remedy for those dealing with emotional stress or hardship. These drops provide gentle support for managing emotions and improving mental well-being.

Spearmint Mental Refresh Tea

INGREDIENTS

- 1 teaspoon dried spearmint leaves
- 1 cup boiling water

PREPARATION

1. Steep spearmint leaves in boiling water for 10 minutes.
2. Strain and drink as needed for mental refreshment.

Benefits: Spearmint helps refresh and clarify the mind, making it a great choice for moments of mental fatigue or stress. This tea is perfect for promoting mental clarity and focus while also calming the nerves.

Wood Betony Mood Stabilizing Infusion

INGREDIENTS

- 1 teaspoon dried wood betony leaves
- 1 cup boiling water

PREPARATION

1. Steep wood betony leaves in boiling water for 10 minutes.
2. Strain and drink daily to stabilize mood.

Benefits: Wood betony is a gentle herb that helps stabilize mood and calm the nervous system. This infusion supports emotional balance and resilience, making it ideal for those dealing with emotional ups and downs.

Hibiscus and Chamomile Relaxation Lotion

INGREDIENTS

- 1 tablespoon dried hibiscus flowers
- 1 tablespoon dried chamomile flowers
- 1/4 cup coconut oil

PREPARATION

1. Infuse hibiscus and chamomile flowers in melted coconut oil for 30 minutes.
2. Strain and pour into a jar.
3. Massage onto the skin as needed to promote relaxation.

Benefits: Hibiscus and chamomile are both known for their relaxing properties. This lotion helps soothe the skin and promote relaxation, making it a perfect remedy for calming the body and mind during stressful times.

BOOK 16

Herbal Support for Fertility and Reproductive Health

Herbs to Support Fertility in Men and Women

NATURAL HERBS FOR ENHANCING FERTILITY IN MEN AND WOMEN

Fertility is influenced by a combination of physical, hormonal, and emotional factors, and for many couples, the journey to conception can be challenging. Herbs offer a natural, supportive approach to enhancing fertility, providing nutrients and compounds that balance hormones, improve reproductive health, and increase the chances of conception. For individuals like Emma, who seek holistic and sustainable ways to support their reproductive health, understanding which herbs are effective for both men and women is essential. Below, we explore several herbs known for their fertility-boosting properties, detailing their benefits and how they can be incorporated into daily routines.

Maca Root: Hormonal Balance and Energy

Maca root, a traditional remedy from the Andes, is widely recognized for its ability to balance hormones in both men and women. It works as an adaptogen, helping the body regulate hormonal imbalances that may interfere with fertility. For women, maca supports the endocrine system, promoting regular ovulation and balancing estrogen levels. For men, it has been shown to enhance libido and improve sperm quality and count, making it a versatile herb for fertility.

Maca can be taken in powder or capsule form, providing flexibility in how it is consumed. For Emma, incorporating maca powder into smoothies or meals offers an easy and effective way to support hormonal health. Its energy-boosting properties also help reduce stress and fatigue, both of which can impact reproductive health. By using maca regularly, Emma and her partner can benefit from its holistic support, enhancing their chances of conception naturally.

Vitex (Chaste Tree Berry): Supporting Female Reproductive Health

Vitex, also known as chaste tree berry, is one of the most effective herbs for female fertility. It works by balancing hormones, particularly progesterone and prolactin, which are crucial for maintaining a regular menstrual cycle. By regulating the luteal phase and supporting ovulation, vitex increases the chances of conception. It is especially beneficial for women experiencing irregular cycles, hormonal imbalances, or conditions like polycystic ovary syndrome (PCOS).

Vitex is typically taken in capsule or tincture form, and its long-term use is safe for most women. For Emma, who may be managing cycle irregularities, using vitex daily can provide a natural and gentle approach to restoring hormonal balance. By incorporating vitex into her routine, she can support her reproductive system, ensuring her body is in an optimal state for conception.

Tribulus Terrestris: Enhancing Male Fertility

Tribulus terrestris is an herb traditionally used to enhance male reproductive health. It boosts testosterone levels, improves sperm count and motility, and increases libido, making it an important herb for men looking to improve their fertility naturally. Tribulus also supports overall reproductive health by enhancing circulation, which is crucial for maintaining healthy sperm production.

Men can take tribulus as a capsule or tincture, making it a convenient addition to their daily routine. For Emma's partner, integrating tribulus into his regimen offers a targeted approach to enhancing fertility, ensuring both partners are actively supporting their reproductive health. By boosting testosterone and improving sperm quality, tribulus plays a vital role in increasing the likelihood of conception.

Red Clover: Nutrient-Rich Support for Women

Red clover is a nutrient-dense herb that provides essential vitamins and minerals needed for reproductive health. It is particularly rich in calcium, magnesium, and phytoestrogens, which help balance hormones and prepare the body for conception. Red clover also acts as a blood purifier, supporting a healthy uterine environment, which is vital for implantation.

Red clover can be consumed as a tea or taken in capsule form. For Emma, drinking red clover tea daily offers a gentle and nourishing way to support her fertility journey. Its calming effects also help reduce stress, ensuring her body remains balanced and receptive to pregnancy. Incorporating red clover into her diet helps create an optimal environment for conception, promoting overall reproductive wellness.

Ashwagandha: Reducing Stress and Supporting Hormonal Balance

Ashwagandha is a powerful adaptogen that supports fertility by reducing stress, balancing hormones, and enhancing overall reproductive health. It is effective for both men and women, making it a versatile herb for couples trying to conceive. For women, ashwagandha helps regulate the menstrual cycle by supporting thyroid function and balancing cortisol levels, both of which are crucial for hormonal stability. For men, it improves sperm quality and motility, contributing to better reproductive outcomes.

Ashwagandha can be taken in capsule or powder form, allowing for flexibility in consumption. For Emma and her partner, incorporating ashwagandha into their daily regimen provides a holistic approach to stress management and hormonal support. By ensuring their bodies are resilient to stress, they enhance their chances of conception, as stress is a significant factor that can affect fertility.

Nettle: Nourishing the Reproductive System

Nettle is an herb rich in vitamins and minerals that support reproductive health, including iron, calcium, and vitamin C. It helps strengthen the uterine lining, making it beneficial for women preparing for pregnancy. Nettle also supports the adrenal glands, which play a role in hormone production and balance. For men, nettle is known to boost testosterone levels and improve sperm health, making it an all-round fertility herb.

Nettle can be consumed as a tea or taken in capsule form. For Emma, drinking nettle tea daily provides a nourishing and gentle way to prepare her body for pregnancy. By ensuring she receives essential nutrients, nettle supports her reproductive system and enhances her overall wellness. Its effects on both partners' fertility make it a valuable addition to their holistic approach to conception.

These herbs provide comprehensive support for fertility in both men and women, addressing hormonal balance, stress management, and nutrient deficiencies naturally. By incorporating these herbs into their daily routines, Emma and her partner can create a supportive environment for conception, aligning with their preference for holistic health solutions.

Natural Remedies for Reproductive Health Conditions

HERBAL REMEDIES FOR ADDRESSING REPRODUCTIVE HEALTH CONDITIONS

Reproductive health conditions, such as polycystic ovary syndrome (PCOS), endometriosis, and hormonal imbalances, can significantly impact fertility and overall well-being. Herbs offer natural solutions that can help manage symptoms, balance hormones, and support reproductive system health. For individuals like Emma, who prefer holistic approaches, understanding these natural remedies provides an opportunity to address reproductive health conditions in a sustainable and effective way. Below, we explore several herbs and their applications for managing these conditions, highlighting how they work and their benefits.

Vitex (Chaste Tree Berry): Balancing Hormones

Vitex, also known as chaste tree berry, is one of the most effective herbs for managing hormonal imbalances, particularly in women with PCOS or irregular menstrual cycles. Vitex works by stimulating the pituitary gland, which helps regulate progesterone and estrogen levels. This is especially important for those with conditions like PCOS, where the balance of these hormones is often disrupted. Vitex also supports the luteal phase of the menstrual cycle, making it beneficial for women experiencing issues with ovulation or irregular periods.

Vitex is usually taken in tincture or capsule form, and it requires consistent use for several months to see results. For Emma, using vitex daily offers a practical and natural solution for managing hormonal imbalances. By regulating her menstrual cycle, vitex can help alleviate symptoms associated with PCOS, such as irregular periods and hormonal acne, improving her overall reproductive health.

Red Raspberry Leaf: Supporting Uterine Health

Red raspberry leaf is a well-known herb for its ability to tone and strengthen the uterine muscles, making it particularly beneficial for women experiencing conditions like endometriosis or menstrual irregularities. The high levels of vitamins and minerals, such as calcium and magnesium, in red raspberry leaf help nourish the reproductive system and support overall uterine health. It also has anti-inflammatory properties that can help reduce the pain and discomfort associated with endometriosis.

Red raspberry leaf is typically consumed as a tea. For Emma, incorporating this tea into her daily routine provides a gentle and supportive way to manage reproductive health. The anti-inflammatory effects of red raspberry leaf help alleviate cramps and pain, while its toning properties promote a healthy menstrual cycle, supporting Emma's holistic approach to reproductive wellness.

Dong Quai: Regulating Menstrual Cycles

Dong quai, often referred to as the "female ginseng," is a traditional Chinese herb used for managing menstrual and reproductive health conditions. It is particularly effective for those experiencing irregular periods or symptoms of menopause, as it helps balance estrogen levels and improves blood flow to the pelvic area. Dong quai also has antispasmodic properties, making it beneficial for alleviating menstrual cramps and other discomforts associated with reproductive health issues.

Dong quai can be taken as a tincture or capsule. For Emma, using dong quai helps regulate her menstrual cycle, ensuring a more consistent and balanced pattern. The herb's ability to promote circulation also supports the overall health of the reproductive organs, making it a valuable remedy for long-term wellness.

Black Cohosh: Alleviating Menopausal Symptoms

Black cohosh is a powerful herb traditionally used to manage symptoms associated with menopause, such as hot flashes, night sweats, and mood swings. It works by mimicking estrogen in the body, which helps stabilize hormone levels and alleviate the discomforts associated with hormonal changes. Additionally, black cohosh is effective in managing symptoms of PCOS by reducing the severity of menstrual cramps and regulating cycles.

Black cohosh is available as a tincture or capsule. For Emma, who may be dealing with perimenopausal symptoms or seeking to manage PCOS, black cohosh offers a natural and effective option for balancing hormones. By integrating this herb into her wellness routine, she can experience relief from common symptoms associated with reproductive health conditions, ensuring she remains comfortable and balanced.

Nettle: Nourishing and Detoxifying the Reproductive System

Nettle is a nutrient-dense herb that offers a range of benefits for reproductive health. Rich in iron, calcium, and vitamins A and C, nettle supports the overall well-being of the reproductive system. It also has anti-inflammatory properties, making it useful for managing symptoms of endometriosis and reducing menstrual pain. Nettle's detoxifying effect helps eliminate toxins from the body, supporting liver function and ensuring hormonal balance.

Nettle can be consumed as a tea or taken as a tincture. For Emma, drinking nettle tea daily provides a simple and effective way to support her reproductive system naturally. Its nourishing properties help alleviate menstrual discomfort and promote regularity, while its detoxifying effects ensure that her body maintains a healthy hormonal balance, essential for managing reproductive health conditions.

Milk Thistle: Supporting Liver Function and Hormone Balance

Milk thistle is a valuable herb for those dealing with hormonal imbalances, as it supports liver function, which is crucial for processing and regulating hormones. Conditions like PCOS or endometriosis can benefit from the detoxifying effects of milk thistle, as a healthy liver ensures that excess hormones are efficiently metabolized. Milk thistle also contains anti-inflammatory properties, which help reduce pain and discomfort associated with these conditions.

Milk thistle is commonly available in capsule or tincture form. For Emma, using milk thistle as part of her wellness plan helps maintain hormone balance naturally. By ensuring her liver functions optimally, she can manage symptoms related to reproductive health conditions more effectively, creating a stable foundation for her overall well-being.

These herbs provide natural solutions for managing reproductive health conditions, supporting hormone balance, and improving overall reproductive wellness. For Emma, integrating these herbs into her daily routine allows her to address her reproductive health holistically, aligning with her preference for natural and sustainable health solutions.

Remedies for Reproductive Wellness

Red Clover Fertility Tea

INGREDIENTS

- 1 teaspoon dried red clover blossoms
- 1 cup boiling water

PREPARATION

1. Steep red clover blossoms in boiling water for 10 minutes.
2. Strain and drink daily to support fertility.

Benefits: Red clover is rich in phytoestrogens that help balance hormones and improve reproductive health. It supports fertility by nourishing the body with essential nutrients and promoting hormonal balance, making it ideal for women trying to conceive.

Chaste Tree (Vitex) Hormonal Balance Capsules

INGREDIENTS

- 1 tablespoon dried chaste tree (Vitex) powder
- Capsule shells

PREPARATION

1. Fill capsule shells with dried chaste tree powder.
2. Take 1-2 capsules daily for hormonal balance.

Benefits: Chaste tree, also known as Vitex, helps regulate hormonal imbalances, particularly in women with irregular cycles or hormonal-related issues. These capsules promote regular menstruation, support fertility, and alleviate PMS symptoms.

Shatavari Reproductive Health Tonic

INGREDIENTS

- 1 tablespoon dried shatavari root powder
- 1 cup warm milk or water

PREPARATION

1. Mix shatavari powder with warm milk or water.
2. Drink daily for reproductive health support.

Benefits: Shatavari is a powerful adaptogenic herb used to support female reproductive health. It helps balance hormones, increase fertility, and support the reproductive system, especially during menopause or postpartum recovery.

Dong Quai Uterine Support Elixir

INGREDIENTS

- 1 tablespoon dried dong quai root
- 1/4 cup alcohol (vodka or glycerin for a non-alcoholic option)

PREPARATION

1. Infuse dong quai root in alcohol or glycerin for 4-6 weeks, shaking occasionally.
2. Strain and take 1-2 droppers daily for uterine support.

Benefits: Dong quai is known for its ability to strengthen the uterus and support overall reproductive health. This elixir promotes hormonal balance, improves circulation to the reproductive organs, and alleviates menstrual cramps.

Maca Root Hormone Regulating Powder

INGREDIENTS

- 1 tablespoon maca root powder
- 1 cup water or smoothie

PREPARATION

1. Mix maca root powder into water or a smoothie.
2. Consume daily for hormone regulation.

Benefits: Maca root is an adaptogen that helps regulate hormonal balance, increase energy, and enhance fertility. It supports both male and female reproductive health by boosting libido and promoting healthy hormone levels.

Black Cohosh Menstrual Relief Capsules

INGREDIENTS

- 1 tablespoon dried black cohosh powder
- Capsule shells

PREPARATION

1. Fill capsule shells with black cohosh powder.
2. Take 1-2 capsules daily to relieve menstrual discomfort.

Benefits: Black cohosh is known for its ability to alleviate menstrual cramps and reduce symptoms of PMS and menopause. These capsules provide relief from pain and discomfort associated with menstruation and help regulate hormonal balance.

Damiana Libido Enhancement Tea

INGREDIENTS

- 1 teaspoon dried damiana leaves
- 1 cup boiling water

PREPARATION

1. Steep damiana leaves in boiling water for 10 minutes.
2. Strain and drink as needed for libido support.

Benefits: Damiana is an aphrodisiac known for enhancing libido and promoting sexual wellness. This tea helps increase sexual desire, support reproductive health, and balance emotions related to sexual well-being.

Raspberry Leaf Pregnancy Support Infusion

INGREDIENTS

- 1 teaspoon dried raspberry leaf
- 1 cup boiling water

PREPARATION

1. Steep raspberry leaf in boiling water for 10 minutes.
2. Strain and drink daily during pregnancy.

Benefits: Raspberry leaf is rich in nutrients that support the uterus and overall pregnancy health. This infusion helps tone the uterus, prepare the body for labor, and provides essential vitamins and minerals during pregnancy.

Nettle Iron-Rich Pregnancy Tonic

INGREDIENTS

- 1 teaspoon dried nettle leaves
- 1 cup boiling water

PREPARATION

1. Steep nettle leaves in boiling water for 10 minutes.
2. Strain and drink daily to boost iron levels during pregnancy.

Benefits: Nettle is packed with iron and essential nutrients, making it a great tonic for supporting pregnancy and preventing anemia. This tonic helps increase energy levels and supports healthy blood production during pregnancy.

Blue Cohosh Birth Preparation Drops

INGREDIENTS

- 1 tablespoon dried blue cohosh root
- 1/4 cup alcohol (vodka or glycerin for a non-alcoholic option)

PREPARATION

1. Infuse blue cohosh root in alcohol or glycerin for 4-6 weeks.
2. Strain and take 1-2 droppers daily in the final weeks of pregnancy to prepare for labor.

Benefits: Blue cohosh helps tone the uterus and prepare the body for labor. These drops are traditionally used during the last few weeks of pregnancy to support a smooth and efficient childbirth process.

Motherwort Menstrual Health Tea

INGREDIENTS

- 1 teaspoon dried motherwort leaves
- 1 cup boiling water

PREPARATION

1. Steep motherwort leaves in boiling water for 10 minutes.
2. Strain and drink daily for menstrual health.

Benefits: Motherwort is known for its ability to relieve menstrual pain, regulate cycles, and support overall reproductive health. This tea helps alleviate PMS symptoms and promotes hormonal balance.

Ashwagandha Fertility Booster Capsules

INGREDIENTS

- 1 tablespoon dried ashwagandha root powder
- Capsule shells

PREPARATION

1. Fill capsule shells with ashwagandha root powder.
2. Take 1-2 capsules daily to boost fertility.

Benefits: Ashwagandha is an adaptogen that supports fertility by balancing hormones, reducing stress, and improving reproductive health. These capsules are beneficial for both men and women seeking to enhance fertility.

Evening Primrose Oil Fertility Support

INGREDIENTS

- 1 teaspoon evening primrose oil

PREPARATION

1. Take 1 teaspoon of evening primrose oil daily.
2. Use during the follicular phase of the menstrual cycle for best results.

Benefits: Evening primrose oil is rich in essential fatty acids that help balance hormones and improve cervical mucus production, promoting fertility. It is commonly used by women trying to conceive.

Sage and Chamomile Menstrual Balance Tea

INGREDIENTS

- 1 teaspoon dried sage leaves
- 1 teaspoon dried chamomile flowers
- 1 cup boiling water

PREPARATION

1. Steep sage leaves and chamomile flowers in boiling water for 10 minutes.
2. Strain and drink daily to support menstrual health.

Benefits: Sage and chamomile work together to relieve menstrual cramps, reduce bloating, and support hormonal balance. This tea helps ease discomfort and promote emotional well-being during menstruation.

Fenugreek Lactation Enhancement Capsules

INGREDIENTS

- 1 tablespoon dried fenugreek seed powder
- Capsule shells

PREPARATION

1. Fill capsule shells with fenugreek seed powder.
2. Take 1-2 capsules daily to enhance lactation.

Benefits: Fenugreek is a well-known galactagogue that helps increase milk production in breastfeeding mothers. These capsules support lactation and ensure a healthy milk supply for nursing mothers.

Yarrow Hormone Support Infusion

INGREDIENTS

- 1 teaspoon dried yarrow flowers
- 1 cup boiling water

PREPARATION

1. Steep yarrow flowers in boiling water for 10 minutes.
2. Strain and drink once daily for hormone support.

Benefits: Yarrow helps regulate hormones, reduce menstrual pain, and support reproductive health. This infusion is beneficial for women dealing with hormonal imbalances, irregular cycles, or menopause symptoms.

Calendula Uterine Healing Tincture

INGREDIENTS

- 1 tablespoon dried calendula flowers
- 1/4 cup alcohol (vodka or glycerin for a non-alcoholic option)

PREPARATION

1. Infuse calendula flowers in alcohol or glycerin for 4-6 weeks.
2. Strain and take 1-2 droppers daily for uterine healing.

Benefits: Calendula is known for its healing properties, particularly in supporting the health of the uterus. This tincture helps reduce inflammation, promote tissue regeneration, and support uterine health, especially after childbirth or surgery.

Lemon Balm PMS Relief Tea

INGREDIENTS

- 1 teaspoon dried lemon balm leaves
- 1 cup boiling water

PREPARATION

1. Steep lemon balm leaves in boiling water for 10 minutes.
2. Strain and drink as needed to relieve PMS symptoms.

Benefits: Lemon balm is known for its calming and mood-lifting properties. This tea helps relieve stress, anxiety, and irritability associated with PMS, while also soothing digestive discomfort that often accompanies hormonal fluctuations.

Moringa Postpartum Health Elixir

INGREDIENTS

- 1 tablespoon dried moringa leaf powder
- 1 cup warm water

PREPARATION

1. Mix moringa powder with warm water and drink once daily during postpartum recovery.

Benefits: Moringa is rich in vitamins, minerals, and antioxidants that support overall health and well-being during postpartum recovery. This elixir helps boost energy levels, support lactation, and replenish vital nutrients lost during childbirth.

Rose Petal Emotional Balance Infusion

INGREDIENTS

- 1 tablespoon dried rose petals
- 1 cup boiling water

PREPARATION

1. Steep rose petals in boiling water for 10 minutes.
2. Strain and drink to promote emotional balance.

Benefits: Rose petals have calming and uplifting properties that help soothe emotions and promote feelings of well-being. This infusion helps relieve emotional stress and anxiety related to reproductive health and hormonal changes.

Marigold Womb Health Capsules

INGREDIENTS

- 1 tablespoon dried marigold flowers
- Capsule shells

PREPARATION

1. Fill capsule shells with dried marigold flower powder.
2. Take 1-2 capsules daily for womb health support.

Benefits: Marigold flowers, also known as calendula, help promote uterine healing and reduce inflammation. These capsules support the overall health of the reproductive system, helping to balance hormones and promote a healthy womb environment.

Angelica Root Reproductive Harmony Drops

INGREDIENTS

- 1 tablespoon dried angelica root
- 1/4 cup alcohol (vodka or glycerin for a non-alcoholic option)

PREPARATION

1. Infuse angelica root in alcohol or glycerin for 4-6 weeks.
2. Strain and take 1-2 droppers daily to promote reproductive harmony.

Benefits: Angelica root helps regulate the menstrual cycle and support overall reproductive health. These drops promote hormonal balance and can help alleviate symptoms of PMS and menopause.

Licorice Hormone Balancing Tincture

INGREDIENTS

- 1 tablespoon dried licorice root
- 1/4 cup alcohol (vodka or glycerin for a non-alcoholic option)

PREPARATION

1. Infuse licorice root in alcohol or glycerin for 4-6 weeks.
2. Strain and take 1-2 droppers daily for hormone balance.

Benefits: Licorice root helps regulate hormone levels and supports adrenal health. This tincture is particularly beneficial for women with hormonal imbalances or adrenal fatigue, promoting overall reproductive wellness.

Nettle and Oatstraw Fertility Tonic

INGREDIENTS

- 1 teaspoon dried nettle leaves
- 1 teaspoon dried oatstraw
- 1 cup boiling water

PREPARATION

1. Steep nettle and oatstraw in boiling water for 10 minutes.
2. Strain and drink daily for fertility support.

Benefits: Nettle and oatstraw are rich in minerals and vitamins that support reproductive health. This tonic nourishes the reproductive system, promotes hormonal balance, and enhances fertility in both men and women.

Dong Quai and Ginseng Fertility Tea

INGREDIENTS

- 1 teaspoon dried dong quai root
- 1 teaspoon dried ginseng root
- 1 cup boiling water

PREPARATION

1. Steep dong quai and ginseng roots in boiling water for 10 minutes.
2. Strain and drink daily to enhance fertility.

Benefits: Dong quai and ginseng are powerful herbs that support fertility by balancing hormones and improving reproductive health. This tea helps enhance libido and promotes a healthy reproductive system.

Holy Basil (Tulsi) Hormonal Harmony Capsules

INGREDIENTS

- 1 tablespoon dried holy basil (tulsi) powder
- Capsule shells

PREPARATION

1. Fill capsule shells with dried holy basil powder.
2. Take 1-2 capsules daily for hormonal balance.

Benefits: Holy basil is an adaptogen that helps balance hormones and reduce stress. These capsules support reproductive health by promoting hormonal harmony and reducing the effects of stress on the body.

Peppermint and Rose Menstrual Cramp Oil

INGREDIENTS

- 10 drops peppermint essential oil
- 10 drops rose essential oil
- 1/4 cup carrier oil (such as coconut oil)

PREPARATION

1. Mix peppermint and rose essential oils with the carrier oil.
2. Massage the oil onto the abdomen during menstruation to relieve cramps.

Benefits: Peppermint and rose essential oils provide a soothing effect on menstrual cramps, helping to relax the muscles and reduce pain. This oil blend helps ease discomfort and promotes a sense of calm during menstruation.

Alfalfa Fertility Support Capsules

INGREDIENTS

- 1 tablespoon dried alfalfa powder
- Capsule shells

PREPARATION

1. Fill capsule shells with dried alfalfa powder.
2. Take 1-2 capsules daily to support fertility.

Benefits: Alfalfa is rich in essential nutrients that support reproductive health and fertility. These capsules provide the body with vital vitamins and minerals that help nourish the reproductive system and promote hormonal balance.

Burdock Root Detox Tea for Women

INGREDIENTS

- 1 teaspoon dried burdock root
- 1 cup boiling water

PREPARATION

1. Steep burdock root in boiling water for 10 minutes.
2. Strain and drink once daily to detoxify the reproductive system.

Benefits: Burdock root is a detoxifying herb that helps cleanse the liver and support reproductive health. This tea promotes hormonal balance, detoxifies the body, and supports overall reproductive wellness.

Thyme Hormone Regulator Tincture

INGREDIENTS

- 1 tablespoon dried thyme leaves
- 1/4 cup alcohol (vodka or glycerin for a non-alcoholic option)

PREPARATION

1. Infuse thyme leaves in alcohol or glycerin for 4-6 weeks.
2. Strain and take 1-2 droppers daily for hormone regulation.

Benefits: Thyme is known for its ability to support the endocrine system and regulate hormone levels. This tincture helps promote hormonal balance and reduce symptoms associated with hormonal fluctuations, such as PMS and menopause.

Chamomile and Ginger Pregnancy Comfort Drops

INGREDIENTS

- 1 teaspoon dried chamomile flowers
- 1 teaspoon grated fresh ginger
- 1/4 cup alcohol (vodka or glycerin for a non-alcoholic option)

PREPARATION

1. Infuse chamomile and ginger in alcohol or glycerin for 4-6 weeks.
2. Strain and take 1-2 droppers daily for pregnancy comfort.

Benefits: Chamomile and ginger are both soothing herbs that help relieve nausea, bloating, and discomfort during pregnancy. These drops provide gentle relief for common pregnancy symptoms, promoting comfort and relaxation.

Hibiscus Fertility Boost Tea

INGREDIENTS

- 1 teaspoon dried hibiscus flowers
- 1 cup boiling water

PREPARATION

1. Steep hibiscus flowers in boiling water for 10 minutes.
2. Strain and drink daily to support fertility.

Benefits: Hibiscus is rich in antioxidants that support reproductive health and boost fertility. This tea helps balance hormones, improve circulation, and promote overall reproductive wellness, making it an excellent choice for those trying to conceive.

Lemon Verbena Lactation Support Infusion

INGREDIENTS

- 1 teaspoon dried lemon verbena leaves
- 1 cup boiling water

PREPARATION

1. Steep lemon verbena leaves in boiling water for 10 minutes.
2. Strain and drink daily to support lactation.

Benefits: Lemon verbena is a calming herb that helps promote lactation and reduce stress in breastfeeding mothers. This infusion supports milk production while providing emotional balance and relaxation.

BOOK 17

Enhancing Hair Health with Herbal Care

Herbs for Strengthening Hair and Scalp Health

NATURAL HERBS FOR STRENGTHENING HAIR AND REVITALIZING SCALP HEALTH

Maintaining strong, healthy hair and a nourished scalp is essential for overall hair vitality. For individuals like Emma, who prefer natural solutions, understanding the benefits of herbs that specifically target hair and scalp health can be transformative. Herbs have long been used to strengthen hair, promote shine, and treat scalp issues such as dryness or dandruff. By incorporating these natural remedies into her routine, Emma can support her hair health in a sustainable and effective manner. Below, we explore several herbs known for their hair and scalp benefits, explaining their properties and applications.

Nettle: A Nutrient-Rich Solution for Hair Health

Nettle is one of the most powerful herbs for hair and scalp health, rich in vitamins A, C, and K, as well as minerals like iron, magnesium, and calcium. These nutrients are essential for promoting hair growth and strengthening the hair shaft. Nettle also contains silica and sulfur, which improve hair texture, reduce breakage, and promote shine.

Nettle can be used as a tea rinse or taken internally as a supplement. For Emma, incorporating nettle tea as a rinse provides a practical and effective way to boost hair strength naturally. By using a nettle rinse after washing her hair, she can enhance the shine and thickness of her hair while nourishing her scalp. Additionally, drinking nettle tea supports overall hair health from within, ensuring her hair receives the nutrients needed for optimal growth and strength.

Rosemary: Stimulating Circulation and Promoting Growth

Rosemary is a well-known herb for hair health, particularly for its ability to stimulate blood circulation in the scalp. Improved circulation ensures that hair follicles receive the oxygen and nutrients they need to grow strong and healthy. Rosemary also has antioxidant properties, which protect the scalp from damage and promote hair growth. Additionally, its antimicrobial benefits help keep the scalp clean and free from dandruff.

Rosemary can be used as an essential oil or as an infusion. For Emma, massaging her scalp with diluted rosemary oil offers an effective way to stimulate hair growth while maintaining a clean and healthy scalp environment. Adding rosemary to her hair care routine not only strengthens her hair but also enhances its natural shine, providing a holistic approach to hair wellness.

Aloe Vera: Hydration and Scalp Soothing

Aloe vera is another versatile herb that is particularly beneficial for the scalp. It has soothing, anti-inflammatory properties that can help reduce scalp irritation, itching, and dandruff. Aloe vera also provides deep hydration, ensuring the scalp remains moisturized, which is essential for healthy hair growth. The enzymes found in aloe vera also help remove dead skin cells from the scalp, promoting a clean and balanced environment for hair follicles.

Aloe vera gel can be applied directly to the scalp as a mask before washing. For Emma, using aloe vera gel weekly as a scalp treatment provides a soothing and moisturizing solution, addressing any dryness or irritation she may experience. By integrating aloe vera into her routine, she ensures her scalp remains hydrated and healthy, which is fundamental for achieving strong, resilient hair.

Horsetail: Silica for Hair Strength

Horsetail is a herb rich in silica, a mineral crucial for strengthening hair and improving its elasticity. Silica helps bond collagen and calcium, which fortify hair strands, reduce breakage, and promote overall hair health. Horsetail also supports the production of keratin, the primary protein in hair, ensuring that each strand remains strong and shiny. Furthermore, horsetail's anti-inflammatory properties benefit the scalp by reducing inflammation and promoting a healthy environment for hair growth.

Horsetail can be consumed as a tea or taken in capsule form. For Emma, drinking horsetail tea offers a convenient and effective way to enhance her hair health from within. The added silica content ensures that her hair remains strong, reducing breakage and improving overall texture. By incorporating horsetail into her routine, she fortifies her hair naturally, supporting long-term hair strength and resilience.

Peppermint: Refreshing Scalp Treatment

Peppermint is another powerful herb for hair and scalp health, known for its cooling and stimulating effects. Peppermint oil increases blood flow to the scalp, which promotes hair growth and strengthens hair follicles. Its antiseptic properties also help reduce dandruff and soothe an itchy scalp, ensuring the scalp remains clean and balanced. The refreshing aroma of peppermint provides an additional benefit, making it a popular choice for invigorating hair treatments.

Peppermint oil can be used as a scalp massage oil when diluted with a carrier oil such as coconut oil. For Emma, massaging her scalp with peppermint oil provides a refreshing and stimulating experience that enhances circulation and supports hair growth. Incorporating peppermint into her hair care routine helps maintain a healthy scalp environment, essential for long-lasting hair vitality.

Sage: Preventing Hair Thinning

Sage is an herb traditionally used to prevent hair thinning and loss. It contains antioxidants that protect hair follicles from damage and stimulate new hair growth. Sage also has astringent properties that help tighten the scalp, improving overall scalp health and reducing hair fall. Its anti-inflammatory effects help manage scalp conditions like dermatitis, ensuring the scalp remains healthy and conducive to hair growth.

Sage can be used as a tea rinse or essential oil. For Emma, incorporating sage tea as a final rinse after washing her hair provides an easy way to support scalp health and strengthen hair. By using sage regularly, she can help prevent hair thinning and maintain her hair's fullness and vibrancy naturally.

These herbs offer a natural and effective approach to enhancing hair and scalp health. By incorporating them into her hair care routine, Emma can achieve strong, healthy hair that aligns with her holistic wellness goals.

Natural Treatments for Hair Growth and Repair

EFFECTIVE HERBAL TREATMENTS FOR HAIR GROWTH AND REPAIR

Hair growth and repair require a holistic approach that not only addresses the health of the scalp but also nurtures the hair follicles and strengthens hair strands. For individuals like Emma, who seek natural, sustainable ways to promote hair growth and repair damage, herbs offer a range of effective solutions. These treatments use the powerful properties of herbs to stimulate growth, nourish the hair, and repair damage caused by environmental factors, styling, or stress. Below, we explore several natural treatments and how they can be incorporated into a daily or weekly hair care routine.

Fenugreek: Stimulating Hair Growth Naturally

Fenugreek seeds are rich in proteins, iron, and nicotinic acid, which are essential for hair growth. They also contain lecithin, a substance that hydrates hair and strengthens roots. Fenugreek helps to prevent hair fall and promotes the growth of new hair by nourishing the hair follicles and increasing blood flow to the scalp. It is especially beneficial for those experiencing thinning hair or hair loss due to stress, hormonal changes, or nutrient deficiencies.

To use fenugreek, the seeds can be soaked overnight and then ground into a paste. This paste can be applied directly to the scalp and hair, left on for 30 minutes, and then rinsed off. For Emma, incorporating a fenugreek hair mask into her weekly routine provides a simple and effective way to stimulate hair growth. The hydrating and nourishing properties of fenugreek ensure that her hair receives essential nutrients, promoting thicker and stronger strands.

Amla (Indian Gooseberry): A Rich Source of Vitamin C

Amla, also known as Indian gooseberry, is a powerful herb for hair growth and repair. It is a rich source of vitamin C and antioxidants, which protect hair from oxidative stress and strengthen the hair shaft. Amla also stimulates hair follicles, promoting the growth of new hair and preventing premature greying. Its anti-inflammatory and antimicrobial properties help keep the scalp healthy, ensuring a supportive environment for hair growth.

Amla powder can be mixed with water or coconut oil to create a paste that can be applied to the scalp and hair. For Emma, using an amla treatment once a week supports both hair growth and scalp health, ensuring her hair remains vibrant and strong. The high vitamin C content in amla also boosts collagen production, which is vital for hair strength and elasticity.

Castor Oil: Enhancing Hair Growth and Repairing Damage

Castor oil is a well-known natural remedy for promoting hair growth and repairing damage. It is rich in ricinoleic acid, which enhances blood circulation to the scalp, stimulating hair growth. Castor oil also contains omega-6 fatty acids that nourish hair and prevent dryness. The thick consistency of the oil forms a protective barrier around hair strands, helping to repair split ends and reduce breakage.

For Emma, applying warm castor oil to her scalp and hair as a pre-wash treatment is an effective way to promote growth and repair. Massaging the oil into the scalp increases circulation, ensuring that hair follicles receive the nutrients needed for optimal growth. The oil can be left on for an hour or overnight for a deeper treatment, providing intense moisture and repair for damaged hair.

Onion Juice: Boosting Hair Follicle Stimulation

Onion juice is another powerful natural remedy for hair growth. Rich in sulfur, onion juice improves blood circulation and promotes collagen production, which supports the health and strength of hair follicles. Sulfur also helps prevent hair thinning and breakage by nourishing the scalp. Additionally, the antibacterial properties of onion juice help keep the scalp free of infections that can impede hair growth.

To use onion juice, onions can be blended and strained to extract the juice, which can then be massaged into the scalp. For Emma, applying onion juice once a week is an effective way to stimulate hair follicles and encourage hair growth. Although the smell may be strong, the benefits of this treatment are significant, making it a potent and cost-effective option for enhancing hair growth and repair.

Hibiscus: Promoting Healthy Hair Growth

Hibiscus is a flower known for its ability to promote hair growth and prevent hair loss. It contains amino acids and vitamin C, which nourish hair follicles and improve hair strength. Hibiscus also helps condition the hair, adding shine and softness while preventing split ends and breakage. Its anti-inflammatory properties help soothe the scalp, making it an excellent option for those with sensitive skin.

Hibiscus flowers can be blended into a paste and applied directly to the scalp and hair. For Emma, incorporating hibiscus into her hair care routine as a mask helps repair damage and promotes growth. The conditioning properties of hibiscus ensure that her hair remains soft and manageable, while its nutrients provide the essential support needed for long-term hair health.

Aloe Vera and Coconut Oil: A Powerful Repairing Combination

Aloe vera is renowned for its hydrating and healing properties, making it an effective treatment for hair repair. It contains enzymes that promote healthy hair growth by reducing inflammation and removing dead skin cells from the scalp. When combined with coconut oil, which is rich in fatty acids that penetrate the hair shaft, aloe vera creates a powerful repairing treatment that nourishes and strengthens hair.

To use this treatment, Emma can mix fresh aloe vera gel with coconut oil and apply it to her scalp and hair as a mask. Leaving the mixture on for 30 minutes before washing it out ensures deep hydration and repair. This combination provides her hair with the moisture it needs, while also improving hair texture and strength, ensuring her hair grows healthier and more resilient.

These natural treatments provide effective and sustainable solutions for enhancing hair growth and repairing damage. For Emma, incorporating these remedies into her hair care regimen allows her to achieve her hair health goals naturally, aligning with her holistic approach to wellness.

Remedies for Hair Care and Healthy Growth

Horsetail Hair Strengthening Rinse

INGREDIENTS

- 1 tablespoon dried horsetail herb
- 1 cup boiling water

PREPARATION

1. Steep horsetail herb in boiling water for 10 minutes.
2. Strain and allow to cool.
3. Pour over hair after shampooing, massaging into the scalp. Leave on for 5 minutes, then rinse.

Benefits: Horsetail is rich in silica, which strengthens hair and promotes growth. This rinse helps improve hair elasticity, reduce breakage, and add shine to dull hair. Regular use supports overall hair health and vitality.

Rosemary Scalp Stimulating Oil

INGREDIENTS

- 10 drops rosemary essential oil
- 1/4 cup carrier oil (such as coconut or olive oil)

PREPARATION

1. Mix rosemary essential oil with the carrier oil.
2. Massage the oil into the scalp for 5-10 minutes.
3. Leave it on for at least 30 minutes or overnight before washing.

Benefits: Rosemary oil stimulates blood circulation to the scalp, promoting hair growth and preventing hair loss. It helps strengthen hair follicles and reduce dandruff, making it a great remedy for improving scalp health.

Nettle Leaf Hair Growth Tea

INGREDIENTS

- 1 teaspoon dried nettle leaves
- 1 cup boiling water

PREPARATION

1. Steep nettle leaves in boiling water for 10 minutes.
2. Strain and drink daily to promote hair growth.

Benefits: Nettle is packed with vitamins and minerals that nourish the scalp and promote hair growth. Drinking nettle tea helps strengthen hair from the inside out, reducing hair loss and promoting thicker, healthier hair.

Aloe Vera Hydrating Hair Mask

INGREDIENTS

- 2 tablespoons fresh aloe vera gel
- 1 tablespoon coconut oil

PREPARATION

1. Mix aloe vera gel with coconut oil.
2. Apply the mixture to damp hair, focusing on the ends.
3. Leave it on for 30 minutes, then rinse thoroughly.

Benefits: Aloe vera hydrates and soothes the scalp, while coconut oil deeply nourishes and strengthens hair. This mask helps combat dryness, reduces frizz, and promotes soft, shiny hair.

Sage and Lavender Anti-Dandruff Rinse

INGREDIENTS

- 1 teaspoon dried sage leaves
- 1 teaspoon dried lavender flowers
- 1 cup boiling water

PREPARATION

1. Steep sage leaves and lavender flowers in boiling water for 10 minutes.
2. Strain and use as a final rinse after shampooing.

Benefits: Sage and lavender have antimicrobial and anti-inflammatory properties that help reduce dandruff and soothe the scalp. This rinse keeps the scalp healthy and promotes shiny, dandruff-free hair.

Marshmallow Root Detangling Spray

INGREDIENTS

- 1 tablespoon dried marshmallow root
- 1 cup water

PREPARATION

1. Simmer marshmallow root in water for 15 minutes.
2. Strain and pour the liquid into a spray bottle.
3. Spray onto damp hair before combing to detangle.

Benefits: Marshmallow root is rich in mucilage, which provides slip and makes it easier to detangle hair. This spray helps prevent breakage and reduces frizz, leaving hair smooth and manageable.

Peppermint Scalp Refreshing Serum

INGREDIENTS

- 10 drops peppermint essential oil
- 1/4 cup jojoba oil

PREPARATION

1. Mix peppermint essential oil with jojoba oil.
2. Massage into the scalp and leave on for 20 minutes before washing.

Benefits: Peppermint oil stimulates blood flow to the scalp, promoting hair growth and reducing itching. This serum provides a refreshing sensation while improving scalp health and hair vitality.

Calendula Hair Shine Infusion

INGREDIENTS

- 1 tablespoon dried calendula flowers
- 1 cup boiling water

PREPARATION

1. Steep calendula flowers in boiling water for 10 minutes.
2. Strain and use as a hair rinse after shampooing.

Benefits: Calendula helps add shine to dull hair while soothing the scalp. This infusion nourishes the hair and promotes softness and luster, making it perfect for revitalizing tired, dry hair.

Burdock Root Hair Growth Capsules

INGREDIENTS

- 1 tablespoon dried burdock root powder
- Capsule shells

PREPARATION

1. Fill capsule shells with burdock root powder.
2. Take 1-2 capsules daily to promote hair growth.

Benefits: Burdock root supports hair growth by nourishing the scalp and improving blood circulation. These capsules strengthen hair follicles and promote healthy, thick hair.

Fenugreek Hair Thickening Oil

INGREDIENTS

- 1 tablespoon fenugreek seeds
- 1/4 cup coconut oil

PREPARATION

1. Infuse fenugreek seeds in coconut oil using a double boiler for 30 minutes.
2. Strain and apply the oil to the scalp and hair. Leave on for at least 30 minutes before washing.

Benefits: Fenugreek seeds are rich in proteins and nicotinic acid, which strengthen hair and promote thicker growth. This oil nourishes the hair shaft, preventing thinning and breakage.

Amla Powder Hair Rejuvenation Mask

INGREDIENTS

- 1 tablespoon amla powder
- 1 tablespoon water

PREPARATION

1. Mix amla powder with water to create a paste.
2. Apply to the scalp and hair, leave for 30 minutes, then rinse.

Benefits: Amla, or Indian gooseberry, is rich in antioxidants and vitamin C, which rejuvenate hair and promote hair growth. This mask helps strengthen roots, reduce hair fall, and enhance natural hair color.

Lemon Peel Hair Lightening Rinse

INGREDIENTS

- Peel of 1 lemon
- 1 cup boiling water

PREPARATION

1. Simmer lemon peel in boiling water for 10 minutes.
2. Strain and use as a final rinse after shampooing.

Benefits: Lemon peel helps naturally lighten hair and add shine. This rinse is perfect for brightening hair and enhancing highlights, especially for those with light-colored hair.

Thyme Hair Loss Prevention Oil

INGREDIENTS

- 10 drops thyme essential oil
- 1/4 cup olive oil

PREPARATION

1. Mix thyme essential oil with olive oil.
2. Massage into the scalp for 5 minutes and leave on for at least 30 minutes before washing.

Benefits: Thyme oil is known for its ability to prevent hair loss by stimulating the scalp and strengthening hair follicles. Regular use can help reduce hair thinning and promote healthy hair growth.

Chamomile Hair Smoothing Serum

INGREDIENTS

- 1 tablespoon chamomile flowers
- 1/4 cup carrier oil (such as almond or jojoba oil)

PREPARATION

1. Infuse chamomile flowers in the carrier oil using a double boiler for 30 minutes.
2. Strain and apply a small amount to damp or dry hair to smooth frizz.

Benefits: Chamomile helps smooth and soften hair, reducing frizz and adding shine. This serum provides a lightweight solution for taming unruly hair and enhancing smoothness.

Hibiscus Hair Repair Mask

INGREDIENTS

- 1 tablespoon dried hibiscus petals
- 1/4 cup yogurt

PREPARATION

1. Blend dried hibiscus petals with yogurt to form a paste.
2. Apply the mixture to the scalp and hair, leave on for 30 minutes, then rinse.

Benefits: Hibiscus strengthens the hair, promotes hair growth, and repairs damaged strands. This mask restores moisture and elasticity to dry, brittle hair, leaving it soft and rejuvenated.

Basil Hair Vitality Tea

INGREDIENTS

- 1 teaspoon dried basil leaves
- 1 cup boiling water

PREPARATION

1. Steep basil leaves in boiling water for 10 minutes.
2. Strain and drink daily to support hair vitality.

Benefits: Basil is known for its ability to improve hair health by nourishing the scalp and promoting circulation. This tea supports hair growth, prevents hair loss, and helps strengthen the hair shaft.

Licorice Root Scalp Treatment Balm

INGREDIENTS

- 1 tablespoon dried licorice root powder
- 1/4 cup shea butter

PREPARATION

1. Mix licorice root powder with melted shea butter.
2. Apply to the scalp and leave on overnight for best results.

Benefits: Licorice root soothes irritated scalps and promotes healthy hair growth. This balm provides deep nourishment to the scalp, helping to reduce dandruff and support hair regeneration.

Mint and Nettle Hair Conditioner

INGREDIENTS

- 1 teaspoon dried mint leaves
- 1 teaspoon dried nettle leaves
- 1 cup boiling water

PREPARATION

1. Steep mint and nettle leaves in boiling water for 10 minutes.
2. Strain and use as a conditioner after shampooing. Leave on for 5 minutes before rinsing.

Benefits: Mint and nettle provide a refreshing and nourishing conditioner that strengthens hair and promotes growth. This conditioner helps reduce hair loss and leaves hair feeling soft and invigorated.

Lavender and Oat Hair Strengthening Infusion

INGREDIENTS

- 1 teaspoon dried lavender flowers
- 1 tablespoon oat straw
- 1 cup boiling water

PREPARATION

1. Steep lavender and oat straw in boiling water for 10 minutes.
2. Strain and use as a final rinse after washing your hair.

Benefits: Lavender soothes the scalp, while oat straw strengthens and nourishes hair. This infusion helps promote healthy hair growth and improves hair texture, making it stronger and more resilient.

Rose Petal Scalp Cooling Tonic

INGREDIENTS

- 1 tablespoon dried rose petals
- 1 cup boiling water

PREPARATION

1. Steep rose petals in boiling water for 10 minutes.
2. Strain and apply to the scalp to cool and refresh. Leave on for 20 minutes before rinsing.

Benefits: Rose petals provide a soothing, cooling effect on the scalp, reducing inflammation and promoting a healthy scalp environment. This tonic also adds shine to the hair and leaves it smelling fragrant.

Gotu Kola Hair Regrowth Capsules

INGREDIENTS

- 1 tablespoon dried gotu kola powder
- Capsule shells

PREPARATION

1. Fill capsule shells with gotu kola powder.
2. Take 1-2 capsules daily to support hair regrowth.

Benefits: Gotu kola stimulates hair growth by improving blood circulation to the scalp. These capsules promote thicker, healthier hair and help prevent hair thinning.

Dandelion Hair Root Strengthening Oil

INGREDIENTS

- 1 tablespoon dried dandelion root
- 1/4 cup olive oil

PREPARATION

1. Infuse dandelion root in olive oil for 30 minutes using a double boiler.
2. Strain and massage the oil into the scalp. Leave on for 30 minutes before washing.

Benefits: Dandelion root nourishes the hair roots, helping to strengthen and fortify hair strands. This oil improves hair structure and reduces breakage, promoting overall hair strength and health.

Birch Leaf Scalp Health Lotion

INGREDIENTS

- 1 tablespoon dried birch leaves
- 1/4 cup water

PREPARATION

1. Steep birch leaves in water for 10 minutes.
2. Strain and apply the liquid to the scalp as a lotion. Leave on for 30 minutes before rinsing.

Benefits: Birch leaves have antibacterial and anti-inflammatory properties that help cleanse the scalp and promote healthy hair growth. This lotion is ideal for soothing irritated scalps and promoting scalp health.

Neem Oil Scalp Treatment Drops

INGREDIENTS

- 10 drops neem oil
- 1 tablespoon carrier oil (such as coconut or jojoba oil)

PREPARATION

1. Mix neem oil with the carrier oil.
2. Massage a few drops into the scalp and leave on for at least 30 minutes before washing.

Benefits: Neem oil has antifungal and antibacterial properties that help treat scalp infections and dandruff. This treatment promotes a healthy scalp environment and reduces hair fall caused by scalp conditions.

Green Tea Hair Antioxidant Rinse

INGREDIENTS

- 1 teaspoon green tea leaves
- 1 cup boiling water

PREPARATION

1. Steep green tea leaves in boiling water for 10 minutes.
2. Strain and use as a final rinse after washing your hair.

Benefits: Green tea is rich in antioxidants that protect hair from damage and promote healthy growth. This rinse helps reduce hair shedding and supports strong, shiny hair.

Black Tea Hair Thickening Wash

INGREDIENTS

- 1 teaspoon black tea leaves
- 1 cup boiling water

PREPARATION

1. Steep black tea leaves in boiling water for 10 minutes.
2. Strain and use as a hair wash. Leave on for 5 minutes before rinsing.

Benefits: Black tea helps thicken hair and reduce hair loss. This wash strengthens hair strands and gives volume to thin or fine hair, leaving it fuller and healthier.

Echinacea Hair Health Serum

INGREDIENTS

- 1 tablespoon echinacea root powder
- 1/4 cup almond oil

PREPARATION

1. Infuse echinacea root powder in almond oil for 30 minutes using a double boiler.
2. Strain and apply the serum to the scalp and hair. Leave on for 30 minutes before rinsing.

Benefits: Echinacea supports scalp health and strengthens hair follicles. This serum helps reduce hair loss, nourish the scalp, and promote stronger, healthier hair.

Yarrow Hair Shine Tea

INGREDIENTS

- 1 teaspoon dried yarrow leaves
- 1 cup boiling water

PREPARATION

1. Steep yarrow leaves in boiling water for 10 minutes.
2. Strain and use as a final rinse after shampooing.

Benefits: Yarrow enhances hair shine and promotes scalp health. This tea helps smooth hair, reduce frizz, and leaves hair looking glossy and well-nourished.

Cucumber and Aloe Hair Hydrating Mask

INGREDIENTS

- 1/2 cucumber, blended
- 2 tablespoons fresh aloe vera gel

PREPARATION

1. Blend cucumber and aloe vera gel together to form a smooth paste.
2. Apply the mixture to the hair and scalp. Leave on for 30 minutes, then rinse thoroughly.

Benefits: Cucumber and aloe vera provide deep hydration to the hair and scalp. This mask helps moisturize dry, damaged hair and soothes the scalp, promoting soft, healthy, and shiny hair.

Clary Sage Hair Growth Capsules

INGREDIENTS

- 1 tablespoon dried clary sage powder
- Capsule shells

PREPARATION

1. Fill capsule shells with dried clary sage powder.
2. Take 1-2 capsules daily to promote hair growth.

Benefits: Clary sage stimulates hair growth by balancing hormones and improving scalp circulation. These capsules help reduce hair loss and promote stronger, thicker hair.

Sea Buckthorn Hair Renewal Oil

INGREDIENTS

- 1 tablespoon sea buckthorn oil
- 1/4 cup carrier oil (such as olive oil or coconut oil)

PREPARATION

1. Mix sea buckthorn oil with the carrier oil.
2. Massage into the scalp and hair, leaving on for 30 minutes before washing.

Benefits: Sea buckthorn oil is rich in vitamins, antioxidants, and essential fatty acids that nourish the scalp and repair damaged hair. This oil helps restore vitality to dull, brittle hair and promotes overall hair renewal and strength.

Chamomile and Apple Cider Vinegar Hair Rinse

INGREDIENTS

- 1 tablespoon dried chamomile flowers
- 1 tablespoon apple cider vinegar
- 1 cup boiling water

PREPARATION

1. Steep chamomile flowers in boiling water for 10 minutes.
2. Strain and mix in the apple cider vinegar.
3. Use as a final rinse after shampooing.

Benefits: Chamomile soothes the scalp and brightens hair, while apple cider vinegar helps balance the scalp's pH and removes product buildup. This rinse leaves hair shiny, smooth, and manageable.

Hibiscus Flower Hair Nourishing Infusion

INGREDIENTS

- 1 tablespoon dried hibiscus flowers
- 1 cup boiling water

PREPARATION

1. Steep hibiscus flowers in boiling water for 10 minutes.
2. Strain and use as a hair rinse or drink as a nourishing tea.

Benefits: Hibiscus is known for its ability to strengthen hair roots, prevent hair fall, and add shine. This infusion helps nourish the hair from the roots, promoting healthy growth and improving overall hair texture.

BOOK 18

Eye Health and Vision Support

Herbal Remedies for Vision Enhancement

NATURAL HERBS FOR ENHANCING VISION AND EYE HEALTH

Maintaining optimal eye health and enhancing vision is crucial, especially as we age or face increased screen time, which can strain our eyes. For individuals like Emma, who seek natural ways to support and improve their vision, herbal remedies offer a range of benefits. These remedies are rich in antioxidants, vitamins, and minerals that protect the eyes, enhance clarity, and reduce the risk of age-related vision problems. Below, we explore several powerful herbs that promote vision enhancement, their properties, and how they can be integrated into a holistic approach to eye health.

Bilberry: Protecting and Strengthening Vision

Bilberry is one of the most effective herbs for eye health, known for its ability to enhance vision, especially night vision. It is rich in anthocyanins, powerful antioxidants that protect the retina and prevent damage from free radicals. These compounds also improve circulation to the eyes, ensuring they receive the necessary nutrients and oxygen for optimal function. Studies have shown that bilberry can reduce eye fatigue, making it particularly useful for individuals who spend long hours in front of screens.

Bilberry can be consumed as a supplement or in tea form. For Emma, taking bilberry capsules daily provides a convenient way to protect her vision and enhance clarity, especially given her screen exposure. Its antioxidant properties ensure her eyes remain healthy, while its ability to improve circulation supports long-term visual acuity.

Eyebright: The Traditional Eye Tonic

Eyebright, as its name suggests, has long been used to support eye health and improve vision. It contains compounds like aucubin, tannins, and flavonoids, which have anti-inflammatory and antioxidant effects. These properties help reduce eye irritation, relieve strain, and improve overall eye clarity. Eyebright is especially beneficial for those experiencing dryness, redness, or inflammation, as it soothes the eyes and supports their natural healing processes.

Eyebright is commonly used as an eye wash or taken in tincture form. For Emma, using eyebright as a daily eye wash provides immediate relief from screen-induced dryness and irritation. Alternatively, taking eyebright tincture supports her eye health from within, ensuring her vision remains sharp and her eyes feel comfortable throughout the day.

Ginkgo Biloba: Enhancing Blood Flow and Protecting Eye Tissues

Ginkgo biloba is a well-known herb for enhancing circulation, and it also plays a crucial role in supporting eye health. By increasing blood flow to the retina, ginkgo ensures that the eyes receive essential nutrients and oxygen, which are vital for maintaining vision. The antioxidants in ginkgo protect eye tissues from oxidative damage, reducing the risk of age-related macular degeneration (AMD) and other vision-related conditions.

Ginkgo biloba can be taken as a supplement or tincture. For Emma, incorporating ginkgo into her daily regimen provides a powerful way to enhance circulation and protect her eyes naturally. By ensuring her eyes are well-nourished, ginkgo helps maintain her vision clarity, even as she ages or deals with prolonged screen exposure.

Fennel: Aiding Eye Health with Antioxidants

Fennel is another herb traditionally used to support eye health. It contains a rich array of antioxidants, such as vitamin C and flavonoids, which protect the eyes from free radical damage. These compounds also strengthen the eye's capillaries and reduce inflammation, promoting overall eye wellness. Fennel seeds have been used to prepare eye washes or teas that soothe irritation and enhance visual clarity.

To use fennel, Emma can prepare a fennel tea and apply it as a compress to her eyes. This practice offers immediate relief from dryness and strain while providing her eyes with essential antioxidants. Additionally, drinking fennel tea supports her vision from within, ensuring her eyes remain protected against oxidative stress.

Turmeric: Reducing Inflammation and Supporting Retinal Health

Turmeric is a powerful anti-inflammatory herb that supports eye health by reducing inflammation and protecting the retina. Curcumin, the active compound in turmeric, has been shown to prevent damage caused by oxidative stress and improve blood circulation to the eyes. This is particularly beneficial for individuals who may be at risk of developing age-related eye conditions like cataracts or macular degeneration.

Turmeric can be consumed as a supplement, tincture, or added to meals. For Emma, integrating turmeric into her diet or using turmeric capsules daily offers a way to protect her eyes naturally. The anti-inflammatory and antioxidant properties of turmeric help maintain her vision clarity, ensuring her eyes remain healthy as she navigates daily stressors and screen use.

Saffron: Enhancing Visual Acuity and Reducing Eye Fatigue

Saffron is a highly valued herb for its vision-enhancing properties. It contains crocin and safranal, compounds that have been shown to improve retinal function and protect photoreceptor cells from damage. Saffron also helps reduce eye fatigue, making it an excellent option for those who experience strain from prolonged screen use or reading. Research suggests that saffron may help slow down the progression of AMD, offering long-term benefits for maintaining visual acuity.

Saffron can be consumed as a tea or taken in capsule form. For Emma, drinking saffron tea regularly provides a simple and luxurious way to support her eye health. The vision-enhancing compounds in saffron ensure that her eyes remain sharp and clear, while its soothing effects help reduce fatigue, making it an ideal addition to her daily wellness routine.

Calendula: Soothing Irritation and Protecting the Eyes

Calendula is known for its anti-inflammatory and healing properties, making it an excellent herb for supporting eye health. It contains flavonoids and carotenoids that protect the eyes from oxidative stress and soothe irritation. Calendula is particularly effective for those dealing with dry eyes or inflammation, as it promotes healing and enhances the overall health of the eye tissues.

Calendula can be used as an eye wash or in tea form. For Emma, using calendula eye drops or compresses provides immediate relief from dryness and irritation, ensuring her eyes remain comfortable and protected. Incorporating calendula into her routine supports her vision enhancement goals, keeping her eyes healthy and resilient.

These herbal remedies provide natural and effective solutions for enhancing vision. For Emma, integrating these herbs into her daily and weekly routines offers a holistic approach to eye health, ensuring her vision remains clear and protected as she navigates the challenges of modern life.

Herbs for Eye Strain and Protection

EFFECTIVE HERBS FOR RELIEVING EYE STRAIN AND ENSURING PROTECTION

In today's digital age, eye strain has become a common issue due to prolonged screen exposure and artificial lighting. For individuals like Emma, who spends extended periods using digital devices, managing eye strain naturally is essential. Fortunately, several herbs offer protective and soothing benefits, helping to alleviate eye strain and support long-term eye health. These herbs, rich in antioxidants and anti-inflammatory compounds, not only relieve discomfort but also provide a protective barrier against damage. Below, we explore some of the most effective herbs for eye strain and protection, detailing their uses and benefits.

Chamomile: Calming Inflammation and Reducing Strain

Chamomile is a well-known herb for its anti-inflammatory and calming properties, making it particularly beneficial for soothing irritated and strained eyes. It contains compounds such as apigenin and chamazulene, which help reduce inflammation and relax the muscles around the eyes. Chamomile is ideal for relieving discomfort caused by prolonged screen use or exposure to harsh lighting.

Chamomile can be used as a warm compress or in tea form. For Emma, placing cooled chamomile tea bags over her closed eyes for 10-15 minutes offers an immediate relief from eye strain, reducing redness and soothing inflammation. Alternatively, she can soak cotton pads in chamomile tea and apply them as a compress. The calming effect of chamomile ensures that her eyes feel refreshed and protected, providing a natural remedy that aligns with her holistic approach to wellness.

Cucumber: A Natural Coolant for Eye Relief

Though not traditionally an herb, cucumber is a natural remedy that has been used for centuries to soothe and hydrate the eyes. Its high water content and cooling properties make it effective for relieving eye strain and reducing puffiness. Cucumber also contains antioxidants like vitamin C, which help protect the delicate tissues around the eyes.

Cucumber slices can be placed directly over closed eyes for 10-15 minutes. For Emma, this simple and refreshing treatment offers a quick and natural way to soothe eye strain after a long day of screen time. The cooling sensation and antioxidants in cucumber provide instant relief, making it a convenient option for maintaining eye comfort.

Eyebright: Traditional Relief for Eye Fatigue

Eyebright (Euphrasia officinalis) has a long history of use in herbal medicine for eye health. Known for its anti-inflammatory and astringent properties, eyebright is effective for reducing eye fatigue and irritation. It contains compounds like flavonoids and tannins that help tighten and tone the eye's blood vessels, improving circulation and relieving redness and swelling.

Eyebright can be used as an eye wash or in tincture form. For Emma, using an eyebright eye wash provides a gentle and effective method for reducing eye strain. By applying eyebright in this way, she can cleanse and refresh her eyes, helping to reduce discomfort and protect against irritation. The herb's traditional reputation for supporting eye health makes it a valuable addition to her daily routine, especially for prolonged screen use.

Green Tea: Antioxidant Protection Against Digital Strain

Green tea is a powerful herb for eye health due to its high content of catechins, which are potent antioxidants that protect the eyes from oxidative damage. These compounds help reduce inflammation and improve circulation around the eyes, which is crucial for maintaining healthy vision. Additionally, the tannins in green tea help soothe puffiness and redness associated with eye strain.

Green tea can be used as an eye compress or consumed as a beverage. For Emma, using cooled green tea bags as a compress provides a quick and effective way to alleviate eye strain. The antioxidants in green tea protect her eyes from the effects of prolonged screen exposure, ensuring her eyes remain healthy and comfortable. Drinking green tea also provides internal benefits, supporting overall eye health from within.

Fennel: Soothing and Hydrating the Eyes

Fennel is an herb known for its anti-inflammatory and hydrating properties, making it an excellent remedy for dry eyes and eye strain. It contains vitamin C and flavonoids, which help protect the eyes from free radical damage and reduce swelling. Fennel's soothing effects help alleviate discomfort caused by dryness and irritation, promoting a balanced and hydrated eye environment.

Fennel seeds can be boiled to create a soothing eye wash. For Emma, using a fennel eye wash offers a natural way to cleanse and hydrate her eyes, reducing strain after hours of screen use. The anti-inflammatory properties of fennel provide immediate relief, ensuring her eyes remain moisturized and protected against further irritation.

Aloe Vera: Hydrating and Healing Support for the Eyes

Aloe vera is another versatile herb beneficial for eye health. It contains enzymes and vitamins, including vitamin A, that support eye tissue health and reduce inflammation. Aloe vera's hydrating properties make it particularly effective for relieving dryness and soothing strained eyes. When applied topically, it can reduce puffiness and improve overall eye comfort.

Aloe vera gel can be applied around the eyes as a mask. For Emma, using a thin layer of fresh aloe vera gel around her eyes provides a cooling and soothing effect, relieving eye strain and ensuring hydration. The natural enzymes in aloe vera promote healing and protect her eyes from further stress, making it a practical solution for maintaining eye wellness.

These herbs provide a range of natural solutions for relieving eye strain and ensuring protection. For Emma, incorporating these remedies into her daily or weekly routine offers a sustainable and holistic approach to maintaining eye health, ensuring that her eyes remain comfortable and resilient even with extended screen exposure.

Remedies for Eye Health and Clarity

Bilberry Vision Enhancing Capsules

INGREDIENTS

- 1 tablespoon dried bilberry powder
- Capsule shells

PREPARATION

1. Fill capsule shells with dried bilberry powder.
2. Take 1-2 capsules daily for vision enhancement.

Benefits: Bilberry is rich in antioxidants, particularly anthocyanins, which improve blood circulation to the eyes and help support overall eye health. These capsules promote better night vision and protect the eyes from age-related conditions.

Eyebright Eye Health Drops

INGREDIENTS

- 1 tablespoon dried eyebright herb
- 1/4 cup distilled water

PREPARATION

1. Simmer eyebright herb in distilled water for 10 minutes.
2. Strain and allow the solution to cool.
3. Use 1-2 drops in each eye as needed for eye comfort and clarity.

Benefits: Eyebright is known for its soothing properties and ability to relieve eye strain and irritation. These drops help reduce redness, improve clarity, and support overall eye health.

Chamomile Eye Comfort Tea

INGREDIENTS

- 1 teaspoon dried chamomile flowers
- 1 cup boiling water

PREPARATION

1. Steep chamomile flowers in boiling water for 10 minutes.
2. Strain and drink to relax eye muscles and reduce strain.

Benefits: Chamomile has anti-inflammatory and calming properties that help relax strained eyes and reduce inflammation. Drinking this tea regularly supports eye comfort and alleviates symptoms of dry or tired eyes.

Goldenseal Eye Wash Solution

INGREDIENTS

- 1 teaspoon dried goldenseal root powder
- 1/4 cup distilled water

PREPARATION

1. Simmer goldenseal root powder in distilled water for 10 minutes.
2. Strain and allow the solution to cool.
3. Use as an eye wash to clean and soothe the eyes.

Benefits: Goldenseal is known for its antimicrobial properties and helps soothe irritated or inflamed eyes. This eye wash is perfect for cleansing the eyes and reducing redness and discomfort.

Blueberry Antioxidant Eye Smoothie

INGREDIENTS

- 1/2 cup fresh blueberries
- 1/2 cup spinach
- 1 cup almond milk
- 1 tablespoon chia seeds

PREPARATION

1. Blend all ingredients until smooth.
2. Drink daily to support eye health.

Benefits: Blueberries are packed with antioxidants that protect the eyes from oxidative stress. This smoothie nourishes the eyes, improves visual clarity, and helps maintain healthy vision over time.

Calendula and Witch Hazel Eye Relief Spray

INGREDIENTS

- 1 tablespoon dried calendula flowers
- 1 tablespoon witch hazel extract
- 1/4 cup distilled water

PREPARATION

1. Steep calendula flowers in boiling water for 10 minutes, then strain.
2. Mix the calendula infusion with witch hazel extract.
3. Spray around the eyes (avoid direct contact) for relief from puffiness and irritation.

Benefits: Calendula soothes and reduces eye inflammation, while witch hazel helps tone the skin around the eyes and reduce puffiness. This spray provides quick relief for tired or irritated eyes.

Dandelion Leaf Vision Support Capsules

INGREDIENTS

- 1 tablespoon dried dandelion leaf powder
- Capsule shells

PREPARATION

1. Fill capsule shells with dried dandelion leaf powder.
2. Take 1-2 capsules daily for vision support.

Benefits: Dandelion leaf is rich in vitamins A and C, which are essential for maintaining healthy vision. These capsules support the retina and help protect the eyes from age-related vision problems.

Rose Petal Eye Refreshing Compress

INGREDIENTS

- 1 tablespoon dried rose petals
- 1/2 cup boiling water

PREPARATION

1. Steep rose petals in boiling water for 10 minutes.
2. Soak a clean cloth in the infusion, wring out excess liquid, and apply to closed eyes for 10 minutes.

Benefits: Rose petals provide a refreshing and cooling effect, reducing eye puffiness and soothing irritated eyes. This compress helps brighten the eyes and reduce redness and swelling.

Cucumber Eye Hydration Gel

INGREDIENTS

- 1/4 cup fresh cucumber juice
- 1 tablespoon aloe vera gel

PREPARATION

1. Blend cucumber juice with aloe vera gel until smooth.
2. Apply gently around the eyes to hydrate and soothe the skin.

Benefits: Cucumber hydrates and refreshes the skin around the eyes, while aloe vera soothes and reduces inflammation. This gel is perfect for reducing puffiness and refreshing tired eyes.

Lavender and Chamomile Eye Pillow

INGREDIENTS

- 1 tablespoon dried lavender flowers
- 1 tablespoon dried chamomile flowers
- Small fabric pouch

PREPARATION

1. Fill the fabric pouch with dried lavender and chamomile flowers.
2. Place the pouch over the eyes while resting for relaxation.

Benefits: Lavender and chamomile help relax the eye muscles and promote restful sleep. This eye pillow reduces tension around the eyes and promotes deep relaxation, perfect for relieving eye strain.

Ginkgo Biloba Visual Clarity Tonic

INGREDIENTS

- 1 teaspoon dried ginkgo biloba leaves
- 1 cup boiling water

PREPARATION

1. Steep ginkgo biloba leaves in boiling water for 10 minutes.
2. Strain and drink daily to improve visual clarity.

Benefits: Ginkgo biloba improves blood flow to the eyes and helps enhance visual clarity. Regular consumption supports eye health, especially for those experiencing visual disturbances or age-related vision decline.

Fennel Seed Eye Strengthening Tea

INGREDIENTS

- 1 teaspoon fennel seeds
- 1 cup boiling water

PREPARATION

1. Steep fennel seeds in boiling water for 10 minutes.
2. Strain and drink daily to strengthen the eyes.

Benefits: Fennel seeds are known to improve eyesight and reduce eye strain. This tea helps strengthen the eye muscles and supports overall eye health.

Carrot and Ginger Eye Health Juice

INGREDIENTS

- 2 medium carrots
- 1-inch piece of fresh ginger
- 1 apple

PREPARATION

1. Juice the carrots, ginger, and apple together.
2. Drink daily to support eye health.

Benefits: Carrots are rich in beta-carotene, which is essential for maintaining good vision. Combined with the anti-inflammatory properties of ginger, this juice supports eye health and protects against vision problems.

Ashwagandha Eye Vitality Capsules

INGREDIENTS

- 1 tablespoon dried ashwagandha root powder
- Capsule shells

PREPARATION

1. Fill capsule shells with dried ashwagandha powder.
2. Take 1-2 capsules daily for eye vitality.

Benefits: Ashwagandha helps reduce oxidative stress and supports healthy vision. These capsules promote overall eye vitality and protect against age-related vision decline.

Marigold (Calendula) Eye Cream

INGREDIENTS

- 1 tablespoon dried calendula flowers
- 1/4 cup coconut oil

PREPARATION

1. Infuse calendula flowers in melted coconut oil for 30 minutes.
2. Strain and pour into a jar. Apply gently around the eyes to soothe and nourish the skin.

Benefits: Calendula is known for its soothing and healing properties. This eye cream helps reduce puffiness, hydrate the skin, and promote a youthful appearance around the eyes.

Aloe Vera Eye Soothing Drops

INGREDIENTS

- 1 tablespoon fresh aloe vera gel
- 1/4 cup distilled water
- Instructions: (#p#)
- Mix aloe vera gel with distilled water.
- Use 1-2 drops in each eye as needed for soothing relief.
- Benefits: Aloe vera soothes and hydrates the eyes, providing relief from dryness and irritation. These drops are perfect for reducing redness and refreshing tired eyes.
- Elderflower Eye Bath Infusion
- Ingredients
- 1 tablespoon dried elderflowers
- 1 cup boiling water

PREPARATION

1. Steep elderflowers in boiling water for 10 minutes.
2. Strain and use the infusion as an eye bath to relieve irritation and discomfort.

Benefits: Elderflower is soothing and anti-inflammatory, making it ideal for reducing eye irritation and discomfort. This infusion gently cleanses the eyes and promotes comfort.

Lemon Balm Eye Protection Tea

INGREDIENTS

- 1 teaspoon dried lemon balm leaves
- 1 cup boiling water

PREPARATION

1. Steep lemon balm leaves in boiling water for 10 minutes.
2. Strain and drink daily to protect and support eye health.

Benefits: Lemon balm is rich in antioxidants, which help protect the eyes from oxidative stress and damage. This tea supports overall eye health and can reduce the risk of age-related eye conditions.

Nettle Vision Support Capsules

INGREDIENTS

- 1 tablespoon dried nettle leaf powder
- Capsule shells

PREPARATION

1. Fill capsule shells with dried nettle leaf powder.
2. Take 1-2 capsules daily to support vision.

Benefits: Nettle is high in nutrients, including vitamins A and C, which are essential for maintaining healthy eyes. These capsules help nourish the eyes and support clear vision.

Mint and Lavender Eye Refresh Mist

INGREDIENTS

- 1 teaspoon dried mint leaves
- 1 teaspoon dried lavender flowers
- 1/4 cup distilled water

PREPARATION

1. Steep mint and lavender in distilled water for 10 minutes, then strain.
2. Pour into a spray bottle and mist lightly around the eyes to refresh.

Benefits: Mint and lavender provide a cooling and

soothing effect, reducing eye strain and fatigue. This mist refreshes tired eyes and leaves the skin around the eyes feeling rejuvenated.

Spearmint Vision-Boosting Infusion

INGREDIENTS

- 1 teaspoon dried spearmint leaves
- 1 cup boiling water

PREPARATION

1. Steep spearmint leaves in boiling water for 10 minutes.
2. Strain and drink daily to boost vision.

Benefits: Spearmint helps improve circulation, which can enhance visual clarity and protect the eyes from strain. This infusion supports overall eye health and helps reduce the effects of visual fatigue.

Turmeric and Honey Eye Compress

INGREDIENTS

- 1 teaspoon turmeric powder
- 1 tablespoon honey
- 1/4 cup warm water

PREPARATION

1. Mix turmeric and honey with warm water to create a solution.
2. Soak a clean cloth in the mixture and apply to closed eyes for 10 minutes.

Benefits: Turmeric reduces inflammation and soothes tired eyes, while honey hydrates and refreshes the skin. This compress helps reduce puffiness and provides relief from irritated eyes.

Sage Eye Comfort Capsules

INGREDIENTS

- 1 tablespoon dried sage powder
- Capsule shells

PREPARATION

1. Fill capsule shells with dried sage powder.
2. Take 1-2 capsules daily for eye comfort and health.

Benefits: Sage is known for its anti-inflammatory properties, making it beneficial for reducing eye strain and supporting overall eye health. These capsules help alleviate discomfort and promote clearer vision.

Mullein Eye Support Drops

INGREDIENTS

- 1 tablespoon dried mullein flowers
- 1/4 cup distilled water

PREPARATION

1. Simmer mullein flowers in distilled water for 10 minutes.
2. Strain and allow to cool before using 1-2 drops in each eye for relief.

Benefits: Mullein soothes irritated eyes and helps relieve redness and discomfort. These drops are particularly useful for those suffering from dry or strained eyes.

Chamomile and Rose Petal Eye Tea

INGREDIENTS

- 1 teaspoon dried chamomile flowers
- 1 teaspoon dried rose petals
- 1 cup boiling water

PREPARATION

1. Steep chamomile and rose petals in boiling water for 10 minutes.
2. Strain and drink daily to soothe the eyes and reduce inflammation.

Benefits: Chamomile and rose petals work together to calm inflammation and reduce redness in the eyes. This tea helps maintain clear vision and promotes overall eye health.

Black Currant Visual Health Smoothie

INGREDIENTS

- 1/2 cup fresh black currants
- 1/2 banana
- 1/2 cup almond milk
- 1 tablespoon flax seeds

PREPARATION

1. Blend all ingredients together until smooth.
2. Drink daily to support visual health.

Benefits: Black currants are rich in antioxidants and vitamins that protect the eyes from oxidative damage. This smoothie helps improve visual acuity and supports the overall health of the eyes.

Green Tea Antioxidant Eye Wash

INGREDIENTS

- 1 teaspoon green tea leaves
- 1/4 cup boiling water

PREPARATION

1. Steep green tea leaves in boiling water for 10 minutes.
2. Strain and allow to cool. Use as an eye wash to cleanse and soothe the eyes.

Benefits: Green tea is rich in antioxidants that protect the eyes from free radical damage. This eye wash helps reduce redness, irritation, and swelling, promoting healthy and refreshed eyes.

Gotu Kola Eye Restoration Capsules

INGREDIENTS

- 1 tablespoon dried gotu kola powder
- Capsule shells

PREPARATION

1. Fill capsule shells with dried gotu kola powder.
2. Take 1-2 capsules daily to restore eye health.

Benefits: Gotu kola improves circulation and supports eye tissue regeneration. These capsules help restore eye health, especially after periods of eye strain or damage.

Burdock Root Eye Comfort Tea

INGREDIENTS

- 1 teaspoon dried burdock root
- 1 cup boiling water

PREPARATION

1. Steep burdock root in boiling water for 10 minutes.
2. Strain and drink daily to soothe eye discomfort.

Benefits: Burdock root helps reduce eye inflammation and irritation, promoting comfort and clear vision. This tea is especially helpful for those dealing with eye strain or tired eyes.

Thyme Eye Health Capsules

INGREDIENTS

- 1 tablespoon dried thyme powder
- Capsule shells

PREPARATION

1. Fill capsule shells with dried thyme powder.
2. Take 1-2 capsules daily to support eye health.

Benefits: Thyme has antioxidant and anti-inflammatory properties that support eye health. These capsules help protect the eyes from oxidative damage and improve visual clarity.

Eyebright and Raspberry Leaf Eye Drops

INGREDIENTS

- 1 teaspoon dried eyebright herb
- 1 teaspoon dried raspberry leaves
- 1/4 cup distilled water

PREPARATION

1. Simmer eyebright and raspberry leaves in distilled water for 10 minutes.
2. Strain and allow to cool. Use 1-2 drops in each eye for clarity and comfort.

Benefits: Eyebright and raspberry leaves help soothe irritated eyes and improve visual clarity. These drops provide gentle relief for red, tired, or strained eyes.

Calendula and Honey Eye Serum

INGREDIENTS

- 1 tablespoon dried calendula flowers
- 1 tablespoon honey
- 1/4 cup coconut oil

PREPARATION

1. Infuse calendula flowers in melted coconut oil for 30 minutes.
2. Strain and stir in honey.
3. Apply gently around the eyes to hydrate and soothe the skin.

Benefits: Calendula and honey provide deep hydration and soothing relief for the skin around the eyes. This serum helps reduce puffiness, fine lines, and dark circles while nourishing the delicate skin.

Hibiscus Vision Clarity Infusion

INGREDIENTS

- 1 teaspoon dried hibiscus flowers
- 1 cup boiling water

PREPARATION

1. Steep hibiscus flowers in boiling water for 10 minutes.
2. Strain and drink daily to improve vision clarity.

Benefits: Hibiscus is rich in antioxidants that support eye health and improve visual clarity. This infusion helps protect the eyes from oxidative stress and promotes clear, sharp vision.

BOOK 19

Detox Strategies for True Wellness

The Science of Detoxification

UNDERSTANDING DETOXIFICATION: HOW THE BODY CLEANSES ITSELF

Detoxification is a fundamental process that the body uses to eliminate toxins and maintain overall health. This natural cleansing mechanism involves multiple organs and systems working together to filter, neutralize, and excrete harmful substances. For individuals like Emma, who seek holistic and sustainable ways to support their wellness journey, understanding the science behind detoxification is essential. By learning how the body detoxifies, Emma can incorporate practices and herbs that enhance and support these natural processes. Below, we explore the main systems involved in detoxification and how they work to maintain balance and health.

The Liver: The Body's Primary Detoxification Organ

The liver plays a central role in detoxification. It is responsible for processing and neutralizing toxins, including chemicals, medications, and metabolic waste. The liver uses two main phases—Phase I and Phase II detoxification—to convert harmful substances into water-soluble compounds that can be excreted through urine or bile.

- **Phase I Detoxification**: In this phase, the liver uses enzymes, particularly the cytochrome P450 enzymes, to break down toxins. These enzymes transform toxins into intermediate compounds, which are often more reactive and potentially harmful if not immediately processed further. This is where antioxidants like glutathione play a crucial role, neutralizing the reactive intermediates produced in Phase I.
- **Phase II Detoxification**: The liver then attaches various molecules (such as amino acids or sulfur compounds) to the intermediate compounds from Phase I, making them water-soluble. This process, known as conjugation, prepares toxins for elimination. Herbs like milk thistle and dandelion are known to support liver function by enhancing these detoxification pathways, ensuring that the liver efficiently processes and excretes toxins.

For Emma, understanding how the liver works highlights the importance of supporting this organ through proper nutrition and herbal remedies. By integrating liver-supportive herbs and foods rich in antioxidants, she can enhance the efficiency of her body's natural detox processes.

The Kidneys: Filtering and Eliminating Waste

The kidneys are essential for filtering blood and removing waste products and toxins from the body through urine. They help maintain the body's balance of electrolytes and regulate blood pressure. The kidneys work continuously to filter out excess water-soluble waste products, including those processed by the liver.

Herbs such as nettle and parsley are known to support kidney function by acting as natural diuretics, promoting urine production and ensuring the efficient removal of toxins. For Emma, including these herbs in her detox regimen offers a natural way to enhance kidney function and promote cleansing.

Drinking adequate water is also crucial for kidney health. Water helps dilute toxins and assists in their removal, emphasizing the importance of hydration in any detoxification strategy. By staying well-hydrated, Emma ensures that her kidneys function optimally, aiding in the effective elimination of toxins.

The Lymphatic System: Transporting and Removing Toxins

The lymphatic system is a network of vessels and nodes that transport lymph fluid throughout the body. It plays a vital role in the immune system and detoxification by collecting toxins, waste, and pathogens from tissues and transporting them to the bloodstream for elimination. Unlike the circulatory system, the lymphatic system does not have a pump like the heart. Instead, it relies on movement and muscle contractions to circulate lymph fluid.

For Emma, engaging in activities that stimulate lymphatic flow, such as exercise, yoga, and dry brushing, can significantly enhance detoxification. Additionally, herbs like cleavers and red clover support lymphatic function, promoting the movement of lymph fluid and aiding in the removal of toxins.

Incorporating these practices ensures that Emma's lymphatic system remains active, allowing it to effectively remove waste and reduce the burden on other detoxification organs.

The Colon: Final Elimination of Toxins

The colon, or large intestine, is the final stage in the body's detoxification process. It is responsible for eliminating solid waste, including undigested food, toxins processed by the liver, and metabolic by-products. A healthy colon ensures that these toxins do not re-enter the bloodstream.

Dietary fiber is essential for maintaining colon health. Fiber binds to toxins and facilitates their movement through the digestive tract. For Emma, including fiber-rich foods like fruits, vegetables, and whole grains supports regular bowel movements, ensuring that her body effectively eliminates waste. Herbs such as psyllium husk and flaxseed also promote colon health by providing additional fiber.

Maintaining a balanced gut microbiome is equally important. Beneficial bacteria help break down toxins and reduce the absorption of harmful compounds. Emma can incorporate probiotic-rich foods, such as yogurt and fermented vegetables, to support her gut health and enhance the detoxification process.

Skin and Lungs: Secondary Detoxification Pathways

In addition to the liver, kidneys, lymphatic system, and colon, the skin and lungs also play a role in detoxification. The skin is the body's largest organ, and it helps eliminate toxins through sweat. Activities like sauna sessions, exercise, and herbal steam baths can promote sweating, helping Emma expel toxins through her skin.

The lungs are responsible for filtering and expelling airborne toxins and carbon dioxide. Deep breathing exercises and respiratory-supporting herbs like eucalyptus and peppermint can enhance lung function, ensuring that Emma's body efficiently expels toxins through respiration.

These organs work in harmony to maintain balance and eliminate waste. Understanding the interconnectedness of these systems allows Emma to approach detoxification holistically, supporting each pathway to enhance overall wellness. By integrating specific herbs and practices that align with these natural processes, Emma can maintain her health and vitality, ensuring her body remains resilient and efficient in its detox efforts.

Herbs for Deep Cleansing and Cellular Renewal

POTENT HERBS FOR DEEP CLEANSING AND CELLULAR RENEWAL

Herbs play a powerful role in detoxification by targeting cellular health and deep cleansing. For Emma, who seeks holistic and effective ways to support her body's natural processes, understanding the properties of these herbs can be transformative. These natural allies assist the body in eliminating toxins, promoting cellular regeneration, and maintaining overall vitality. Below, we explore several herbs that are particularly effective for deep cleansing and cellular renewal, detailing their properties, applications, and benefits.

Dandelion Root: Supporting Liver Function and Cleansing

Dandelion root is one of the most effective herbs for supporting the liver, the body's main detoxification organ. It is rich in antioxidants and nutrients that aid the liver in filtering toxins and waste from the bloodstream. Dandelion root enhances bile production, which is essential for digesting fats and eliminating toxins. By promoting efficient liver function, this herb ensures that the body's natural cleansing processes remain robust.

Dandelion root can be consumed as a tea, tincture, or supplement. For Emma, incorporating dandelion root tea into her daily routine offers a simple way to support her liver's detoxification efforts. Its diuretic properties also promote the elimination of waste through the kidneys, ensuring a comprehensive approach to cleansing. The antioxidants in dandelion root help protect liver cells, fostering an environment conducive to cellular renewal.

Milk Thistle: Regenerating and Protecting Liver Cells

Milk thistle is another essential herb for liver health, known for its ability to protect and regenerate liver cells. The active compound in milk thistle, silymarin, is a potent antioxidant that defends the liver against toxins and supports its ability to repair and regenerate. Milk thistle's anti-inflammatory properties also reduce liver inflammation, making it particularly useful for those exposed to environmental toxins or stress.

For Emma, taking milk thistle as a daily supplement or tincture enhances her liver's ability to cleanse the body and renew cells. By supporting the liver's regenerative functions, milk thistle helps ensure that the body's detox pathways remain efficient, promoting overall wellness. This herb's long-standing reputation in herbal medicine makes it a reliable choice for maintaining cellular health.

Burdock Root: Blood Cleansing and Cellular Detoxification

Burdock root is a powerful blood purifier that helps the body remove toxins at the cellular level. It supports the liver and kidneys, ensuring that toxins are efficiently processed and eliminated. Rich in antioxidants, burdock root also fights free radicals, protecting cells from damage and supporting cellular regeneration. Its anti-inflammatory properties make it beneficial for skin health, as it helps clear toxins that can manifest as skin issues.

Burdock root can be used as a tea or added to soups and stews. For Emma, drinking burdock root tea provides a consistent source of antioxidants that cleanse her blood and promote cellular renewal. This herb's gentle yet effective action ensures that her body maintains a balanced and clean internal environment, supporting her holistic approach to detoxification.

Cilantro: Binding and Eliminating Heavy Metals

Cilantro, a common culinary herb, is also a powerful detoxifier, especially effective for eliminating heavy metals like mercury and lead. It contains compounds that bind to these metals, making them easier for the body to eliminate. This process is crucial for deep cleansing, as heavy metal buildup can lead to cellular damage and compromise detox pathways.

Cilantro can be added to smoothies, salads, or taken as an extract. For Emma, using cilantro in her meals regularly ensures a steady intake of this detoxifying herb. By supporting the removal of heavy metals, cilantro helps protect her cells from damage, promoting long-term health and cellular vitality.

Red Clover: Enhancing Lymphatic Cleansing

Red clover is an herb known for its ability to cleanse the lymphatic system, which plays a vital role in detoxification. The lymphatic system removes toxins and waste products from tissues, preventing them from accumulating in the body. Red clover supports lymphatic flow, ensuring that toxins are efficiently transported to the bloodstream for elimination. It also contains isoflavones, which have antioxidant properties that protect cells and support renewal.

Red clover can be consumed as a tea or tincture. For Emma, incorporating red clover tea into her routine promotes lymphatic cleansing and cellular health. The herb's gentle action helps maintain a balanced internal environment, supporting her detoxification efforts holistically. By enhancing the flow of lymph fluid, red clover ensures that toxins do not stagnate, reducing the burden on other detox organs.

Schisandra: Supporting Cellular Health and Liver Function

Schisandra is an adaptogenic herb that supports liver function and promotes cellular regeneration. It is rich in lignans, compounds that protect liver cells and enhance detoxification enzymes. Schisandra also improves the body's resistance to stress, which can compromise detox pathways and cellular health. Its adaptogenic properties help balance the body's response to toxins, supporting overall wellness.

Schisandra can be taken as a tincture, supplement, or tea. For Emma, using schisandra as part of her detox regimen provides a dual benefit: supporting liver health while enhancing her body's resilience to stress. The herb's ability to protect and regenerate cells ensures that her detoxification efforts lead to lasting wellness.

Cleavers: Promoting Lymphatic Drainage and Skin Health

Cleavers is a valuable herb for detoxification, particularly in supporting the lymphatic system and skin health. It promotes lymphatic drainage, which helps flush toxins from the body and reduces inflammation.

Cleavers can be consumed as a tea or tincture. For Emma, using cleavers tea provides an effective way to support her lymphatic system and promote skin health. The herb's gentle detoxifying properties ensure a comprehensive cleanse, targeting both deep cellular health and surface-level toxins, which aligns with her holistic approach to wellness.

These herbs provide powerful tools for deep cleansing and cellular renewal, supporting the body's natural detox pathways. For Emma, incorporating these herbs into her wellness routine allows her to engage in a holistic approach to detoxification, ensuring that her body remains resilient, balanced, and healthy.

Detox Remedies for Whole Body Health

Dandelion Root Detox Tea

INGREDIENTS

- 1 teaspoon dried dandelion root
- 1 cup boiling water

PREPARATION

1. Steep dried dandelion root in boiling water for 10 minutes.
2. Strain and drink daily to support detoxification.

Benefits: Dandelion root is a powerful liver detoxifier that helps stimulate bile production and eliminate toxins from the body. This tea supports liver health, aids digestion, and promotes overall detoxification.

Burdock and Milk Thistle Liver Cleanse Capsules

INGREDIENTS

- 1 tablespoon dried burdock root powder
- 1 tablespoon dried milk thistle seed powder
- Capsule shells

PREPARATION

1. Fill capsule shells with equal parts of burdock root and milk thistle seed powders.
2. Take 1-2 capsules daily for liver support and detoxification.

Benefits: Burdock root and milk thistle are known for their liver-cleansing properties. These capsules help detoxify the liver, protect it from toxins, and promote overall liver function.

Chicory Root Digestive Cleanse Drink

INGREDIENTS

- 1 tablespoon dried chicory root
- 1 cup boiling water

PREPARATION

1. Steep chicory root in boiling water for 10 minutes.
2. Strain and drink to support digestion and detoxification.

Benefits: Chicory root is a natural prebiotic that promotes healthy digestion and supports liver detoxification. This drink helps cleanse the digestive system, improve gut health, and remove toxins from the body.

Nettle Leaf Blood Purifying Infusion

INGREDIENTS

- 1 teaspoon dried nettle leaves
- 1 cup boiling water

PREPARATION

1. Steep nettle leaves in boiling water for 10 minutes.
2. Strain and drink daily to purify the blood.

Benefits: Nettle leaf is rich in vitamins and minerals that help cleanse the blood and promote overall health. This infusion supports the elimination of toxins and improves circulation, aiding in detoxification.

Beetroot and Ginger Detox Smoothie

INGREDIENTS

- 1 small beetroot, peeled and chopped
- 1-inch piece of fresh ginger
- 1 cup water
- 1 tablespoon honey (optional)

PREPARATION

1. Blend beetroot, ginger, and water until smooth.
2. Strain or drink as is, adding honey if desired.

Benefits: Beetroot is a natural liver detoxifier, while ginger promotes digestion and immune support. This smoothie helps cleanse the body, improve digestion, and boost energy levels.

Echinacea Immune Detox Drops

INGREDIENTS

- 1 tablespoon dried echinacea root
- 1/4 cup alcohol (vodka or glycerin for a non-alcoholic option)

PREPARATION

1. Infuse echinacea root in alcohol or glycerin for 4-6 weeks.
2. Strain and take 1-2 droppers daily to detoxify and support immune function.

Benefits: Echinacea boosts the immune system and helps the body eliminate toxins. These drops support overall detoxification while strengthening the body's defenses against infections.

Lemon Peel and Cayenne Detox Drink

INGREDIENTS

- Peel of 1 lemon
- 1 pinch cayenne pepper
- 1 cup warm water

PREPARATION

1. Steep lemon peel in warm water for 10 minutes.
2. Add a pinch of cayenne pepper and stir well.
3. Drink daily to promote detoxification.

Benefits: Lemon peel is rich in antioxidants and helps cleanse the liver, while cayenne pepper boosts metabolism and stimulates digestion. This drink supports overall detoxification and boosts energy.

Aloe Vera Digestive Detox Gel

INGREDIENTS

- 2 tablespoons fresh aloe vera gel
- 1 cup water

PREPARATION

1. Blend fresh aloe vera gel with water until smooth.
2. Drink daily to support digestion and detoxification.

Benefits: Aloe vera soothes the digestive system and helps remove toxins from the intestines. This gel supports healthy digestion, promotes regularity, and aids in detoxifying the gut.

Turmeric and Black Pepper Detox Paste

INGREDIENTS

- 1 tablespoon ground turmeric
- 1/4 teaspoon black pepper
- 1/4 cup water

PREPARATION

1. Mix turmeric and black pepper with water to form a paste.
2. Consume 1 teaspoon daily or add to food and drinks to support detoxification.

Benefits: Turmeric is a powerful anti-inflammatory and antioxidant, while black pepper enhances its absorption. This paste helps cleanse the liver, reduce inflammation, and promote whole-body detoxification.

Green Tea and Lemongrass Detox Infusion

INGREDIENTS

- 1 teaspoon green tea leaves
- 1 teaspoon dried lemongrass
- 1 cup boiling water

PREPARATION

1. Steep green tea and lemongrass in boiling water for 5-7 minutes.
2. Strain and drink daily to support detoxification.

Benefits: Green tea is rich in antioxidants that help detoxify the body, while lemongrass supports digestion and liver function. This infusion helps cleanse the body and promotes overall wellness.

Schisandra Berry Cleansing Capsules

INGREDIENTS

- 1 tablespoon dried schisandra berry powder
- Capsule shells

PREPARATION

1. Fill capsule shells with dried schisandra berry powder.
2. Take 1-2 capsules daily for whole-body detoxification.

Benefits: Schisandra berries are known for their detoxifying properties, particularly in supporting liver function. These capsules help cleanse the body of toxins and promote energy and vitality.

Calendula Flower Skin Detox Bath

INGREDIENTS

- 1/4 cup dried calendula flowers
- 1 muslin bag or cloth

PREPARATION

1. Place calendula flowers in a muslin bag and tie securely.
2. Add the bag to a warm bath and soak for 20 minutes.

Benefits: Calendula has anti-inflammatory and detoxifying properties that soothe the skin and promote healing. This bath helps detoxify the skin and reduces inflammation, leaving the skin feeling refreshed and rejuvenated.

Artichoke Leaf Gallbladder Cleanse Tea

INGREDIENTS

- 1 teaspoon dried artichoke leaf
- 1 cup boiling water

PREPARATION

1. Steep artichoke leaf in boiling water for 10 minutes.
2. Strain and drink daily to support gallbladder health and detoxification.

Benefits: Artichoke leaf supports the liver and gallbladder, promoting bile production and aiding in the elimination of toxins. This tea helps cleanse the liver and gallbladder, supporting overall digestive health.

Yellow Dock Blood Purifier Capsules

INGREDIENTS

- 1 tablespoon dried yellow dock root powder
- Capsule shells

PREPARATION

1. Fill capsule shells with dried yellow dock root powder.
2. Take 1-2 capsules daily to purify the blood.

Benefits: Yellow dock is a powerful blood purifier that supports the liver and digestive system. These capsules help detoxify the blood, improve circulation, and support overall health.

Cilantro Heavy Metal Detox Drops

INGREDIENTS

- 1 tablespoon fresh cilantro leaves
- 1/4 cup alcohol (vodka or glycerin for a non-alcoholic option)

PREPARATION

1. Infuse fresh cilantro leaves in alcohol or glycerin for 4-6 weeks.
2. Strain and take 1-2 droppers daily to help eliminate heavy metals.

Benefits: Cilantro is known for its ability to bind to heavy metals and help remove them from the body. These drops support detoxification of heavy metals, particularly from the liver and kidneys (#ni#)

Cabbage Leaf Detox Wrap

INGREDIENTS

- 4 large cabbage leaves

PREPARATION

1. Soften cabbage leaves by steaming for 2-3 minutes.
2. Wrap them around the abdomen and leave for 20-30 minutes to detoxify.

Benefits: Cabbage leaves have anti-inflammatory and detoxifying properties that help draw out toxins and reduce bloating. This detox wrap supports lymphatic drainage and promotes digestive health.

Holy Basil (Tulsi) Antioxidant Detox Tea

INGREDIENTS

- 1 teaspoon dried holy basil (tulsi) leaves
- 1 cup boiling water

PREPARATION

1. Steep holy basil leaves in boiling water for 10 minutes.
2. Strain and drink daily for antioxidant support and detoxification.

Benefits: Holy basil is a powerful adaptogen that helps the body eliminate toxins and reduce oxidative stress. This tea supports overall detoxification and promotes balance and wellness.

Ginger and Lemon Immune Detox Elixir

INGREDIENTS

- 1-inch piece of fresh ginger
- Juice of 1 lemon
- 1 tablespoon honey
- 1 cup warm water

PREPARATION

1. Grate the ginger and add it to warm water.
2. Stir in the lemon juice and honey until well mixed.
3. Drink daily for detoxification and immune support.

Benefits: Ginger and lemon are both powerful detoxifiers that help cleanse the body, boost the immune system, and improve digestion. This elixir supports overall detoxification and promotes a healthy immune response.

Red Clover Lymphatic Detox Infusion

INGREDIENTS

- 1 teaspoon dried red clover flowers
- 1 cup boiling water

PREPARATION

1. Steep red clover flowers in boiling water for 10 minutes.
2. Strain and drink daily to support lymphatic detoxification.

Benefits: Red clover is known for its ability to cleanse the lymphatic system and promote the removal of toxins from the body. This infusion supports the body's natural detox processes and helps maintain lymphatic health.

Yarrow and Mint Digestive Detox Capsules

INGREDIENTS

- 1 tablespoon dried yarrow powder
- 1 tablespoon dried mint powder
- Capsule shells

PREPARATION

1. Fill capsule shells with equal parts yarrow and mint powder.
2. Take 1-2 capsules daily to support digestive detoxification.

Benefits: Yarrow and mint work together to soothe the digestive system and promote the elimination of toxins. These capsules help cleanse the gut, reduce bloating, and support digestive wellness.

Cranberry Kidney Cleanse Drink

INGREDIENTS

- 1/2 cup fresh cranberries
- 1 cup water
- 1 tablespoon honey (optional)

PREPARATION

1. Blend cranberries with water until smooth.
2. Strain and add honey if desired.
3. Drink daily to support kidney health and detoxification.

Benefits: Cranberries are known for their ability to cleanse the kidneys and urinary tract. This drink supports kidney health, promotes urinary function, and helps eliminate toxins from the body.

Fennel Seed Digestive Detox Tea

INGREDIENTS

- 1 teaspoon fennel seeds
- 1 cup boiling water

PREPARATION

1. Steep fennel seeds in boiling water for 10 minutes.
2. Strain and drink daily to promote digestive detoxification.

Benefits: Fennel seeds are known for their digestive benefits, helping to cleanse the digestive tract, reduce bloating, and eliminate toxins. This tea supports overall digestive health and promotes detoxification.

Milk Thistle Liver Support Capsules

INGREDIENTS

- 1 tablespoon dried milk thistle seed powder
- Capsule shells

PREPARATION

1. Fill capsule shells with dried milk thistle powder.
2. Take 1-2 capsules daily for liver detoxification.

Benefits: Milk thistle is well-known for its liver-protecting and detoxifying properties. These capsules support liver function, aid in the removal of toxins, and promote overall liver health.

Ginger and Orange Detox Bath Salts

INGREDIENTS

- 1 cup Epsom salts
- 1 tablespoon dried ginger powder
- Zest of 1 orange

PREPARATION

1. Mix Epsom salts, ginger powder, and orange zest together.
2. Add the mixture to a warm bath and soak for 20 minutes to detoxify.

Benefits: Ginger and orange work together to stimulate circulation and detoxify the skin. This bath promotes relaxation, reduces inflammation, and helps the body release toxins through the skin.

Chlorella Heavy Metal Detox Capsules

INGREDIENTS

- 1 tablespoon dried chlorella powder
- Capsule shells

PREPARATION

1. Fill capsule shells with chlorella powder.
2. Take 1-2 capsules daily to support heavy metal detoxification.

Benefits: Chlorella is a powerful detoxifier that helps bind to heavy metals and remove them from the body. These capsules support overall detoxification, particularly for those exposed to environmental toxins.

Lemon Verbena Skin Detox Lotion

INGREDIENTS

- 1 tablespoon dried lemon verbena leaves
- 1/4 cup coconut oil

PREPARATION

1. Infuse lemon verbena leaves in melted coconut oil for 30 minutes.
2. Strain and pour into a jar. Apply the lotion to the skin daily to detoxify and hydrate.

Benefits: Lemon verbena helps detoxify the skin while providing soothing hydration. This lotion promotes healthy skin, reduces inflammation, and supports the skin's natural detox process.

Pine Needle Immune Support Tea

INGREDIENTS

- 1 tablespoon fresh pine needles
- 1 cup boiling water

PREPARATION

1. Steep pine needles in boiling water for 10 minutes.
2. Strain and drink daily to support the immune system and detoxification.

Benefits: Pine needles are rich in antioxidants and vitamin C, which support the immune system and help cleanse the body of toxins. This tea strengthens immune function and promotes overall wellness.

Peppermint and Thyme Detox Drink

INGREDIENTS

- 1 teaspoon dried peppermint leaves
- 1 teaspoon dried thyme leaves
- 1 cup boiling water

PREPARATION

1. Steep peppermint and thyme leaves in boiling water for 10 minutes.
2. Strain and drink daily to support detoxification and digestion.

Benefits: Peppermint and thyme help cleanse the digestive system and promote the elimination of toxins. This drink soothes the stomach, supports digestion, and promotes overall detoxification.

Marshmallow Root Digestive Soothing Elixir

INGREDIENTS

- 1 tablespoon dried marshmallow root
- 1 cup water

PREPARATION

1. Simmer marshmallow root in water for 15 minutes.
2. Strain and drink to soothe the digestive system and support detoxification.

Benefits: Marshmallow root soothes the digestive tract and helps reduce inflammation, promoting healthy digestion and detoxification. This elixir is perfect for calming digestive discomfort and supporting gut health.

Barberry Bark Liver Detox Tincture

INGREDIENTS

- 1 tablespoon dried barberry bark
- 1/4 cup alcohol (vodka or glycerin for a non-alcoholic option)

PREPARATION

1. Infuse barberry bark in alcohol or glycerin for 4-6 weeks.
2. Strain and take 1-2 droppers daily to support liver detoxification.

Benefits: Barberry bark promotes liver function and supports the elimination of toxins. This tincture helps cleanse the liver, improve digestion, and enhance overall detoxification.

Triphala Ayurvedic Digestive Detox Capsules

INGREDIENTS

- 1 tablespoon dried triphala powder
- Capsule shells

PREPARATION

1. Fill capsule shells with dried triphala powder.
2. Take 1-2 capsules daily to support digestive detoxification.

Benefits: Triphala is an ancient Ayurvedic remedy that supports digestive health and detoxification. These capsules help cleanse the digestive tract, promote regularity, and improve overall digestion.

Cinnamon and Honey Detox Tonic

INGREDIENTS

- 1 teaspoon ground cinnamon
- 1 tablespoon honey
- 1 cup warm water

PREPARATION

1. Mix cinnamon and honey into warm water until well combined.
2. Drink daily to promote detoxification and support digestion.

Benefits: Cinnamon and honey work together to stimulate digestion and cleanse the body of toxins. This tonic supports digestive health, boosts metabolism, and promotes overall detoxification.

Clover and Dandelion Root Detox Infusion

INGREDIENTS

- 1 teaspoon dried clover flowers
- 1 teaspoon dried dandelion root
- 1 cup boiling water

PREPARATION

1. Steep clover flowers and dandelion root in boiling water for 10 minutes.
2. Strain and drink daily to support detoxification.

Benefits: Clover and dandelion root promote detoxification by supporting liver and kidney function. This infusion helps cleanse the blood, improve circulation, and support the body's natural detox processes.

BOOK 20

Anti-Inflammatory Herbal Solutions

Understanding Chronic Inflammation

EXPLORING THE NATURE AND IMPACT OF CHRONIC INFLAMMATION

Chronic inflammation is a persistent, low-grade inflammatory response that can occur within the body over an extended period. Unlike acute inflammation, which is the body's immediate response to injury or infection and typically resolves once healing begins, chronic inflammation is prolonged, often lasting months or years. This ongoing inflammatory state can silently damage tissues, organs, and cells, leading to a range of health issues. Understanding the underlying mechanisms and triggers of chronic inflammation is essential for individuals like Emma, who aim to adopt holistic, natural strategies for reducing inflammation and promoting overall well-being.

The Body's Inflammatory Response: From Acute to Chronic

Inflammation is the body's natural defense mechanism against injury, infection, and toxins. When the immune system detects a threat, it triggers the release of pro-inflammatory molecules like cytokines and white blood cells to the affected area. This process is designed to protect and heal tissues by eliminating harmful agents and initiating repair. In the case of acute inflammation, this response is short-lived and resolves once the threat is neutralized. Signs of acute inflammation often include redness, swelling, heat, and pain, all of which are part of the body's efforts to contain and repair damage.

However, chronic inflammation occurs when this response does not resolve, and the immune system remains in a constant state of alert. This may result from unresolved infections, exposure to environmental toxins, ongoing stress, or an autoimmune disorder where the immune system mistakenly attacks healthy tissues. The continuous production of inflammatory molecules can begin to cause damage rather than promote healing. This chronic state disrupts normal cellular function, leading to tissue degradation, fibrosis, and even the formation of plaques, contributing to various chronic conditions such as cardiovascular diseases, arthritis, diabetes, and neurodegenerative disorders.

Factors Contributing to Chronic Inflammation

Chronic inflammation is often driven by a combination of lifestyle, environmental, and genetic factors. Recognizing these contributors helps individuals like Emma identify areas where they can make changes to reduce inflammation naturally.

- **Diet**: A significant contributor to chronic inflammation is an unhealthy diet, particularly one high in refined sugars, processed foods, trans fats, and an imbalance of omega-6 to omega-3 fatty acids. These foods promote the release of pro-inflammatory molecules, perpetuating the inflammatory cycle. On the other hand, a diet rich in anti-inflammatory foods like leafy greens, fatty fish, nuts, and herbs can help counteract this effect.
- **Stress:** Chronic stress is another major factor that keeps the body in a prolonged inflammatory state.

When an individual experiences stress, the body releases cortisol, a hormone meant to modulate the immune response. However, with persistent stress, cortisol levels remain elevated, weakening its ability to regulate inflammation effectively, leading to a chronic inflammatory response.

- **Toxins and Environmental Exposure**: Long-term exposure to pollutants, heavy metals, and toxins in the environment can also trigger chronic inflammation. These substances can accumulate in the body, activating the immune system continuously as it attempts to eliminate them, which over time contributes to cellular damage and inflammation.
- **Sedentary Lifestyle**: Lack of physical activity is closely linked to increased inflammation. Regular movement helps modulate the inflammatory response by reducing adipose tissue, which is a source of pro-inflammatory cytokines. For Emma, incorporating gentle exercises like yoga, walking, or stretching can significantly aid in reducing inflammation.
- **Genetics and Autoimmune Conditions**: For some, chronic inflammation is tied to genetic predispositions or autoimmune diseases like rheumatoid arthritis or lupus, where the immune system mistakenly attacks healthy tissues. These conditions require a tailored approach to manage inflammation, often incorporating both herbal support and lifestyle modifications.

The Long-Term Impact of Chronic Inflammation

Left unchecked, chronic inflammation can lead to severe health complications. Continuous inflammation degrades tissues and disrupts the balance of the body's internal systems, contributing to a wide range of illnesses. For instance:

- **Cardiovascular Disease**: Chronic inflammation can damage blood vessels, leading to the formation of plaques and increasing the risk of heart disease and stroke. Elevated levels of inflammatory markers, such as C-reactive protein (CRP), are often associated with higher cardiovascular risks.
- **Metabolic Disorders**: Inflammation is closely linked with insulin resistance, which can develop into metabolic syndrome or type 2 diabetes. High levels of pro-inflammatory cytokines interfere with insulin signaling, affecting how the body regulates glucose and fat.
- **Neurodegenerative Diseases**: Chronic inflammation is also implicated in neurodegenerative diseases like Alzheimer's and Parkinson's. Inflammatory responses in the brain can damage neurons and disrupt normal cognitive functions, leading to memory loss and decline in motor skills.
- **Digestive and Autoimmune Conditions**: In the digestive system, chronic inflammation can manifest as conditions like Crohn's disease or ulcerative colitis. In autoimmune conditions, persistent inflammation causes the immune system to target healthy cells, leading to ongoing tissue damage.

Recognizing and Addressing Chronic Inflammation

For individuals like Emma, understanding the signs and implications of chronic inflammation is the first step toward addressing it. Symptoms such as persistent fatigue, joint pain, digestive issues, or unexplained weight gain can be indicators of an underlying inflammatory process. By identifying these early, Emma can take proactive steps to manage and reduce inflammation naturally, incorporating anti-inflammatory herbs, dietary changes, and stress management techniques.

Incorporating herbs like turmeric, ginger, and green tea, which contain anti-inflammatory compounds such as curcumin and polyphenols, can help modulate the body's response. These herbs work by reducing the levels of pro-inflammatory molecules, providing a natural and effective approach to managing chronic inflammation. For Emma, aligning her lifestyle and diet with anti-inflammatory principles offers a sustainable path to wellness, ensuring that her body remains balanced and resilient.

Top Herbs for Reducing Inflammation Naturally

EFFECTIVE HERBAL ALLIES FOR NATURAL INFLAMMATION REDUCTION

Inflammation is a natural response that can become problematic when it persists over time. For individuals like Emma, who aim to manage inflammation without relying on pharmaceuticals, herbs provide powerful, natural solutions. Rich in anti-inflammatory compounds, these herbs can be integrated into daily routines to reduce inflammation and support overall wellness. Below, we explore some of the most effective herbs known for their anti-inflammatory properties and their applications.

Turmeric: The Golden Healer

Turmeric is one of the most well-known herbs for reducing inflammation, particularly due to its active compound, curcumin. Curcumin has been extensively studied for its anti-inflammatory and antioxidant effects. It works by inhibiting molecules like NF-kB, which play a central role in inflammation. Turmeric is especially effective in managing inflammation associated with conditions like arthritis, digestive issues, and cardiovascular diseases.

Turmeric can be consumed in various forms, including capsules, tinctures, or as a spice added to meals. For Emma, incorporating turmeric into her daily diet—whether as a golden milk latte or a supplement—ensures that she benefits from its potent anti-inflammatory properties. The versatility of turmeric makes it an easy addition to her wellness routine, providing a consistent source of support for her body's natural inflammatory responses.

Ginger: The Versatile Anti-Inflammatory Root

Ginger is another powerful anti-inflammatory herb, frequently used in traditional medicine to reduce pain and inflammation. The compounds gingerol and shogaol, found in ginger, have potent anti-inflammatory effects that help reduce pain and swelling, particularly in conditions like osteoarthritis and digestive inflammation. Ginger also supports overall immune health, making it an excellent herb for Emma's holistic health approach.

Ginger can be consumed fresh, as a tea, or in powdered form. For Emma, drinking ginger tea daily not only offers relief from inflammation but also provides warmth and digestive support, enhancing her overall well-being. Fresh ginger slices added to meals or smoothies also provide a convenient way to incorporate this versatile herb into her diet.

Boswellia: The Ancient Remedy for Joint Health

Boswellia, also known as frankincense, has a long history of use in Ayurvedic medicine for managing inflammation, particularly in joints. The active compounds in boswellia, called boswellic acids, inhibit the production of pro-inflammatory enzymes, reducing inflammation and pain. This makes it especially effective for individuals dealing with chronic inflammatory conditions like arthritis.

Boswellia is commonly available as a capsule or tincture. For Emma, taking boswellia daily helps manage joint inflammation, ensuring her mobility and comfort. Its long-standing reputation as a natural anti-inflammatory remedy makes boswellia a reliable ally for reducing chronic inflammation and supporting long-term joint health.

Green Tea: Antioxidant-Rich Inflammation Fighter

Green tea is not only a popular beverage but also a powerful anti-inflammatory herb. It contains catechins, a type of antioxidant that reduces inflammation and protects cells from damage. The most potent of these catechins is epigallocatechin-3-gallate (EGCG), which has been shown to inhibit inflammatory pathways and reduce the risk of chronic diseases, including heart disease and cancer.

For Emma, drinking green tea daily provides an easy and refreshing way to incorporate anti-inflammatory benefits into her lifestyle. Green tea can be consumed hot or cold, and matcha—an even more concentrated form—offers additional benefits. This flexibility allows Emma to adapt green tea to her preferences while ensuring she consistently supports her body's natural anti-inflammatory mechanisms.

Holy Basil (Tulsi): The Adaptogenic Inflammation Reducer

Holy basil, or tulsi, is an adaptogenic herb known for its ability to modulate the body's stress response while reducing inflammation. The eugenol and other compounds in holy basil have anti-inflammatory effects, particularly in the respiratory system and joints. By balancing stress hormones like cortisol, which can exacerbate inflammation, tulsi offers a dual approach to managing inflammation and stress.

Emma can incorporate holy basil into her wellness routine by drinking tulsi tea or taking it as a supplement. The herb's adaptogenic properties make it particularly suitable for Emma, who may encounter stressors that could trigger inflammation. Tulsi's calming effect supports her overall well-being, ensuring her body remains resilient and balanced.

Rosemary: Protecting Cells and Reducing Inflammation

Rosemary is a common culinary herb with powerful anti-inflammatory properties. Its active compounds, such as rosmarinic acid, have been shown to reduce inflammation and oxidative stress, particularly in the brain and joints. Rosemary's ability to protect cells from damage makes it an excellent herb for individuals aiming to manage chronic inflammation.

Rosemary can be used fresh in cooking or taken as a tea or essential oil. For Emma, using rosemary in her meals provides a flavorful way to gain its anti-inflammatory benefits. Drinking rosemary tea or using rosemary-infused oil for massages can further enhance her inflammation management strategy. The herb's versatility and accessibility make it a valuable component of Emma's holistic approach.

Ashwagandha: The Adaptogen for Balancing Inflammation

Ashwagandha is another adaptogenic herb known for balancing the body's inflammatory response, particularly during times of stress. It contains withanolides, which have anti-inflammatory effects and help modulate the immune system. Ashwagandha is effective in reducing inflammation related to stress, autoimmune conditions, and chronic fatigue, providing broad-spectrum support for overall health.

Ashwagandha can be taken as a powder, capsule, or tincture. For Emma, adding ashwagandha to her morning smoothie or taking it as a supplement provides a steady source of anti-inflammatory support. Its adaptogenic properties also ensure that her body remains balanced and resilient, addressing inflammation both directly and indirectly through stress reduction.

These herbs offer Emma a range of options for managing inflammation naturally. By integrating them into her daily routine, she can reduce chronic inflammation, protect her cells from damage, and enhance her overall well-being. Each herb provides unique benefits, ensuring a comprehensive approach to managing and reducing inflammation holistically.

Remedies for Combating Inflammation

Turmeric and Ginger Anti-Inflammatory Tea

INGREDIENTS

- 1 teaspoon ground turmeric
- 1/2 teaspoon fresh grated ginger
- 1 cup boiling water
- 1 teaspoon honey (optional)

PREPARATION

1. Steep turmeric and ginger in boiling water for 10 minutes.
2. Strain and add honey if desired.
3. Drink daily for inflammation support.

Benefits: Turmeric and ginger are potent anti-inflammatory herbs that help reduce inflammation throughout the body. This tea is excellent for soothing joint pain, improving digestion, and boosting overall immunity.

Ashwagandha Inflammation Control Capsules

INGREDIENTS

- 1 tablespoon dried ashwagandha root powder
- Capsule shells

PREPARATION

1. Fill capsule shells with dried ashwagandha root powder.
2. Take 1-2 capsules daily to reduce inflammation.

Benefits: Ashwagandha is an adaptogen that helps balance stress and reduce inflammation. These capsules support overall body health by targeting inflammation, particularly in joints and muscles.

Boswellia Joint Relief Capsules

INGREDIENTS

- 1 tablespoon dried boswellia resin powder
- Capsule shells

PREPARATION

1. Fill capsule shells with dried boswellia resin powder.

2. Take 1-2 capsules daily for joint relief and anti-inflammatory support.

Benefits: Boswellia is known for its anti-inflammatory properties, particularly in reducing joint pain and swelling. These capsules are ideal for individuals suffering from arthritis or other inflammatory joint conditions.

White Willow Bark Pain Relief Tea

INGREDIENTS

- 1 teaspoon dried white willow bark
- 1 cup boiling water

PREPARATION

1. Steep white willow bark in boiling water for 10 minutes.
2. Strain and drink to relieve pain and reduce inflammation.

Benefits: White willow bark contains salicin, a natural pain reliever, and anti-inflammatory agent. This tea helps reduce headaches, joint pain, and inflammation without the side effects of synthetic painkillers.

Chamomile and Lavender Inflammatory Balm

INGREDIENTS

- 1 tablespoon dried chamomile flowers
- 1 tablespoon dried lavender flowers
- 1/4 cup coconut oil

PREPARATION

1. Infuse chamomile and lavender in melted coconut oil for 30 minutes.
2. Strain and pour into a container. Apply to inflamed areas as needed.

Benefits: Chamomile and lavender are known for their soothing and anti-inflammatory properties. This balm helps reduce skin irritation, inflammation, and pain when applied topically.

Devil's Claw Anti-Arthritis Capsules

INGREDIENTS

- 1 tablespoon dried devil's claw root powder
- Capsule shells

PREPARATION

1. Fill capsule shells with dried devil's claw root powder.
2. Take 1-2 capsules daily to alleviate arthritis symptoms and inflammation.

Benefits: Devil's claw is a natural anti-inflammatory herb commonly used to relieve arthritis pain and reduce joint inflammation. These capsules promote joint health and mobility.

Pine Bark Extract Anti-Inflammatory Serum

INGREDIENTS

- 1 tablespoon pine bark extract
- 1/4 cup carrier oil (such as jojoba oil)

PREPARATION

1. Mix pine bark extract with carrier oil.
2. Apply to inflamed areas of the skin daily.

Benefits: Pine bark extract is rich in antioxidants and

helps reduce inflammation when applied topically. This serum promotes skin healing, reduces redness, and supports overall skin health.

Ginseng Inflammation Support Elixir

INGREDIENTS

- 1 teaspoon dried ginseng root
- 1 cup boiling water

PREPARATION

1. Steep ginseng root in boiling water for 10 minutes.
2. Strain and drink daily to reduce inflammation.

Benefits: Ginseng helps regulate immune function and reduce chronic inflammation. This elixir supports overall health by boosting energy levels and reducing inflammatory responses in the body.

Moringa Leaf Anti-Inflammatory Infusion

INGREDIENTS

- 1 teaspoon dried moringa leaf
- 1 cup boiling water

PREPARATION

1. Steep moringa leaves in boiling water for 10 minutes.
2. Strain and drink daily to combat inflammation.

Benefits: Moringa is packed with antioxidants and anti-inflammatory compounds that help reduce inflammation throughout the body. This infusion promotes joint health, reduces pain, and improves overall wellness.

Holy Basil (Tulsi) Joint Pain Relief Tea

INGREDIENTS

- 1 teaspoon dried holy basil leaves
- 1 cup boiling water

PREPARATION

1. Steep holy basil leaves in boiling water for 10 minutes.
2. Strain and drink to relieve joint pain and inflammation.

Benefits: Holy basil is an adaptogen with powerful anti-inflammatory properties. This tea helps relieve joint pain, reduce inflammation, and improve overall health.

Yarrow and Thyme Anti-Inflammatory Drops

INGREDIENTS

- 1 tablespoon dried yarrow flowers
- 1 tablespoon dried thyme leaves
- 1/4 cup alcohol (vodka or glycerin for a non-alcoholic option)

PREPARATION

1. Infuse yarrow and thyme in alcohol or glycerin for 4-6 weeks.
2. Strain and take 1-2 droppers daily to reduce inflammation.

Benefits: Yarrow and thyme are both known for their anti-inflammatory and antimicrobial properties. These drops help reduce inflammation and support the immune system, especially during colds and flu.

Rosehip Antioxidant Tea

INGREDIENTS

- 1 tablespoon dried rosehips
- 1 cup boiling water

PREPARATION

1. Steep rosehips in boiling water for 10 minutes.
2. Strain and drink daily for anti-inflammatory support.

Benefits: Rosehips are rich in vitamin C and antioxidants, which help reduce inflammation and support immune function. This tea promotes overall health and helps combat chronic inflammation.

Goldenrod Joint Support Tincture

INGREDIENTS

- 1 tablespoon dried goldenrod
- 1/4 cup alcohol (vodka or glycerin for a non-alcoholic option)

PREPARATION

1. Infuse goldenrod in alcohol or glycerin for 4-6 weeks.
2. Strain and take 1-2 droppers daily to support joint health and reduce inflammation.

Benefits: Goldenrod is an anti-inflammatory herb that helps reduce joint pain and swelling. This tincture supports healthy joints and promotes mobility, especially for those with arthritis.

Ginger and Lemon Anti-Inflammatory Drink

INGREDIENTS

- 1 teaspoon fresh grated ginger
- Juice of 1 lemon
- 1 cup warm water

PREPARATION

1. Mix ginger and lemon juice into warm water.
2. Drink daily for anti-inflammatory support.

Benefits: Ginger and lemon work together to reduce inflammation and support immune health. This drink soothes digestive inflammation and promotes whole-body wellness.

Burdock Root Blood Cleansing Capsules

INGREDIENTS

- 1 tablespoon dried burdock root powder
- Capsule shells

PREPARATION

1. Fill capsule shells with dried burdock root powder.
2. Take 1-2 capsules daily to cleanse the blood and reduce inflammation.

Benefits: Burdock root is a natural blood purifier and anti-inflammatory herb that supports liver health. These capsules help cleanse the body of toxins and reduce chronic inflammation.

Comfrey Anti-Inflammatory Poultice

INGREDIENTS

- 1 tablespoon dried comfrey leaves
- 1/4 cup water

PREPARATION

1. Mix comfrey leaves with water to create a paste.

Apply the paste to inflamed areas and cover with a cloth. Leave on for 20 minutes before rinsing.

Benefits: Comfrey is known for its ability to reduce inflammation and promote healing. This poultice is ideal for treating joint pain, swelling, and bruises.

Clove and Peppermint Pain Relief Balm

INGREDIENTS

- 1 tablespoon dried clove powder
- 10 drops peppermint essential oil
- 1/4 cup coconut oil

PREPARATION

1. Mix clove powder and peppermint oil into melted coconut oil.
2. Apply to painful or inflamed areas for relief.

Benefits: Clove and peppermint work together to reduce pain and inflammation. This balm is perfect for soothing muscle aches, joint pain, and headaches.

Meadowsweet Joint Health Capsules

INGREDIENTS

- 1 tablespoon dried meadowsweet powder
- Capsule shells

PREPARATION

1. Fill capsule shells with dried meadowsweet powder.
2. Take 1-2 capsules daily for joint health and inflammation relief.

Benefits: Meadowsweet is a natural anti-inflammatory herb that helps reduce pain and swelling in the joints. These capsules are ideal for individuals suffering from arthritis or joint discomfort.

Blue Vervain Inflammation Reduction Tea

INGREDIENTS

- 1 teaspoon dried blue vervain leaves
- 1 cup boiling water

PREPARATION

1. Steep blue vervain leaves in boiling water for 10 minutes.
2. Strain and drink daily to reduce inflammation.

Benefits: Blue vervain is known for its anti-inflammatory and relaxing properties. This tea helps reduce stress-related inflammation and soothes tension in the body.

Calendula Inflammatory Control Wash

INGREDIENTS

- 1 tablespoon dried calendula flowers
- 1 cup boiling water

PREPARATION

1. Steep calendula flowers in boiling water for 10 minutes.
2. Strain and use the liquid as a wash for inflamed skin.

Benefits: Calendula is a gentle anti-inflammatory herb that soothes irritated and inflamed skin. This wash promotes healing and reduces redness, making it perfect for sensitive skin conditions.

Eucalyptus Inflammation Support Steam

INGREDIENTS

- 10 drops eucalyptus essential oil
- 1 bowl of hot water

PREPARATION

1. Add eucalyptus oil to hot water.
2. Inhale the steam for 10-15 minutes to reduce inflammation in the respiratory system.

Benefits: Eucalyptus oil helps clear the airways and reduce inflammation in the respiratory tract. This steam is ideal for relieving congestion, sinus inflammation, and respiratory discomfort.

Oregano Oil Anti-Inflammatory Capsules

INGREDIENTS

- 10 drops oregano essential oil
- Capsule shells

PREPARATION

1. Fill capsule shells with oregano oil.
2. Take 1-2 capsules daily to reduce inflammation and support immune health.

Benefits: Oregano oil has strong anti-inflammatory and antimicrobial properties. These capsules help combat infections and reduce inflammation, particularly in the digestive tract and respiratory system.

St. John's Wort Inflammatory Control Capsules

INGREDIENTS

- 1 tablespoon dried St. John's wort powder
- Capsule shells

PREPARATION

1. Fill capsule shells with dried St. John's wort powder.
2. Take 1-2 capsules daily to support inflammation control.

Benefits: St. John's wort is known for its anti-inflammatory and mood-lifting properties. These capsules help reduce inflammation while supporting mental well-being.

Nettle Leaf Inflammation Reducing Tea

INGREDIENTS

- 1 teaspoon dried nettle leaves
- 1 cup boiling water

PREPARATION

1. Steep nettle leaves in boiling water for 10 minutes.
2. Strain and drink daily to reduce inflammation.

Benefits: Nettle leaf is a powerful anti-inflammatory herb that helps reduce swelling and pain, especially in the joints. This tea promotes joint health and supports detoxification.

Echinacea Anti-Inflammatory Infusion

INGREDIENTS

- 1 teaspoon dried echinacea root
- 1 cup boiling water

PREPARATION

1. Steep echinacea root in boiling water for 10 minutes.
2. Strain and drink to reduce inflammation and support immune function.

Benefits: Echinacea helps reduce inflammation and boost the immune system. This infusion is ideal for relieving inflammatory conditions while supporting overall immune health.

Sage and Rosemary Inflammatory Relief Oil

INGREDIENTS

- 1 tablespoon dried sage leaves
- 1 tablespoon dried rosemary leaves
- 1/4 cup olive oil

PREPARATION

1. Infuse sage and rosemary in olive oil using a double boiler for 30 minutes.
2. Strain and apply the oil to inflamed areas of the skin or joints.

Benefits: Sage and rosemary are both anti-inflammatory herbs that help reduce pain and swelling. This oil is ideal for massaging into sore joints or inflamed skin to promote healing and relief.

Lemon Balm Inflammation Support Drops

INGREDIENTS

- 1 tablespoon dried lemon balm leaves
- 1/4 cup alcohol (vodka or glycerin for a non-alcoholic option)

PREPARATION

1. Infuse lemon balm leaves in alcohol or glycerin for 4-6 weeks.
2. Strain and take 1-2 droppers daily to reduce inflammation.

Benefits: Lemon balm is known for its calming and anti-inflammatory properties. These drops help reduce inflammation, particularly in the digestive system, while promoting relaxation.

Ginger Root Inflammation Support Capsules

INGREDIENTS

- 1 tablespoon dried ginger root powder
- Capsule shells

PREPARATION

1. Fill capsule shells with dried ginger root powder.
2. Take 1-2 capsules daily to reduce inflammation and support digestion.

Benefits: Ginger root is a powerful anti-inflammatory herb that supports digestive health and reduces overall inflammation in the body. These capsules are ideal for reducing pain and promoting wellness.

Thyme and Honey Anti-Inflammatory Elixir

INGREDIENTS

- 1 teaspoon dried thyme leaves
- 1 tablespoon honey
- 1 cup warm water

PREPARATION

1. Steep thyme leaves in warm water for 10 minutes, then strain.
2. Stir in honey and drink daily to reduce inflammation.

Benefits: Thyme is a natural anti-inflammatory herb, and when combined with honey, this elixir soothes inflammation, particularly in the throat and respiratory system.

Ginkgo Biloba Inflammation Support Tea

INGREDIENTS

- 1 teaspoon dried ginkgo biloba leaves
- 1 cup boiling water

PREPARATION

1. Steep ginkgo biloba leaves in boiling water for 10 minutes.
2. Strain and drink daily to support inflammation control.

Benefits: Ginkgo biloba helps improve circulation and reduce inflammation, particularly in the cardiovascular and nervous systems. This tea promotes brain health and reduces inflammation throughout the body.

Marshmallow Root Inflammation Control Capsules

INGREDIENTS

- 1 tablespoon dried marshmallow root powder
- Capsule shells

PREPARATION

1. Fill capsule shells with dried marshmallow root powder.
2. Take 1-2 capsules daily to soothe inflammation.

Benefits: Marshmallow root is known for its soothing and anti-inflammatory effects, particularly in the digestive tract. These capsules help reduce inflammation and promote digestive health.

Licorice Root Anti-Inflammatory Tincture

INGREDIENTS

- 1 tablespoon dried licorice root
- 1/4 cup alcohol (vodka or glycerin for a non-alcoholic option)

PREPARATION

1. Infuse licorice root in alcohol or glycerin for 4-6 weeks.
2. Strain and take 1-2 droppers daily to reduce inflammation.

Benefits: Licorice root is a potent anti-inflammatory herb that helps reduce inflammation, particularly in the digestive system. This tincture supports digestive health and soothes inflamed tissues.

Elderberry Inflammatory Support Syrup

INGREDIENTS

- 1/2 cup dried elderberries
- 1 cup water
- 1/4 cup honey

PREPARATION

1. Simmer elderberries in water for 20 minutes, then strain.
2. Stir in honey and store in a jar. Take 1 tablespoon daily to reduce inflammation.

Benefits: Elderberries are rich in antioxidants and have strong anti-inflammatory properties. This syrup helps reduce inflammation, boost immune function, and support respiratory health.

BOOK 21

Herbal Support for Weight Management

Herbs That Aid Metabolism and Fat Burning

BOOSTING METABOLISM AND ENHANCING FAT BURNING WITH HERBAL ALLIES

Managing weight effectively often involves enhancing metabolism and promoting fat burning. For individuals like Emma, who seek natural and sustainable methods, herbs provide a powerful, holistic approach to supporting these processes. Many herbs possess thermogenic and metabolic-boosting properties, helping the body burn calories efficiently and mobilize stored fat. Below, we explore several herbs renowned for their ability to aid metabolism and fat burning, offering practical ways to incorporate them into a daily wellness routine.

Green Tea: A Thermogenic Powerhouse

Green tea is one of the most well-researched herbs for weight management. Its primary active compound, EGCG (epigallocatechin gallate), has been shown to boost metabolism and promote fat oxidation. By increasing the body's heat production (thermogenesis), green tea helps burn more calories, even at rest. Studies suggest that combining green tea consumption with physical activity can further enhance fat-burning effects, making it a valuable tool in weight management strategies.

Emma can incorporate green tea into her daily routine as a hot beverage or in powdered matcha form. Drinking two to three cups of green tea daily provides a steady source of EGCG, helping her body burn fat more efficiently. The mild caffeine content in green tea also contributes to increased energy levels, supporting her overall activity and exercise efforts.

Cayenne Pepper: Igniting Thermogenesis

Cayenne pepper, known for its spicy kick, contains capsaicin, a compound that boosts metabolism by increasing the body's thermogenic activity. Capsaicin enhances calorie burning by raising the body's temperature, which, in turn, requires more energy to cool down. This process not only supports fat burning but also aids in appetite suppression, making cayenne pepper a multifaceted herb for weight management.

Emma can easily add cayenne pepper to her meals or take it in capsule form if she prefers a non-spicy option. Incorporating cayenne pepper into soups, stews, or smoothies provides a simple and effective way to increase her metabolism naturally. The spice's heat helps keep her metabolism active, especially when combined with regular movement or exercise.

Ginger: Enhancing Digestion and Metabolism

Ginger is another powerful herb for boosting metabolism and supporting fat burning. It contains gingerol, an active compound that not only aids in digestion but also has thermogenic properties. By enhancing digestion, ginger helps the body break down and utilize nutrients more efficiently, while its metabolism-boosting effects increase the number of calories burned throughout the day.

Emma can use ginger in various forms—fresh, dried, or as a tea. Drinking ginger tea before meals can stimulate digestion and increase metabolic activity. Additionally, adding fresh ginger to smoothies or meals provides a flavorful and convenient way to incorporate its benefits. The versatility of ginger makes it a practical option for Emma's holistic approach to weight management.

Ginseng: Supporting Metabolic Health and Energy Levels

Ginseng, particularly Panax ginseng, is a renowned adaptogenic herb that not only helps the body adapt to stress but also boosts metabolism and supports fat burning. Ginseng has been shown to improve insulin sensitivity and stabilize blood sugar levels, which are crucial for maintaining a healthy metabolism. By enhancing the body's energy levels, ginseng supports physical activity, which is essential for burning fat effectively.

Emma can take ginseng as a supplement or incorporate it into her diet through tea. Consuming ginseng in the morning helps sustain her energy levels throughout the day, promoting an active lifestyle that supports her weight management goals. By balancing her metabolism and energy, ginseng ensures that her body remains efficient in burning fat and maintaining overall health.

Cinnamon: Regulating Blood Sugar and Boosting Metabolism

Cinnamon is an excellent herb for weight management due to its ability to regulate blood sugar levels and increase metabolism. By stabilizing blood glucose, cinnamon helps prevent insulin spikes, which can lead to fat storage. The herb's active compounds, including cinnamaldehyde, also promote thermogenesis, enhancing the body's ability to burn fat.

Emma can add cinnamon to her diet in several ways, such as sprinkling it on oatmeal, adding it to smoothies, or incorporating it into teas. The sweet, warming flavor makes cinnamon an enjoyable and easy addition to meals, supporting her metabolic health without any drastic dietary changes. Its ability to balance blood sugar levels also helps control cravings, further aiding her weight management efforts.

Fenugreek: Boosting Metabolism and Reducing Appetite

Fenugreek is an herb traditionally used in various cultures for its numerous health benefits, including its ability to support metabolism and aid in weight management. Rich in soluble fiber, fenugreek helps control appetite by creating a sense of fullness, while its compounds support fat metabolism. Studies suggest that fenugreek may also reduce dietary fat absorption, making it a valuable tool for weight management.

Emma can consume fenugreek seeds soaked in water or as a tea. Taking fenugreek before meals helps her feel full faster, reducing her overall calorie intake while boosting her metabolism. This simple, natural approach aligns with her holistic wellness philosophy, supporting her weight management goals sustainably.

Dandelion: A Natural Diuretic and Metabolism Booster

Dandelion is a versatile herb known for its diuretic properties and its ability to support liver function. The liver plays a critical role in metabolizing fats, and a well-functioning liver ensures that the body processes and burns fat efficiently. Additionally, dandelion helps reduce water retention, providing a natural way to manage weight without harsh diuretics.

Emma can drink dandelion tea or take it in supplement form to enjoy its benefits. Incorporating dandelion tea into her daily routine helps keep her metabolism active while supporting her body's natural detoxification processes. Its mild, earthy flavor makes it an easy and pleasant addition to her holistic wellness plan.

These herbs offer Emma a range of options for naturally boosting her metabolism and supporting fat burning. By integrating them into her daily routine, she can achieve her weight management goals sustainably, ensuring her body remains efficient and balanced in its metabolic processes. The versatility and accessibility of these herbs make them valuable allies for Emma's holistic journey toward health and wellness.

Balancing Appetite and Cravings with Natural Solutions

NATURAL HERBS AND METHODS TO CONTROL APPETITE AND CURB CRAVINGS

Balancing appetite and managing cravings is a critical component of sustainable weight management. For individuals like Emma, who seek natural ways to maintain control over their eating habits, herbs and natural solutions offer effective and holistic methods to regulate hunger and reduce the urge for unhealthy snacks. By incorporating these remedies into her routine, Emma can align her wellness journey with a balanced approach to nutrition, ensuring she stays on track without feeling deprived or stressed. Below, we explore several herbs and strategies designed to help manage appetite and cravings naturally.

Fenugreek: A Fiber-Rich Appetite Suppressant

Fenugreek seeds are rich in soluble fiber, which plays a vital role in appetite regulation. When consumed, the seeds swell in the stomach, forming a gel-like substance that promotes a feeling of fullness. This action helps reduce overall calorie intake, making it easier to manage portions and avoid overeating. The seeds also help stabilize blood sugar levels, preventing spikes that can lead to cravings for sugary foods.

For Emma, incorporating fenugreek into her meals or taking it as a supplement can be an effective way to control her appetite naturally. Drinking fenugreek tea before meals or adding ground seeds to smoothies can create a sense of satiety, ensuring she consumes fewer calories while maintaining her energy levels. This practical, natural solution aligns with Emma's preference for simple, integrative wellness strategies.

Gymnema Sylvestre: Reducing Sugar Cravings

Gymnema Sylvestre, a herb often used in traditional Ayurvedic medicine, is known for its ability to suppress sugar cravings. The active compounds in gymnema can block the sugar receptors on the taste buds, reducing the sweet taste sensation. This effect not only decreases the desire for sugary foods but also supports balanced blood glucose levels, which is essential for managing appetite and preventing energy crashes.

Emma can use gymnema as a tea or in capsule form, taking it before meals to reduce the likelihood of reaching for sweet treats afterward. Incorporating gymnema into her daily routine helps her maintain control over her cravings, particularly when she feels the urge for sugar-rich snacks. This herb's long-standing reputation as a natural appetite suppressant makes it a reliable ally in her weight management plan.

Hoodia Gordonii: A Traditional Appetite Suppressant

Hoodia Gordonii, a succulent plant from Africa, has been traditionally used to suppress appetite. It contains a compound called P57, which is believed to influence the hypothalamus—the part of the brain responsible for hunger signals. By tricking the brain into feeling full, hoodia can help reduce overall food intake, making it a valuable tool for those aiming to control their appetite naturally.

For Emma, taking hoodia in supplement form provides an easy and effective way to manage hunger. By using hoodia as a natural appetite suppressant, she can focus on balanced meals without the distraction of constant hunger or cravings. This approach allows her to stick to her wellness goals while still feeling satisfied.

Cinnamon: Stabilizing Blood Sugar and Reducing Cravings

Cinnamon is a versatile herb that not only adds flavor to meals but also helps manage cravings. Its ability to stabilize blood sugar levels ensures that Emma's energy remains steady, reducing the likelihood of sudden hunger pangs. By regulating insulin sensitivity, cinnamon prevents the spikes and crashes that often lead to cravings for high-sugar or high-fat foods.

Emma can add cinnamon to her daily diet by sprinkling it on oatmeal, blending it into smoothies, or incorporating it into tea. These small dietary adjustments allow her to enjoy the flavor and benefits of cinnamon without making drastic changes to her routine. This natural approach helps her maintain control over her appetite, supporting her journey toward balanced nutrition.

Fennel Seeds: Calming Digestion and Managing Hunger

Fennel seeds are traditionally used to aid digestion and reduce appetite. The seeds contain essential oils that have a calming effect on the digestive system, helping to relieve bloating and discomfort, which can sometimes be mistaken for hunger. Additionally, fennel's mild diuretic properties help eliminate water retention, promoting a feeling of lightness and satiety.

For Emma, chewing on fennel seeds between meals or drinking fennel tea offers a simple way to manage her appetite. The seeds' natural properties ensure that she feels satisfied without reaching for unnecessary snacks, making it easier for her to maintain a balanced diet. This herb's accessibility and effectiveness make it a convenient choice for Emma's holistic weight management plan.

Garcinia Cambogia: Supporting Appetite Control

Garcinia cambogia is a tropical fruit known for its weight management properties, particularly its ability to suppress appetite. The active ingredient in garcinia cambogia, hydroxycitric acid (HCA), is believed to increase serotonin levels in the brain, which can help reduce emotional eating and cravings. By influencing mood and hunger signals, this herb provides a comprehensive approach to managing appetite.

Emma can take garcinia cambogia as a supplement to enhance her ability to resist cravings and emotional eating triggers. This natural solution aligns with her preference for sustainable, herbal remedies that support her weight management journey. By incorporating garcinia cambogia into her routine, Emma can maintain balance in her diet, ensuring that she sticks to her wellness goals without feeling deprived.

Psyllium Husk: Promoting Fullness and Digestive Health

Psyllium husk, a natural fiber, is another effective tool for appetite management. When consumed with water, psyllium expands in the stomach, creating a sense of fullness that reduces hunger. This fiber also supports digestive health, ensuring that nutrients are absorbed efficiently while waste is eliminated. By promoting regularity, psyllium helps Emma feel lighter and more satisfied throughout the day.

Emma can add psyllium husk to her smoothies, oatmeal, or take it as a supplement. Drinking it with plenty of water ensures she gets the full benefits of this appetite-regulating fiber. By incorporating psyllium into her daily routine, she can naturally manage her appetite while supporting her digestive system, aligning with her holistic approach to wellness.

These herbs and natural solutions offer Emma a range of tools to manage her appetite and cravings effectively. By integrating these herbs into her routine, she can maintain control over her eating habits, supporting her weight management goals sustainably and naturally. This comprehensive approach ensures that her wellness journey remains balanced, fulfilling, and aligned with her values.

Remedies for Weight Control and Metabolic Health

Garcinia Cambogia Appetite Suppressant Capsules

INGREDIENTS

- 1 tablespoon dried garcinia cambogia powder
- Capsule shells

PREPARATION

1. Fill capsule shells with dried garcinia cambogia powder.
2. Take 1-2 capsules daily to suppress appetite and support weight management.

Benefits: Garcinia cambogia helps reduce appetite by increasing serotonin levels, which can lead to reduced cravings and improved mood. It supports weight loss by preventing fat storage and controlling hunger.

Green Tea Metabolism Boosting Infusion

INGREDIENTS

- 1 teaspoon green tea leaves
- 1 cup boiling water

PREPARATION

1. Steep green tea leaves in boiling water for 5-7 minutes.
2. Strain and drink daily to boost metabolism.

Benefits: Green tea contains catechins and caffeine, which help increase metabolic rate and fat oxidation. Drinking this infusion regularly supports weight loss and helps improve energy levels.

Dandelion Root Diuretic Tea

INGREDIENTS

- 1 teaspoon dried dandelion root
- 1 cup boiling water

PREPARATION

1. Steep dried dandelion root in boiling water for 10 minutes.
2. Strain and drink to support water weight reduction.

Benefits: Dandelion root is a natural diuretic that helps the body eliminate excess water and toxins. It promotes healthy liver function and aids in reducing bloating and water retention.

Fennel Seed Digestive and Weight Control Tea

INGREDIENTS

- 1 teaspoon fennel seeds
- 1 cup boiling water

PREPARATION

1. Steep fennel seeds in boiling water for 10 minutes.
2. Strain and drink to support digestion and weight control.

Benefits: Fennel seeds help improve digestion, reduce bloating, and suppress appetite. This tea supports weight management by promoting healthy digestion and reducing cravings.

Yerba Mate Energy-Boosting Drink

INGREDIENTS

- 1 teaspoon yerba mate leaves
- 1 cup boiling water

PREPARATION

1. Steep yerba mate leaves in boiling water for 5 minutes.
2. Strain and drink for an energy boost and weight support.

Benefits: Yerba mate is a natural stimulant that increases energy and supports fat metabolism. It helps reduce fatigue, curb appetite, and promotes weight loss.

Cayenne Pepper Fat Burning Tincture

INGREDIENTS

- 1 teaspoon cayenne pepper powder
- 1/4 cup alcohol (vodka or glycerin for a non-alcoholic option)

PREPARATION

1. Infuse cayenne pepper in alcohol or glycerin for 4-6 weeks.
2. Strain and take 1-2 droppers daily to boost fat burning.

Benefits: Cayenne pepper contains capsaicin, which helps boost metabolism and increase fat burning. This tincture supports weight loss by enhancing thermogenesis and promoting fat breakdown.

Licorice Root Craving Control Capsules

INGREDIENTS

- 1 tablespoon dried licorice root powder
- Capsule shells

PREPARATION

1. Fill capsule shells with dried licorice root powder.
2. Take 1-2 capsules daily to control cravings and support digestion.

Benefits: Licorice root helps balance blood sugar levels and reduce cravings for sweets. It also supports digestion, which aids in weight management by promoting a healthier metabolism.

Cinnamon and Honey Weight Management Elixir

INGREDIENTS

- 1 teaspoon ground cinnamon
- 1 tablespoon honey
- 1 cup warm water

PREPARATION

1. Mix cinnamon and honey in warm water until well combined.
2. Drink daily to support weight management.

Benefits: Cinnamon helps regulate blood sugar levels and improve insulin sensitivity, while honey provides a natural energy boost. This elixir helps reduce cravings and supports a balanced metabolism.

Gymnema Leaf Sugar Balance Capsules

INGREDIENTS

- 1 tablespoon dried gymnema leaf powder
- Capsule shells

PREPARATION

1. Fill capsule shells with dried gymnema leaf powder.
2. Take 1-2 capsules daily to balance blood sugar levels.

Benefits: Gymnema leaf is known for its ability to reduce sugar absorption and balance blood sugar levels. These capsules help control sugar cravings and support healthy weight management.

Lemon and Ginger Detox Drink

INGREDIENTS

- Juice of 1 lemon
- 1-inch piece fresh ginger, grated
- 1 cup warm water

PREPARATION

1. Mix lemon juice and grated ginger in warm water.
2. Drink daily to detoxify and support weight management.

Benefits: Lemon and ginger both promote detoxification and boost metabolism. This drink helps cleanse the digestive system, reduce bloating, and supports weight loss.

Holy Basil (Tulsi) Weight Control Tea

INGREDIENTS

- 1 teaspoon dried holy basil (tulsi) leaves
- 1 cup boiling water

PREPARATION

1. Steep holy basil leaves in boiling water for 10 minutes.
2. Strain and drink to support weight control.

Benefits: Holy basil is an adaptogen that helps balance stress hormones and support weight management. This tea reduces stress-related eating and helps balance metabolism.

Bitter Melon Blood Sugar Balancing Capsules

INGREDIENTS

- 1 tablespoon dried bitter melon powder
- Capsule shells

PREPARATION

1. Fill capsule shells with dried bitter melon powder.
2. Take 1-2 capsules daily to balance blood sugar levels and support weight control.

Benefits: Bitter melon helps regulate blood sugar levels and improve insulin sensitivity. These capsules are beneficial for individuals looking to manage their weight by controlling sugar levels.

Nettle and Mint Detox Tea

INGREDIENTS

- 1 teaspoon dried nettle leaves
- 1 teaspoon dried mint leaves
- 1 cup boiling water

PREPARATION

1. Steep nettle and mint leaves in boiling water for 10 minutes.
2. Strain and drink daily to detoxify and support weight loss.

Benefits: Nettle and mint promote detoxification, improve digestion, and help reduce water retention. This tea supports weight loss by cleansing the body and improving metabolic function.

Ginseng Metabolic Stimulation Capsules

INGREDIENTS

- 1 tablespoon dried ginseng root powder
- Capsule shells

PREPARATION

1. Fill capsule shells with dried ginseng powder.
2. Take 1-2 capsules daily to boost metabolism and energy.

Benefits: Ginseng is a natural stimulant that boosts energy levels and supports metabolic function. These capsules help increase calorie burn and reduce fatigue, making them beneficial for weight management.

Hibiscus Fat Metabolism Tea

INGREDIENTS

- 1 teaspoon dried hibiscus flowers
- 1 cup boiling water

PREPARATION

1. Steep hibiscus flowers in boiling water for 10 minutes.
2. Strain and drink daily to support fat metabolism.

Benefits: Hibiscus is rich in antioxidants and helps improve fat metabolism, making it an excellent choice for weight loss. This tea helps reduce fat storage and supports healthy digestion.

Psyllium Husk Digestive Support Drink

INGREDIENTS

- 1 tablespoon psyllium husk powder
- 1 cup water

PREPARATION

1. Mix psyllium husk powder into water and drink immediately.
2. Drink daily to support digestion and weight control.

Benefits: Psyllium husk provides soluble fiber that supports digestive health, promotes regularity, and helps control appetite. This drink is beneficial for weight management by improving digestion and promoting satiety.

Fenugreek Appetite Control Capsules

INGREDIENTS

- 1 tablespoon dried fenugreek seed powder
- Capsule shells

PREPARATION

1. Fill capsule shells with dried fenugreek seed powder.
2. Take 1-2 capsules daily to control appetite and support weight management.

Benefits: Fenugreek seeds help control appetite by promoting a feeling of fullness. These capsules are an excellent tool for reducing overeating and supporting weight loss efforts.

Apple Cider Vinegar and Honey Tonic

INGREDIENTS

- 1 tablespoon apple cider vinegar
- 1 teaspoon honey
- 1 cup warm water

PREPARATION

1. Mix apple cider vinegar and honey in warm water.
2. Drink daily, preferably before meals, to support weight management.

Benefits: Apple cider vinegar helps control appetite, regulate blood sugar levels, and improve digestion. When combined with honey, this tonic provides a natural energy boost while supporting metabolism and fat loss.

Burdock Root Weight Balance Capsules

INGREDIENTS

- 1 tablespoon dried burdock root powder
- Capsule shells

PREPARATION

1. Fill capsule shells with dried burdock root powder.
2. Take 1-2 capsules daily to balance weight and detoxify the body.

Benefits: Burdock root is known for its detoxifying properties, supporting liver function, and improving digestion. These capsules promote weight balance by helping the body eliminate toxins and reducing inflammation.

Peppermint Digestive Support Drops

INGREDIENTS

- 1 tablespoon dried peppermint leaves
- 1/4 cup alcohol (vodka or glycerin for a non-alcoholic option)

PREPARATION

1. Infuse dried peppermint leaves in alcohol or glycerin for 4-6 weeks.
2. Strain and take 1-2 droppers daily to support digestion and reduce bloating.

Benefits: Peppermint helps improve digestion, reduce bloating, and relieve digestive discomfort. These drops promote healthy digestion and support weight management by improving nutrient absorption and reducing overeating.

Guarana Metabolic Boost Tea

INGREDIENTS

- 1 teaspoon dried guarana powder
- 1 cup boiling water

PREPARATION

1. Steep guarana powder in boiling water for 5 minutes.
2. Strain and drink daily to boost metabolism and energy levels.

Benefits: Guarana is a natural stimulant that boosts metabolism and energy. This tea helps increase calorie burning and reduces fatigue, making it an excellent choice for weight management.

White Tea Appetite Suppressant Infusion

INGREDIENTS

- 1 teaspoon white tea leaves
- 1 cup boiling water

PREPARATION

1. Steep white tea leaves in boiling water for 5 minutes.
2. Strain and drink daily to help suppress appetite.

Benefits: White tea is rich in antioxidants and helps reduce appetite, making it a great addition to any weight management routine. It also supports fat burning and boosts metabolism.

Black Seed Oil Weight Loss Capsules

INGREDIENTS

- 1 tablespoon black seed oil
- Capsule shells

PREPARATION

1. Fill capsule shells with black seed oil.
2. Take 1-2 capsules daily to promote weight loss and support digestion.

Benefits: Black seed oil has been shown to aid in weight loss by reducing appetite and improving fat metabolism. It also supports digestive health and promotes overall well-being.

Spirulina Energy Smoothie

INGREDIENTS

- 1 tablespoon spirulina powder
- 1/2 banana
- 1/2 cup almond milk
- 1 tablespoon chia seeds

PREPARATION

1. Blend all ingredients until smooth.
2. Drink as a meal replacement or energy boost to support weight loss.

Benefits: Spirulina is a nutrient-dense superfood that helps boost energy, reduce hunger, and support fat loss. This smoothie is perfect as a low-calorie meal replacement that keeps you feeling full and energized.

Turmeric and Black Pepper Metabolism Booster

INGREDIENTS

- 1 teaspoon ground turmeric
- 1/4 teaspoon black pepper
- 1 cup warm water

PREPARATION

1. Mix turmeric and black pepper into warm water.
2. Drink daily to boost metabolism and reduce inflammation.

Benefits: Turmeric and black pepper work together to enhance fat burning, reduce inflammation, and improve metabolic function. This drink supports weight loss by boosting digestion and fat metabolism.

Ginger and Lemon Weight Loss Elixir

INGREDIENTS

- 1 teaspoon grated ginger
- Juice of 1 lemon
- 1 cup warm water

PREPARATION

1. Mix grated ginger and lemon juice in warm water.
2. Drink daily to support weight loss and improve digestion.

Benefits: Ginger and lemon are both powerful detoxifiers that boost metabolism and support fat loss. This elixir helps improve digestion, reduce bloating, and promote overall weight management.

Triphala Ayurvedic Weight Control Capsules

INGREDIENTS

- 1 tablespoon dried triphala powder
- Capsule shells

PREPARATION

1. Fill capsule shells with dried triphala powder.
2. Take 1-2 capsules daily to support digestive health and weight control.

Benefits: Triphala is an Ayurvedic blend that supports digestion, promotes detoxification, and aids in weight loss. These capsules help balance metabolism and support healthy weight management.

Rooibos Digestive Support Tea

INGREDIENTS

- 1 teaspoon dried rooibos leaves
- 1 cup boiling water

PREPARATION

1. Steep rooibos leaves in boiling water for 10 minutes.
2. Strain and drink to support digestion and reduce bloating.

Benefits: Rooibos is a caffeine-free tea that helps improve digestion, reduce bloating, and support weight loss. Its natural antioxidants promote overall health and wellness while aiding in weight control.

Aloe Vera Digestive Health Juice

INGREDIENTS

- 2 tablespoons fresh aloe vera gel
- 1 cup water

PREPARATION

1. Blend fresh aloe vera gel with water until smooth.
2. Drink daily to support digestion and weight management.

Benefits: Aloe vera is known for its soothing and detoxifying properties. This juice helps improve digestion, reduce inflammation, and support weight management by promoting healthy gut function.

Dandelion and Lemon Detox Water

INGREDIENTS

- 1 teaspoon dried dandelion root
- Juice of 1 lemon
- 1 cup water

PREPARATION

1. Steep dandelion root in water for 10 minutes, then strain.
2. Add lemon juice and stir well. Drink daily to detoxify and support weight loss.

Benefits: Dandelion root is a natural diuretic that helps reduce water retention, while lemon boosts digestion and detoxification. This detox water supports weight loss by cleansing the body and reducing bloating.

Clove and Cumin Digestive Balance Capsules

INGREDIENTS

- 1/2 tablespoon ground clove
- 1/2 tablespoon ground cumin
- Capsule shells

PREPARATION

1. Fill capsule shells with equal parts clove and cumin powder.
2. Take 1-2 capsules daily to support digestion and weight balance.

Benefits: Clove and cumin both promote digestion, reduce bloating, and improve nutrient absorption. These capsules help balance digestive health and support weight management by reducing overeating.

Spearmint and Fennel Slimming Tea

INGREDIENTS

- 1 teaspoon dried spearmint leaves
- 1 teaspoon fennel seeds
- 1 cup boiling water

PREPARATION

1. Steep spearmint and fennel in boiling water for 10 minutes.
2. Strain and drink daily to support slimming and digestion.

Benefits: Spearmint and fennel both aid in digestion, reduce bloating, and promote fat metabolism. This tea helps support weight loss and maintain a balanced digestive system.

Sage Weight Balance Tincture

INGREDIENTS

- 1 tablespoon dried sage leaves
- 1/4 cup alcohol (vodka or glycerin for a non-alcoholic option)

PREPARATION

Infuse sage leaves in alcohol or glycer

1. in for 4-6 weeks.
2. Strain and take 1-2 droppers daily to support weight balance.

Benefits: Sage is known for its ability to balance hormones and reduce stress-related weight gain. This tincture helps support metabolism, reduce cravings, and promote weight loss.

BOOK 22

Strengthening Bone Health

Herbal Calcium and Mineral Sources

NATURAL SOURCES OF CALCIUM AND ESSENTIAL MINERALS FOR BONE HEALTH

Maintaining strong and healthy bones requires an adequate intake of calcium and other essential minerals. While dairy is often highlighted as a primary source of calcium, there are numerous herbal and plant-based alternatives that can provide the necessary nutrients for bone health, especially for those like Emma who prefer natural or non-dairy options. These herbs not only offer calcium but also a range of minerals like magnesium, silica, and phosphorus, which work synergistically to strengthen bones and support overall skeletal health. Below, we explore some of the most effective herbal sources of calcium and essential minerals that Emma can integrate into her wellness routine.

Nettle: A Calcium and Mineral Powerhouse

Nettle (Urtica dioica) is a nutrient-dense herb that is rich in calcium, magnesium, iron, and silica—key minerals for bone health. Nettle's high mineral content makes it an excellent choice for those looking to supplement their diet with natural calcium. The bioavailability of minerals in nettle ensures that they are easily absorbed and utilized by the body, supporting bone density and overall skeletal integrity.

For Emma, incorporating nettle into her routine is simple. Nettle can be taken as a tea, tincture, or infusion, providing a versatile way to benefit from its rich mineral profile. Drinking nettle tea daily or adding dried nettle leaves to soups and stews can enhance her calcium intake without relying on dairy. This aligns with Emma's preference for accessible, herbal solutions that fit seamlessly into her lifestyle.

Horsetail: A Rich Source of Silica

Horsetail (Equisetum arvense) is another valuable herb for bone health due to its high silica content. Silica is a crucial mineral for collagen production, which forms the foundation of bone and connective tissues. By supporting collagen synthesis, silica ensures that bones remain flexible and strong. In addition to silica, horsetail also contains calcium and magnesium, making it a comprehensive herb for bone health.

Emma can take horsetail as an infusion or a capsule. Drinking horsetail tea daily provides her with a steady source of silica, which complements other minerals in her diet, promoting optimal bone density. For those concerned about bone fragility, horsetail's unique mineral combination offers a powerful, natural solution.

Oat Straw: Building and Maintaining Bone Mass

Oat straw (Avena sativa) is an excellent herb for those seeking a plant-based source of calcium. It also contains magnesium, which works in conjunction with calcium to maintain bone density and strength. The combination of these minerals makes oat straw an effective herb for preventing bone loss, particularly as individuals age.

Additionally, its high levels of silica support the regeneration of bone tissue, ensuring that bones remain resilient.

For Emma, consuming oat straw tea or tincture regularly provides a simple and effective way to support her bone health. Oat straw can be easily integrated into her daily routine, and its mild, grassy flavor pairs well with other herbal infusions. By adding oat straw, Emma ensures she gets a balanced intake of essential minerals crucial for bone development and maintenance.

Red Clover: Supporting Hormonal Balance and Bone Health

Red clover (Trifolium pratense) is a unique herb that not only provides calcium but also contains phytoestrogens, which are beneficial for bone health, especially in women. As estrogen levels decline with age, bone density can decrease, leading to conditions like osteoporosis. Red clover's phytoestrogens mimic estrogen in the body, helping to protect bone density and support the absorption of calcium.

Emma can incorporate red clover into her wellness plan by drinking it as tea or taking it as a supplement. Regular use of red clover tea provides her with both calcium and plant-based estrogens, promoting bone health and preventing age-related bone loss. This herb's dual action ensures that Emma's bones remain strong while also supporting her hormonal balance.

Alfalfa: A Comprehensive Mineral Provider

Alfalfa (Medicago sativa) is a nutrient-rich herb that offers not only calcium but also magnesium, phosphorus, and vitamin K—all of which are vital for bone health. Vitamin K plays a critical role in binding calcium to the bone matrix, ensuring that the calcium is effectively utilized by the body. Alfalfa's mineral-rich profile makes it a valuable addition to any bone-strengthening regimen.

For Emma, alfalfa can be consumed as tea, juice, or capsules. The herb's mild flavor makes it a versatile option for teas and smoothies. Drinking alfalfa tea regularly provides her with a broad spectrum of minerals necessary for bone health. Alfalfa's bioavailability ensures that Emma's body can easily absorb and benefit from its mineral content, supporting her holistic approach to wellness.

Dandelion Greens: Calcium and Liver Support

Dandelion greens (Taraxacum officinale) are a natural source of calcium and also provide other bone-supporting minerals like magnesium and potassium. Dandelion not only strengthens bones but also supports liver function, which is essential for processing and metabolizing nutrients. A healthy liver ensures that minerals are properly absorbed and utilized, enhancing the effectiveness of any bone-supporting regimen.

Emma can add dandelion greens to her salads or consume them as a tea or tincture. Incorporating dandelion into her meals allows her to benefit from its calcium content while also promoting liver health, ensuring that her body remains efficient in absorbing and utilizing nutrients. This herb's versatility makes it a convenient and effective choice for Emma's comprehensive bone health strategy.

Amaranth: A Calcium-Rich Grain Alternative

Amaranth is not only a nutrient-dense grain but also an excellent source of calcium, magnesium, and phosphorus. These minerals are crucial for maintaining bone density and preventing bone loss. In addition to its mineral content, amaranth is also high in protein, which supports the building blocks needed for collagen and bone tissue.

Emma can incorporate amaranth into her diet as a breakfast porridge or use it as a grain substitute in various dishes. Its mild flavor and texture make it a versatile option that fits well into her holistic approach to nutrition. By adding amaranth to her meals, Emma ensures a consistent intake of calcium and other essential minerals necessary for strong bones.

These herbal and plant-based sources of calcium provide Emma with a range of options for naturally supporting her bone health. By integrating these herbs into her routine, she can maintain strong and resilient bones, ensuring her overall health and vitality.

Preventing Osteoporosis Naturally

NATURAL APPROACHES TO OSTEOPOROSIS PREVENTION

Osteoporosis, a condition characterized by reduced bone density and increased fracture risk, often affects individuals as they age, particularly women. However, Emma, like many others who prefer a holistic and proactive approach to wellness, can take advantage of natural strategies to prevent osteoporosis and maintain strong bones. By integrating herbal remedies, nutrient-rich foods, and lifestyle modifications, Emma can build a resilient foundation for her bone health while aligning with her preference for natural solutions.

Calcium and Magnesium: The Foundation for Strong Bones

Ensuring adequate calcium intake is essential for preventing osteoporosis. However, calcium works best when paired with magnesium, a mineral that facilitates calcium absorption and utilization in the body. Without enough magnesium, calcium can deposit in soft tissues instead of bones, leading to imbalances. Incorporating both of these minerals into Emma's diet is crucial for maintaining bone density and strength.

Herbs like nettle and oat straw are excellent sources of calcium and magnesium. Regular consumption of nettle tea or oat straw infusions provides a bioavailable source of these minerals. Emma can drink these infusions daily to ensure she meets her calcium and magnesium needs naturally, without relying solely on supplements. This approach fits her preference for integrating practical and accessible herbal remedies into her daily routine.

Vitamin D and K: Essential for Bone Mineralization

Vitamin D plays a critical role in calcium absorption, while vitamin K is essential for binding calcium to the bone matrix. Without adequate levels of these vitamins, the body struggles to maintain healthy bones, increasing the risk of osteoporosis. While Emma can obtain some vitamin D through sun exposure, she might also consider using herbs that help enhance the body's natural absorption processes.

Herbs like alfalfa and horsetail are valuable because they support the body's ability to utilize calcium effectively, enhancing the overall impact of dietary vitamin D and K intake. Emma can include these herbs as teas or supplements, which provide a synergistic effect with other bone-building nutrients. Additionally, vitamin K-rich foods such as leafy greens, including kale and parsley, can be easily incorporated into her meals, providing natural sources that align with her dietary preferences.

Adaptogenic Herbs: Supporting Hormonal Balance for Bone Health

Hormonal changes, especially a decline in estrogen levels during menopause, can significantly impact bone density. Estrogen is vital for maintaining bone health, and its reduction can accelerate bone loss, leading to osteoporosis. For Emma, balancing hormones naturally is crucial in her prevention strategy.

Adaptogenic herbs like red clover and black cohosh contain phytoestrogens—plant-based compounds that mimic estrogen in the body. These herbs help stabilize hormone levels, reducing the impact of hormonal fluctuations on bone health. By drinking red clover tea or using black cohosh supplements, Emma can support her hormonal balance, protecting her bones as she ages. This approach provides a gentle, natural alternative to hormone replacement therapy, aligning with Emma's holistic lifestyle.

Anti-Inflammatory Herbs: Reducing Bone Loss

Chronic inflammation is another contributing factor to osteoporosis, as it can accelerate bone loss. Herbs with anti-inflammatory properties, such as turmeric and ginger, not only reduce inflammation but also support overall bone health. Turmeric, with its active compound curcumin, is particularly effective in mitigating inflammation and has been shown to promote bone density.

Emma can incorporate turmeric into her diet by adding it to soups, smoothies, or teas. Drinking turmeric tea daily not only supports bone health but also aligns with her preference for using simple, herbal solutions in her wellness routine. Ginger, similarly, can be taken as tea or added to meals, providing an accessible way to incorporate anti-inflammatory benefits into her everyday life.

Silica and Boron: Enhancing Bone Density Naturally

Silica and boron are two essential minerals that play a significant role in maintaining bone density. Silica supports collagen production, which forms the foundation for bone structure, while boron enhances calcium absorption and retention. Herbs such as horsetail and dandelion are rich in these minerals, making them valuable allies in the fight against osteoporosis.

Horsetail, for example, is one of the best plant sources of silica. Emma can drink horsetail tea or take it as a supplement, ensuring that her bones receive the collagen support needed for strength and flexibility. Dandelion greens, rich in both silica and boron, can be added to salads or consumed as tea, providing a natural, nutrient-dense option that fits Emma's holistic lifestyle.

Weight-Bearing Exercise: A Natural Boost for Bone Strength

Alongside dietary and herbal strategies, weight-bearing exercises play a crucial role in preventing osteoporosis. Physical activities such as walking, yoga, and resistance training stimulate bone remodeling and strengthen the skeletal system. These exercises promote bone density, ensuring that the body continually regenerates and maintains strong bones.

Emma can incorporate regular movement into her routine by choosing exercises that suit her lifestyle, such as yoga or pilates, which not only build strength but also enhance flexibility and balance. These practices align with her holistic approach, offering both physical and mental benefits that contribute to overall well-being. Combining exercise with her herbal regimen provides a comprehensive and effective strategy for long-term bone health.

Herbal Infusions and Diet: Creating a Balanced Approach

To maximize bone health, Emma can create a balanced approach by combining herbal infusions, nutrient-rich foods, and physical activity. Herbal infusions such as nettle, red clover, and horsetail provide a steady source of essential minerals, while a diet rich in leafy greens, seeds, and whole grains ensures she meets her vitamin and mineral needs. This integrative approach supports her preference for natural, accessible, and sustainable solutions.

By maintaining a daily regimen that includes these herbs and dietary changes, Emma can naturally fortify her bones, preventing osteoporosis without the need for synthetic supplements. This approach empowers her to take control of her health, aligning with her values and lifestyle.

Remedies for Bone Strength and Joint Care

Horsetail Bone Strength Infusion

INGREDIENTS

- 1 teaspoon dried horsetail
- 1 cup boiling water

PREPARATION

1. Steep horsetail in boiling water for 10 minutes.
2. Strain and drink daily to strengthen bones.

Benefits: Horsetail is rich in silica, a mineral essential for bone strength. Regular consumption of this infusion supports bone density and helps in the repair and maintenance of bones.

Nettle Leaf Calcium Boost Capsules

INGREDIENTS

- 1 tablespoon dried nettle leaf powder
- Capsule shells

PREPARATION

1. Fill capsule shells with dried nettle leaf powder.
2. Take 1-2 capsules daily to boost calcium intake.

Benefits: Nettle leaf is a natural source of calcium and other minerals essential for bone health. These capsules support bone density and help prevent bone-related issues like osteoporosis.

Alfalfa Bone Support Tea

INGREDIENTS

- 1 teaspoon dried alfalfa leaves
- 1 cup boiling water

PREPARATION

1. Steep alfalfa leaves in boiling water for 10 minutes.
2. Strain and drink to support bone health.

Benefits: Alfalfa is packed with vitamins and minerals that are vital for maintaining strong and healthy bones. This tea helps improve bone density and supports overall skeletal health.

Red Clover Mineral-Rich Infusion

INGREDIENTS

- 1 tablespoon dried red clover blossoms
- 1 cup boiling water

PREPARATION

1. Steep red clover blossoms in boiling water for 10 minutes.
2. Strain and drink to provide essential minerals for bone health.

Benefits: Red clover is rich in calcium, magnesium, and other minerals that support bone density and help prevent bone loss. Regular consumption of this infusion strengthens the skeletal system.

Dandelion and Burdock Root Bone Health Tonic

INGREDIENTS

- 1 teaspoon dried dandelion root
- 1 teaspoon dried burdock root
- 1 cup boiling water

PREPARATION

1. Steep dandelion and burdock roots in boiling water for 10 minutes.
2. Strain and drink to support bone health and detoxify the body.

Benefits: Dandelion and burdock roots help detoxify the body while providing nutrients that strengthen bones. This tonic supports liver health and promotes better absorption of essential minerals.

Oatstraw Calcium-Rich Capsules

INGREDIENTS

- 1 tablespoon dried oatstraw powder
- Capsule shells

PREPARATION

1. Fill capsule shells with dried oatstraw powder.
2. Take 1-2 capsules daily to support bone health.

Benefits: Oatstraw is rich in calcium and magnesium, which are crucial for maintaining bone density and preventing fractures. These capsules are a convenient way to support bone health naturally.

Black Cohosh Bone Support Elixir

INGREDIENTS

- 1 tablespoon dried black cohosh root
- 1/4 cup alcohol (vodka or glycerin for a non-alcoholic option)

PREPARATION

1. Infuse black cohosh root in alcohol or glycerin for 4-6 weeks.
2. Strain and take 1-2 droppers daily to support bone health.

Benefits: Black cohosh is known for its bone-supporting properties, particularly for post-menopausal women. This elixir helps maintain bone density and supports hormonal balance, which is crucial for bone health.

Comfrey Joint and Bone Health Balm

INGREDIENTS

- 1 tablespoon dried comfrey leaves
- 1/4 cup coconut oil

PREPARATION

1. Infuse comfrey leaves in melted coconut oil for 30 minutes.
2. Strain and store in a jar. Apply to joints and bones as needed.

Benefits: Comfrey is known for its ability to promote bone healing and reduce inflammation. This balm is perfect for soothing joint pain and supporting bone health, especially in cases of fractures or arthritis.

Licorice Root Calcium Support Capsules

INGREDIENTS

- 1 tablespoon dried licorice root powder
- Capsule shells

PREPARATION

1. Fill capsule shells with dried licorice root powder.
2. Take 1-2 capsules daily to support calcium absorption and bone health.

Benefits: Licorice root helps improve calcium absorption in the body, supporting stronger bones and preventing bone loss. These capsules are a great addition to a bone health regimen.

Chamomile Anti-Inflammatory Bone Tea

INGREDIENTS

- 1 teaspoon dried chamomile flowers
- 1 cup boiling water

PREPARATION

1. Steep chamomile flowers in boiling water for 10 minutes.
2. Strain and drink daily to reduce inflammation and support bone health.

Benefits: Chamomile has anti-inflammatory properties that help reduce bone and joint inflammation. This tea soothes aches and promotes better bone health by reducing inflammation around joints.

Meadowsweet Joint and Bone Strength Tea

INGREDIENTS

- 1 teaspoon dried meadowsweet leaves
- 1 cup boiling water

PREPARATION

1. Steep meadowsweet leaves in boiling water for 10 minutes.
2. Strain and drink daily to support joint and bone strength.

Benefits: Meadowsweet contains salicylates, which help reduce joint inflammation and support bone health. This tea is particularly beneficial for individuals suffering from arthritis or joint pain.

Seaweed Calcium Supplement Capsules

INGREDIENTS

- 1 tablespoon dried seaweed powder
- Capsule shells

PREPARATION

1. Fill capsule shells with dried seaweed powder.
2. Take 1-2 capsules daily to support calcium levels and bone health.

Benefits: Seaweed is rich in calcium and other minerals that promote bone density. These capsules are a natural and effective way to boost calcium intake and strengthen bones.

Sage Bone Fortification Tincture

INGREDIENTS

- 1 tablespoon dried sage leaves
- 1/4 cup alcohol (vodka or glycerin for a non-alcoholic option)

PREPARATION

1. Infuse sage leaves in alcohol or glycerin for 4-6 weeks.
2. Strain and take 1-2 droppers daily to support bone strength.

Benefits: Sage is known for its ability to support hormonal balance, which is crucial for bone health, especially in women. This tincture helps strengthen bones and supports overall skeletal health.

White Willow Bark Bone Pain Relief Oil

INGREDIENTS

- 1 tablespoon dried white willow bark
- 1/4 cup olive oil

PREPARATION

1. Infuse white willow bark in olive oil using a double boiler for 30 minutes.
2. Strain and store in a jar. Massage into painful areas as needed.

Benefits: White willow bark is a natural pain reliever that helps reduce bone and joint pain. This oil can be applied to sore areas to relieve discomfort and promote faster healing.

Marshmallow Root Bone Health Elixir

INGREDIENTS

- 1 tablespoon dried marshmallow root
- 1/4 cup water

PREPARATION

1. Simmer marshmallow root in water for 10 minutes.
2. Strain and drink to soothe inflammation and support bone health.

Benefits: Marshmallow root has anti-inflammatory properties that help reduce inflammation in the joints and bones. This elixir is perfect for soothing bone pain and promoting overall bone health.

Ginger and Turmeric Bone Support Infusion

INGREDIENTS

- 1 teaspoon grated fresh ginger
- 1 teaspoon turmeric powder
- 1 cup boiling water

PREPARATION

1. Steep ginger and turmeric in boiling water for 10 minutes.

Strain and drink daily to reduce inflammation and support bone health. (#ol#)

Benefits: Ginger and turmeric are powerful anti-inflammatory herbs that help reduce joint pain and promote bone health. This infusion supports the body's ability to maintain strong, healthy bones.

Gotu Kola Joint Health Capsules

INGREDIENTS

- 1 tablespoon dried gotu kola powder
- Capsule shells

PREPARATION

1. Fill capsule shells with dried gotu kola powder.
2. Take 1-2 capsules daily to support joint health and reduce inflammation.

Benefits: Gotu kola helps improve circulation and reduce joint inflammation, making it an excellent herb for supporting joint health. These capsules promote flexibility and joint strength.

Fenugreek Bone Strength Powder

INGREDIENTS

- 1 tablespoon dried fenugreek seed powder

PREPARATION

1. Mix 1 teaspoon of fenugreek powder into warm water or juice.
2. Consume daily to support bone strength.

Benefits: Fenugreek is rich in calcium and other essential minerals that help strengthen bones and improve bone density. Regular intake supports healthy bones, especially for women at risk of osteoporosis.

Rose Hip Bone and Joint Tonic

INGREDIENTS

- 1 tablespoon dried rose hips
- 1 cup boiling water

PREPARATION

1. Steep rose hips in boiling water for 10 minutes.
2. Strain and drink daily to support bone and joint health.

Benefits: Rose hips are high in vitamin C and antioxidants, which help strengthen bones and reduce inflammation in the joints. This tonic promotes healthy connective tissues and supports joint mobility.

Burdock and Red Raspberry Leaf Infusion

INGREDIENTS

- 1 teaspoon dried burdock root
- 1 teaspoon dried red raspberry leaf
- 1 cup boiling water

PREPARATION

1. Steep burdock root and red raspberry leaf in boiling water for 10 minutes.
2. Strain and drink daily for bone health support.

Benefits: Burdock and red raspberry leaf are packed with minerals that support healthy bones. This infusion helps promote bone density and provides essential nutrients for overall skeletal health.

Calendula Calcium Support Capsules

INGREDIENTS

- 1 tablespoon dried calendula flower powder
- Capsule shells

PREPARATION

1. Fill capsule shells with dried calendula powder.
2. Take 1-2 capsules daily to support calcium absorption.

Benefits: Calendula is known for its anti-inflammatory properties and supports calcium absorption, helping to strengthen bones and reduce inflammation in joints.

Ashwagandha Bone Health Drops

INGREDIENTS

- 1 tablespoon dried ashwagandha root
- 1/4 cup alcohol (vodka or glycerin for a non-alcoholic option)

PREPARATION

1. Infuse ashwagandha root in alcohol or glycerin for 4-6 weeks.
2. Strain and take 1-2 droppers daily to support bone health.

Benefits: Ashwagandha is an adaptogen that supports bone strength, especially during times of stress. These drops help improve bone density and promote overall skeletal health.

Yarrow Bone Fortification Capsules

INGREDIENTS

- 1 tablespoon dried yarrow powder
- Capsule shells

PREPARATION

1. Fill capsule shells with dried yarrow powder.
2. Take 1-2 capsules daily to support bone fortification.

Benefits: Yarrow is rich in minerals that help support bone strength and fortification. These capsules help maintain healthy bones and reduce the risk of fractures.

Pine Bark Joint Strength Infusion

INGREDIENTS

- 1 teaspoon dried pine bark
- 1 cup boiling water

PREPARATION

1. Steep pine bark in boiling water for 10 minutes.
2. Strain and drink daily to support joint strength.

Benefits: Pine bark is a powerful antioxidant that helps protect joints and promote healthy cartilage. This infusion supports joint mobility and reduces inflammation in the joints.

Elderberry Joint Health Capsules

INGREDIENTS

- 1 tablespoon dried elderberry powder
- Capsule shells

PREPARATION

1. Fill capsule shells with dried elderberry powder.
2. Take 1-2 capsules daily to promote joint health.

Benefits: Elderberry is rich in antioxidants and anti-inflammatory compounds that support joint health. These capsules help reduce joint pain and stiffness while promoting flexibility.

Clary Sage Bone and Joint Support Tincture

INGREDIENTS

- 1 tablespoon dried clary sage leaves
- 1/4 cup alcohol (vodka or glycerin for a non-alcoholic option)

PREPARATION

1. Infuse clary sage leaves in alcohol or glycerin for 4-6 weeks.
2. Strain and take 1-2 droppers daily to support bones and joints.

Benefits: Clary sage helps balance hormones, which is vital for bone health. This tincture supports bone density and joint mobility, especially in post-menopausal women.

Peppermint and Licorice Bone Strength Tea

INGREDIENTS

- 1 teaspoon dried peppermint leaves
- 1 teaspoon dried licorice root
- 1 cup boiling water

PREPARATION

1. Steep peppermint and licorice root in boiling water for 10 minutes.
2. Strain and drink daily to support bone strength.

Benefits: Peppermint and licorice work together to support healthy bones by reducing inflammation and promoting calcium absorption. This tea helps improve bone density and joint health.

Lemon Balm Bone Health Lotion

INGREDIENTS

- 1 tablespoon dried lemon balm leaves
- 1/4 cup coconut oil

PREPARATION

1. Infuse lemon balm in melted coconut oil for 30 minutes.
2. Strain and store in a jar. Apply to joints and bones as needed.

Benefits: Lemon balm has anti-inflammatory properties that soothe bone and joint pain. This lotion helps reduce swelling and promotes bone health when applied topically.

Sage and Lavender Joint Support Balm

INGREDIENTS

- 1 tablespoon dried sage leaves
- 1 tablespoon dried lavender flowers
- 1/4 cup coconut oil

PREPARATION

1. Infuse sage and lavender in melted coconut oil for 30 minutes.
2. Strain and store in a jar. Apply to joints as needed for relief.

Benefits: Sage and lavender both have anti-inflammatory properties that help soothe joint pain and reduce swelling. This balm supports joint flexibility and comfort.

Echinacea Bone Recovery Capsules

INGREDIENTS

- 1 tablespoon dried echinacea root powder
- Capsule shells

PREPARATION

1. Fill capsule shells with dried echinacea root powder.
2. Take 1-2 capsules daily to support bone recovery.

Benefits: Echinacea supports the immune system and promotes faster recovery of bones after injury or surgery. These capsules are ideal for supporting bone healing and reducing inflammation.

Milk Thistle Bone Health Infusion

INGREDIENTS

- 1 teaspoon dried milk thistle seeds
- 1 cup boiling water

PREPARATION

1. Steep milk thistle seeds in boiling water for 10 minutes.
2. Strain and drink daily to support bone health and detoxify the body.

Benefits: Milk thistle helps detoxify the liver, which is crucial for proper calcium absorption and bone health. This infusion supports strong bones and overall detoxification.

Chamomile and Ginger Bone Strength Capsules

INGREDIENTS

- 1 tablespoon dried chamomile flowers
- 1 tablespoon dried ginger root powder
- Capsule shells

PREPARATION

1. Fill capsule shells with equal parts chamomile and ginger powder.
2. Take 1-2 capsules daily to reduce inflammation and support bone strength.

Benefits: Chamomile and ginger work together to reduce bone inflammation and support overall bone health. These capsules are ideal for maintaining strong and healthy bones.

Aloe Vera Joint Health Elixir

INGREDIENTS

- 2 tablespoons fresh aloe vera gel
- 1 cup water

PREPARATION

1. Blend fresh aloe vera gel with water until smooth.
2. Drink daily to support joint health and reduce inflammation.

Benefits: Aloe vera is known for its soothing and anti-inflammatory properties. This elixir helps reduce joint inflammation and promotes healthy joint function, making it ideal for those with arthritis or joint pain.

BOOK 23

Herbal Allies for Diabetes Support

Managing Blood Sugar Levels with Herbs

NATURAL HERBAL SOLUTIONS FOR BLOOD SUGAR MANAGEMENT

Managing blood sugar levels naturally is essential for individuals like Emma who seek holistic approaches to support their health and prevent complications associated with diabetes. Herbs have long been used in traditional medicine to regulate glucose levels, enhance insulin function, and maintain overall metabolic balance. Integrating these herbs into her daily routine can offer Emma a natural and effective way to manage her blood sugar levels, complementing her dietary and lifestyle practices. Here, we explore some of the most effective herbs for blood sugar management and how Emma can incorporate them into her wellness journey.

Bitter Melon: A Natural Glucose Regulator

Bitter melon (Momordica charantia) is a powerful herb traditionally used in Ayurvedic and Chinese medicine for its blood sugar-lowering properties. It contains compounds such as charantin and polypeptide-p, which mimic insulin's action, helping to lower blood glucose levels. Bitter melon also enhances glucose uptake in the cells, which can be beneficial for those with insulin resistance.

Emma can consume bitter melon as a juice, in capsule form, or even cooked in meals. While the taste may be bitter, its effects on blood sugar are profound, making it a worthwhile addition to her regimen. Incorporating bitter melon juice into her morning routine, for example, can help regulate her blood sugar levels throughout the day. This aligns with her preference for natural solutions that offer tangible results.

Fenugreek Seeds: Supporting Insulin Function

Fenugreek seeds are rich in soluble fiber and contain compounds that slow carbohydrate digestion and absorption, thereby reducing post-meal blood sugar spikes. The seeds also improve insulin sensitivity, making it easier for the body to regulate glucose levels naturally. Fenugreek's ability to lower fasting blood sugar levels has been well-documented, making it an essential herb for diabetes support.

Emma can incorporate fenugreek into her diet by adding the seeds to her meals or drinking fenugreek tea. Soaking the seeds overnight and consuming them on an empty stomach is a traditional practice known to stabilize blood sugar levels effectively. For those like Emma who appreciate simple and natural approaches, fenugreek offers an accessible way to manage glucose fluctuations.

Cinnamon: Enhancing Glucose Metabolism

Cinnamon (Cinnamomum verum) is a well-known spice with significant blood sugar-regulating properties. It works by improving insulin sensitivity and increasing glucose uptake by cells. Studies have shown that cinnamon can reduce fasting blood sugar levels and improve hemoglobin A1c, a marker of long-term glucose control.

Its active compound, cinnamaldehyde, plays a crucial role in enhancing insulin function.

For Emma, adding cinnamon to her diet is straightforward. She can sprinkle cinnamon powder on her oatmeal, blend it into smoothies, or enjoy it as a tea. This flexibility makes cinnamon an easy and pleasant addition to her daily routine, supporting her holistic approach to managing blood sugar naturally. The sweet, warming flavor of cinnamon also makes it a comforting, sustainable choice.

Gymnema Sylvestre: The Sugar Destroyer

Gymnema Sylvestre, often called the "sugar destroyer," is another potent herb for managing blood sugar levels. Gymnemic acids, its active compounds, reduce the absorption of sugar in the intestines and enhance insulin function. By suppressing the taste of sweetness, gymnema can also help curb sugar cravings, making it easier for individuals like Emma to maintain a balanced diet without the temptation of sugary foods.

Emma can take gymnema in capsule form or as a tea before meals to maximize its effects. Using gymnema regularly helps regulate her blood sugar levels while supporting her long-term wellness goals. Its dual action—reducing sugar absorption and suppressing sugar cravings—aligns perfectly with Emma's holistic lifestyle, providing her with a comprehensive approach to blood sugar management.

Berberine: A Plant Compound for Blood Sugar Control

Berberine is an alkaloid found in various plants like goldenseal and barberry. It has been widely studied for its blood sugar-lowering properties, comparable to some pharmaceutical treatments. Berberine activates an enzyme called AMP-activated protein kinase (AMPK), which plays a crucial role in regulating metabolism and maintaining blood sugar levels. It also enhances insulin sensitivity, promoting better glucose uptake and utilization.

Emma can take berberine as a supplement, ensuring she follows the recommended dosage, as it can be quite potent. Including berberine in her routine offers a natural, evidence-based solution for managing blood sugar. This approach fits her preference for using well-researched, natural methods that support her body's metabolic processes.

Holy Basil: An Adaptogen for Blood Sugar Balance

Holy basil (Ocimum sanctum), also known as tulsi, is an adaptogenic herb that supports the body's stress response while regulating blood sugar levels. Chronic stress can lead to elevated blood sugar, as stress hormones like cortisol promote glucose release into the bloodstream. Holy basil helps balance these hormones, reducing stress-induced glucose spikes. Additionally, it has been shown to enhance insulin function and lower fasting blood sugar levels.

Emma can include holy basil as a tea, tincture, or capsule. Drinking holy basil tea throughout the day provides her with both stress relief and blood sugar support. By addressing the root causes of elevated blood sugar, holy basil offers a holistic solution that fits Emma's wellness philosophy, ensuring her approach is both proactive and comprehensive.

Aloe Vera: Promoting Insulin Sensitivity

Aloe vera is not only known for its skin-healing properties but also for its potential to lower blood sugar levels. The gel from aloe vera leaves contains compounds that improve insulin sensitivity and help reduce fasting blood sugar levels. For Emma, incorporating aloe vera juice into her daily routine offers an easy and hydrating way to support her blood sugar management.

Consuming aloe vera juice in the morning, ideally before meals, can help stabilize blood sugar throughout the day. This simple addition to her diet complements her holistic approach to wellness, providing her with a natural and effective means of maintaining balance.

These herbs provide Emma with a wide array of options to manage her blood sugar levels naturally. By integrating these remedies into her lifestyle, she can take control of her health and reduce her reliance on conventional medications, aligning with her preference for sustainable and holistic solutions. This comprehensive approach ensures that she not only manages her blood sugar levels but also supports her overall well-being, fostering a balanced and fulfilling wellness journey.

Herbs for Insulin Sensitivity and Pancreatic Health

NATURAL HERBS FOR ENHANCING INSULIN SENSITIVITY AND PANCREATIC HEALTH

Maintaining proper insulin sensitivity and supporting pancreatic function are crucial for individuals managing diabetes naturally. Emma, like many who prefer holistic approaches, can benefit from herbs that enhance insulin efficiency and promote pancreatic health. These herbs not only support the regulation of blood sugar levels but also contribute to overall well-being, ensuring a balanced and sustainable approach to managing diabetes. Below, we explore some of the most effective herbs that enhance insulin sensitivity and support pancreatic health.

Fenugreek: A Time-Tested Insulin Enhancer

Fenugreek (Trigonella foenum-graecum) is a well-known herb in traditional medicine, particularly in Ayurvedic practices, for its ability to improve insulin sensitivity. The seeds contain soluble fiber and compounds such as 4-hydroxyisoleucine, which enhance insulin release and improve glucose metabolism. This makes fenugreek a powerful ally for Emma as she seeks to stabilize her blood sugar levels through natural means.

For Emma, integrating fenugreek into her diet is straightforward. She can consume the seeds soaked in water, as a tea, or in powdered form. Soaking a teaspoon of fenugreek seeds overnight and consuming them in the morning offers a simple and effective method to boost insulin sensitivity. This approach aligns with her preference for easily accessible herbal solutions that fit seamlessly into her daily routine.

Berberine: Nature's Powerful Insulin Activator

Berberine is an active compound found in several plants, such as goldenseal, Oregon grape, and barberry. It has gained attention for its potent ability to improve insulin sensitivity and promote pancreatic health. Berberine activates an enzyme known as AMP-activated protein kinase (AMPK), which plays a significant role in regulating glucose uptake and metabolism, much like the mechanism of some pharmaceutical treatments for diabetes.

Emma can incorporate berberine as a supplement, ensuring that she follows the recommended dosage, as it can be quite potent. Regular use of berberine not only enhances insulin function but also protects pancreatic cells from damage, promoting overall health. This herb's scientific backing provides Emma with confidence in its effectiveness, aligning with her preference for well-researched, evidence-based natural therapies.

Bitter Melon: Supporting Pancreatic Function

Bitter melon (Momordica charantia) is a traditional herb used for managing diabetes in many cultures, including Chinese and Ayurvedic medicine. It contains compounds like charantin and polypeptide-p, which act similarly to insulin, helping to lower blood sugar levels naturally. Furthermore, bitter melon supports pancreatic health by enhancing insulin production and improving the regeneration of beta cells—the cells responsible for insulin secretion.

For Emma, consuming bitter melon juice or capsules before meals can help stabilize her blood sugar levels throughout the day. Though the taste may be bitter, the herb's profound effects on insulin sensitivity and pancreatic function make it a valuable addition to her routine. Its ability to support insulin production while also enhancing sensitivity ensures that Emma's body remains efficient in regulating glucose levels.

Holy Basil: An Adaptogen for Insulin and Pancreatic Support

Holy basil (Ocimum sanctum), also known as tulsi, is an adaptogenic herb that not only helps manage stress but also enhances insulin sensitivity. Chronic stress can lead to elevated cortisol levels, which negatively impact insulin function and blood sugar regulation. Holy basil works to balance stress hormones, indirectly improving insulin function and protecting pancreatic health.

Emma can incorporate holy basil as a tea, tincture, or supplement. Drinking holy basil tea daily provides her with a dual benefit: reducing stress and enhancing insulin sensitivity. By using an adaptogen like holy basil, Emma can address multiple aspects of her health, ensuring that her approach to managing diabetes is both comprehensive and holistic.

Gymnema Sylvestre: The Pancreatic Protector

Gymnema Sylvestre is often referred to as the "sugar destroyer" due to its ability to block the taste of sweetness and reduce sugar cravings. More importantly, gymnema has shown to enhance insulin production and promote the regeneration of pancreatic beta cells. These actions make it a crucial herb for improving insulin sensitivity and protecting pancreatic health, especially for individuals managing diabetes.

Emma can take gymnema as a tea or in capsule form. Consuming gymnema before meals can help reduce her body's absorption of sugar while supporting insulin function. The herb's protective effects on the pancreas make it an essential component of Emma's natural diabetes management plan, ensuring she has a balanced approach to both blood sugar control and pancreatic health.

Turmeric: Reducing Inflammation for Better Insulin Function

Turmeric (Curcuma longa) is widely recognized for its anti-inflammatory properties, which are essential in managing diabetes. Chronic inflammation can interfere with insulin function, making it difficult for the body to regulate glucose levels effectively. Curcumin, the active compound in turmeric, has been shown to reduce inflammation and enhance insulin sensitivity, making it a valuable herb for those managing diabetes.

Emma can consume turmeric as a tea, in her meals, or in supplement form. By incorporating turmeric into her daily diet, she not only supports insulin function but also protects her pancreas from inflammation-related damage. Turmeric's versatility and accessibility align with Emma's preference for integrating practical and effective herbal solutions into her lifestyle.

Cinnamon: A Metabolic Booster for Insulin Efficiency

Cinnamon (Cinnamomum verum) is another potent herb known for its effects on insulin sensitivity and glucose metabolism. It enhances insulin function by improving glucose uptake in the cells, making it an effective tool for managing blood sugar levels. The active compounds in cinnamon, such as cinnamaldehyde, help the body respond better to insulin, promoting healthier blood sugar regulation.

Emma can add cinnamon to her meals, beverages, or take it as a tea. Its sweet and warming flavor makes it an enjoyable and easy herb to include in her daily routine. Regular use of cinnamon not only supports insulin sensitivity but also aligns with Emma's preference for simple, accessible, and effective natural remedies.

These herbs provide Emma with a range of natural solutions to enhance insulin sensitivity and protect pancreatic health. By integrating these options into her daily wellness practices, she can manage her blood sugar levels effectively while adhering to her holistic approach to health. This comprehensive strategy ensures that Emma has the tools she needs to maintain balance and support her body's natural functions, reinforcing her commitment to sustainable and natural wellness.

Remedies for Diabetes and Blood Sugar Control

Bitter Melon Blood Sugar Balance Capsules

INGREDIENTS

- 1 tablespoon dried bitter melon powder
- Capsule shells

PREPARATION

1. Fill capsule shells with dried bitter melon powder.
2. Take 1-2 capsules daily to support blood sugar balance.

Benefits: Bitter melon helps reduce blood sugar levels by improving insulin sensitivity and glucose metabolism. It is particularly beneficial for managing diabetes and preventing blood sugar spikes.

Cinnamon and Clove Blood Sugar Tea

INGREDIENTS

- 1 teaspoon ground cinnamon
- 1/2 teaspoon whole cloves
- 1 cup boiling water

PREPARATION

1. Steep cinnamon and cloves in boiling water for 10 minutes.
2. Strain and drink daily to support balanced blood sugar levels.

Benefits: Cinnamon is known to improve insulin sensitivity and reduce blood sugar levels, while cloves offer additional antioxidant support. This tea is a natural way to control blood sugar and enhance metabolic health.

Fenugreek Seed Insulin Support Capsules

INGREDIENTS

- 1 tablespoon dried fenugreek seed powder
- Capsule shells

PREPARATION

1. Fill capsule shells with dried fenugreek seed powder.
2. Take 1-2 capsules daily to support insulin function and blood sugar control.

Benefits: Fenugreek seeds help regulate insulin production and improve glucose metabolism, making them highly effective in managing diabetes and reducing blood sugar spikes.

Gymnema Leaf Sugar Craving Control Tea

INGREDIENTS

- 1 teaspoon dried gymnema leaves
- 1 cup boiling water

PREPARATION

1. Steep gymnema leaves in boiling water for 10 minutes.
2. Strain and drink to curb sugar cravings and regulate blood sugar levels.

Benefits: Gymnema has the unique ability to block the taste of sugar and reduce cravings. It also helps improve insulin function, making it an excellent choice for people managing diabetes.

Nettle Leaf Blood Sugar Control Infusion

INGREDIENTS

- 1 teaspoon dried nettle leaves
- 1 cup boiling water

PREPARATION

1. Steep nettle leaves in boiling water for 10 minutes.
2. Strain and drink daily to support blood sugar control.

Benefits: Nettle is a nutrient-dense herb that helps regulate blood sugar levels and improve insulin sensitivity. This infusion provides support for diabetes management and overall metabolic health.

Dandelion Root Diabetic Support Capsules

INGREDIENTS

- 1 tablespoon dried dandelion root powder
- Capsule shells

PREPARATION

1. Fill capsule shells with dried dandelion root powder.
2. Take 1-2 capsules daily to support diabetic health.

Benefits: Dandelion root supports liver function and helps detoxify the body, both of which are essential for healthy blood sugar levels. These capsules are a beneficial addition to a diabetes management regimen.

Lemon Balm Sugar Regulation Tincture

INGREDIENTS

- 1 tablespoon dried lemon balm leaves
- 1/4 cup alcohol (vodka or glycerin for a non-alcoholic option)

PREPARATION

1. Infuse lemon balm leaves in alcohol or glycerin for 4-6 weeks.
2. Strain and take 1-2 droppers daily to regulate blood sugar levels.

Benefits: Lemon balm helps reduce stress, which can have a positive impact on blood sugar levels. This tincture supports balanced glucose levels while promoting relaxation.

Holy Basil (Tulsi) Diabetic Health Elixir

INGREDIENTS

- 1 teaspoon dried holy basil (tulsi) leaves
- 1 cup boiling water

PREPARATION

1. Steep holy basil leaves in boiling water for 10 minutes.
2. Strain and drink daily to support diabetic health.

Benefits: Holy basil is an adaptogen that helps manage stress and improve insulin sensitivity. This elixir supports blood sugar balance and overall well-being, making it ideal for managing diabetes.

Aloe Vera Sugar Control Gel

INGREDIENTS

- 2 tablespoons fresh aloe vera gel
- 1 cup water

PREPARATION

1. Blend fresh aloe vera gel with water until smooth.
2. Drink daily to support blood sugar regulation.

Benefits: Aloe vera helps reduce blood sugar levels by improving insulin sensitivity and promoting glucose metabolism. This gel supports overall diabetic health and helps manage blood sugar.

Goat's Rue Insulin Support Capsules

INGREDIENTS

- 1 tablespoon dried goat's rue powder
- Capsule shells

PREPARATION

1. Fill capsule shells with dried goat's rue powder.
2. Take 1-2 capsules daily to support insulin sensitivity and glucose metabolism.

Benefits: Goat's rue is known for its ability to improve insulin function and support healthy glucose levels. These capsules are a natural way to enhance insulin sensitivity and manage diabetes.

Blueberry Leaf Blood Sugar Tea

INGREDIENTS

- 1 teaspoon dried blueberry leaves
- 1 cup boiling water

PREPARATION

1. Steep blueberry leaves in boiling water for 10 minutes.
2. Strain and drink daily to regulate blood sugar.

Benefits: Blueberry leaves help reduce blood sugar levels and improve insulin sensitivity. This tea provides antioxidant support while promoting balanced glucose levels in diabetics.

Hibiscus Blood Pressure Control Tea

INGREDIENTS

- 1 teaspoon dried hibiscus flowers
- 1 cup boiling water

PREPARATION

1. Steep hibiscus flowers in boiling water for 10 minutes.
2. Strain and drink daily to support blood pressure and blood sugar control.

Benefits: Hibiscus helps lower blood pressure and supports cardiovascular health, both of which are crucial for individuals managing diabetes. This tea helps promote overall well-being by regulating blood sugar and blood pressure.

Ginger and Turmeric Sugar Balance Infusion

INGREDIENTS

- 1 teaspoon grated fresh ginger
- 1/2 teaspoon turmeric powder
- 1 cup boiling water

PREPARATION

1. Steep ginger and turmeric in boiling water for 10 minutes.
2. Strain and drink daily to support blood sugar balance.

Benefits: Ginger and turmeric are powerful anti-inflammatory agents that help regulate blood sugar and improve insulin sensitivity. This infusion is beneficial for managing diabetes and promoting metabolic health.

Ginseng Glucose Control Capsules

INGREDIENTS

- 1 tablespoon dried ginseng root powder
- Capsule shells

PREPARATION

1. Fill capsule shells with dried ginseng root powder.
2. Take 1-2 capsules daily to regulate glucose levels.

Benefits: Ginseng is known to improve insulin function and help regulate blood sugar. These capsules support balanced blood glucose levels and promote overall metabolic health.

Oregano Leaf Blood Sugar Regulation Oil

INGREDIENTS

- 1 tablespoon dried oregano leaves
- 1/4 cup olive oil

PREPARATION

1. Infuse oregano leaves in olive oil for 2 weeks.
2. Strain and use 1 teaspoon of the oil daily to support blood sugar regulation.

Benefits: Oregano oil has been shown to improve insulin sensitivity and support balanced blood sugar levels. This oil helps manage glucose levels naturally and promotes healthy metabolic function.

Bay Leaf Diabetic Support Tea

INGREDIENTS

- 1 teaspoon dried bay leaves
- 1 cup boiling water

PREPARATION

1. Steep bay leaves in boiling water for 10 minutes.
2. Strain and drink daily to support diabetic health.

Benefits: Bay leaves help regulate blood sugar and improve insulin sensitivity. This tea is beneficial for individuals managing diabetes as it supports overall metabolic health and balanced glucose levels.

Sage Glucose Balance Capsules

INGREDIENTS

- 1 tablespoon dried sage leaf powder
- Capsule
- shells

PREPARATION

1. Fill capsule shells with dried sage powder.
2. Take 1-2 capsules daily to support glucose balance.

Benefits: Sage has been shown to improve insulin sensitivity and regulate blood sugar levels. These capsules support glucose balance and promote overall health in diabetics.

Echinacea Immune Support Capsules for Diabetics

INGREDIENTS

- Echinacea root powder
- Empty vegetable capsules

PREPARATION

1. Fill the empty vegetable capsules with echinacea root powder using a capsule filler or by hand.
2. Store the filled capsules in a cool, dry place.
3. Take one capsule daily or as recommended by a healthcare professional.

Benefits: Echinacea is known for its immune-boosting properties, which are particularly beneficial for diabetics who may experience weakened immune systems. This remedy helps strengthen the immune response, reducing the likelihood of infections and improving overall health. Additionally, echinacea has anti-inflammatory properties that may support better blood sugar control and enhance overall wellness in those managing diabetes.

Yarrow Blood Sugar Management Infusion

INGREDIENTS

- 1 teaspoon dried yarrow leaves
- 1 cup hot water

PREPARATION

1. Add the dried yarrow leaves to a cup of hot water.
2. Steep for 10 minutes, then strain the infusion.
3. Drink once daily, preferably in the morning.

Benefits: Yarrow is traditionally used for its anti-inflammatory and blood sugar-regulating properties. It may help stabilize blood sugar levels, making it beneficial for individuals managing diabetes. Additionally, yarrow supports circulation and reduces inflammation, contributing to overall metabolic health.

Rosemary Blood Pressure and Sugar Control Drops

INGREDIENTS

- Fresh rosemary leaves
- Vodka or apple cider vinegar (for tincture base)

PREPARATION

1. Place fresh rosemary leaves in a jar and cover them with vodka or apple cider vinegar.
2. Seal the jar and let it sit for 4-6 weeks, shaking occasionally.
3. Strain the mixture and store it in a dropper bottle.
4. Take 15-20 drops daily in water.

Benefits: Rosemary is known for its ability to support cardiovascular health by improving circulation and lowering blood pressure, both crucial for managing diabetes. Its antioxidant properties also help regulate blood sugar levels and reduce inflammation, enhancing overall health.

Chamomile Blood Glucose Support Tea

INGREDIENTS

- 1 teaspoon dried chamomile flowers
- 1 cup hot water

PREPARATION

1. Add chamomile flowers to hot water and steep for 5-10 minutes.
2. Strain the tea and drink it warm.

Benefits: Chamomile tea is not only calming but also effective in managing blood sugar levels. Its anti-inflammatory and antioxidant properties help reduce blood glucose levels, providing a natural way to manage diabetes. Additionally, it aids in digestive health and relaxation, which is beneficial for overall wellness.

Licorice Root Sugar Level Control Capsules

INGREDIENTS

- Licorice root powder
- Empty vegetable capsules

PREPARATION

1. Fill vegetable capsules with licorice root powder.
2. Store capsules in a cool, dry place.
3. Take one capsule daily as directed by a healthcare provider.

Benefits: Licorice root contains compounds that can help balance blood sugar levels and improve insulin resistance, making it beneficial for diabetics. It also has anti-inflammatory and antioxidant properties that support the immune system and overall metabolic health.

Mulberry Leaf Blood Sugar Support Tea

INGREDIENTS

- 1 teaspoon dried mulberry leaves
- 1 cup hot water

PREPARATION

1. Add the dried mulberry leaves to a cup of hot water.
2. Steep for 5-7 minutes, then strain.
3. Drink once or twice daily.

Benefits: Mulberry leaves contain compounds that help regulate blood sugar levels and improve insulin sensitivity. Drinking this tea regularly can assist in maintaining stable glucose levels, supporting a diabetic-friendly lifestyle. Additionally, it offers antioxidants that protect against cell damage and inflammation.

Dandelion and Peppermint Sugar Balance Capsules

INGREDIENTS

- Dried dandelion root powder
- Dried peppermint leaf powder
- Empty vegetable capsules

PREPARATION

1. Mix the dandelion root powder and peppermint leaf powder.
2. Fill vegetable capsules with the mixture.
3. Store capsules in a cool, dry place.
4. Take one capsule daily.

Benefits: Dandelion and peppermint work synergistically to promote healthy blood sugar levels and improve digestion. Dandelion supports liver function and detoxification, while peppermint aids in digestion and helps reduce inflammation. Together, they enhance metabolic health and support blood sugar balance.

Lemon Verbena Insulin Support Tea

INGREDIENTS

- 1 teaspoon dried lemon verbena leaves
- 1 cup hot water

PREPARATION

1. Steep lemon verbena leaves in hot water for 5-10 minutes.
2. Strain the tea and drink it warm.

Benefits: Lemon verbena has natural properties that may enhance insulin sensitivity, making it a beneficial herb for managing blood sugar levels. It also offers calming effects, which help reduce stress—a factor that can influence blood glucose levels. Regular consumption may support balanced insulin and glucose levels.

Burdock Root Diabetic Health Capsules

INGREDIENTS

- Burdock root powder
- Empty vegetable capsules

PREPARATION

1. Fill capsules with burdock root powder.
2. Store capsules in a dry, cool environment.
3. Take one capsule daily.

Benefits: Burdock root is known for its detoxifying properties and its ability to support liver health, which is crucial for managing blood sugar levels. Its anti-inflammatory and antioxidant effects help improve insulin sensitivity and reduce complications related to diabetes.

Goldenseal Sugar Regulation Drops

INGREDIENTS

- Goldenseal root
- Vodka or apple cider vinegar (for tincture)

PREPARATION

1. Place goldenseal root in a jar and cover with vodka or apple cider vinegar.
2. Let it steep for 4-6 weeks, shaking occasionally.
3. Strain and store in a dropper bottle.
4. Take 15-20 drops daily in water.

Benefits: Goldenseal contains berberine, a compound known to help regulate blood sugar levels. It also has antimicrobial properties that strengthen the immune system, which is especially important for diabetics. This tincture supports both sugar balance and overall health.

Milk Thistle Blood Sugar Detox Tea

INGREDIENTS

- 1 teaspoon milk thistle seeds
- 1 cup hot water

PREPARATION

1. Crush the milk thistle seeds and add them to hot water.
2. Steep for 10 minutes, then strain.
3. Drink once daily.

Benefits: Milk thistle supports liver health, which plays a key role in regulating blood sugar levels. Its detoxifying properties aid in cleansing the liver, helping improve insulin function and glucose metabolism. It is a valuable ally in managing diabetes and maintaining overall metabolic health.

Spearmint Blood Glucose Balance Infusion

INGREDIENTS

- 1 teaspoon dried spearmint leaves
- 1 cup hot water

PREPARATION

1. Add dried spearmint leaves to hot water and steep for 5 minutes.
2. Strain and enjoy warm or cold.

Benefits: Spearmint is known for its digestive benefits and its ability to regulate blood sugar levels. Drinking spearmint infusion can help maintain balanced glucose levels, while its calming effects aid in reducing stress—a factor that can influence blood sugar.

Linden Flower Diabetic Support Capsules

INGREDIENTS

- Dried linden flowers
- Empty vegetable capsules

PREPARATION

1. Grind dried linden flowers into a fine powder.
2. Fill capsules with the powder.
3. Store in a cool, dry place.
4. Take one capsule daily.

Benefits: Linden flowers help manage blood sugar levels and reduce inflammation, supporting diabetics in maintaining stable glucose levels. They also promote relaxation, which can be beneficial in managing stress-related spikes in blood sugar.

Triphala Ayurvedic Sugar Balance Capsules

INGREDIENTS

- Triphala powder
- Empty vegetable capsules

PREPARATION

1. Fill capsules with triphala powder.
2. Store in a cool, dry place.
3. Take one capsule daily before meals.

Benefits: Triphala, a blend of three fruits, is an ancient Ayurvedic remedy known for its blood sugar balancing and digestive health benefits. It supports insulin sensitivity and reduces blood sugar levels, making it a powerful supplement for diabetes management.

Red Clover Diabetic Health Infusion

INGREDIENTS

- 1 teaspoon dried red clover flowers
- 1 cup hot water

PREPARATION

1. Steep red clover flowers in hot water for 10 minutes.
2. Strain and drink warm.

Benefits: Red clover has anti-inflammatory properties that help manage blood sugar levels and reduce the risk of complications in diabetics. Its phytoestrogens also support cardiovascular health, making it a valuable addition to a diabetic's wellness regimen.

Olive Leaf Blood Sugar Capsules

INGREDIENTS

- Olive leaf powder
- Empty vegetable capsules

PREPARATION

1. Fill capsules with olive leaf powder.
2. Store capsules in a cool, dry place.
3. Take one capsule daily.

Benefits: Olive leaf is known for its ability to lower blood sugar levels and improve insulin sensitivity. Its antioxidant properties also help reduce inflammation and protect against diabetic complications, supporting overall health and wellness.

BOOK 24

Boosting Cognitive Function Naturally

Herbs for Memory and Brain Performance

ENHANCING MEMORY AND BRAIN PERFORMANCE WITH HERBAL REMEDIES

Cognitive function and memory are central to our daily lives, influencing everything from problem-solving to creativity and long-term learning. For those like Emma, who seek to boost brain performance while maintaining a natural and holistic lifestyle, certain herbs offer profound benefits. By incorporating these herbs into her daily routine, Emma can enhance her cognitive abilities and memory retention, supporting her goals of staying mentally sharp and focused. Below, we explore several herbs that have proven effective in enhancing brain function, improving memory, and sustaining cognitive health.

Ginkgo Biloba: The Ancient Memory Booster

Ginkgo biloba, one of the oldest known medicinal plants, has been used for centuries in traditional Chinese medicine to enhance memory and mental clarity. It works primarily by improving blood circulation to the brain, ensuring that neurons receive ample oxygen and nutrients. This increased blood flow supports cognitive function, sharpens focus, and improves memory retention.

For Emma, taking ginkgo biloba as a supplement or tea can be an effective way to integrate its benefits into her daily routine. Ginkgo's antioxidants also help protect brain cells from oxidative stress, a critical factor in maintaining long-term brain health. Its dual action—improving circulation and protecting neurons—makes it a valuable herb for those who prioritize both immediate cognitive enhancement and long-term brain wellness.

Bacopa Monnieri: The Herb of Longevity

Known as a potent adaptogen and brain tonic in Ayurveda, Bacopa monnieri, or brahmi, is another powerful herb for boosting cognitive performance and memory. Bacopa has been shown to enhance communication between neurons, supporting memory retention and learning abilities. It contains bacosides, compounds that help repair damaged neurons and enhance synaptic communication, making it an effective solution for those seeking to improve both short-term and long-term memory.

Emma can consume Bacopa monnieri as a supplement, tincture, or tea. Regular use of this herb supports her goal of achieving a balanced and efficient cognitive function. Bacopa's ability to reduce anxiety and stress further enhances its benefits, as a calm mind is better able to absorb and retain information. For Emma, who values practical, multi-benefit remedies, bacopa provides a comprehensive approach to cognitive wellness.

Rosemary: The Aromatic Brain Stimulant

Rosemary (Rosmarinus officinalis) is not just a kitchen herb; it has significant cognitive-enhancing properties as well. Inhaling rosemary's aroma has been shown to improve memory performance and increase alertness. The active compound, 1,8-cineole, is believed to interact with brain chemistry, boosting levels of neurotransmitters like acetylcholine, which play a crucial role in learning and memory.

Emma can use rosemary in various ways—adding it to meals, using rosemary essential oil for aromatherapy, or even drinking it as an herbal tea. Incorporating rosemary oil into her daily routine, whether by diffusing it in her workspace or applying it topically, provides her with an accessible and effective method to enhance cognitive function naturally. This aligns with her preference for integrating easily available herbs into her holistic lifestyle.

Gotu Kola: The Mind-Calming Brain Tonic

Gotu kola (Centella asiatica) is another revered herb in Ayurvedic and traditional Chinese medicine for its cognitive-enhancing properties. Often called the "herb of longevity," gotu kola is known to improve memory, reduce mental fatigue, and support overall brain health. It enhances blood flow to the brain, similar to ginkgo biloba, but also has adaptogenic properties, helping to calm the nervous system.

Emma can take gotu kola as a tea or in capsule form to reap its benefits. Its calming effects make it ideal for reducing stress, which can often impair memory and focus. By promoting both relaxation and cognitive enhancement, gotu kola fits seamlessly into Emma's holistic regimen, providing her with a natural, well-rounded solution for mental clarity and memory support.

Sage: The Herb for Mental Clarity

Sage (Salvia officinalis) is well-regarded not only for its culinary uses but also for its powerful effects on memory and brain performance. Research suggests that sage can inhibit the breakdown of acetylcholine, a neurotransmitter critical for learning and memory. Sage's antioxidant properties also help protect the brain from free radical damage, which is crucial for long-term cognitive health.

Emma can incorporate sage into her routine by drinking sage tea or using sage essential oil for aromatherapy. Consuming sage regularly supports both her immediate memory retention and her overall cognitive wellness, offering her a simple and effective way to stay mentally sharp. Its dual ability to enhance clarity and protect the brain aligns perfectly with her goals of maintaining cognitive function naturally.

Lion's Mane Mushroom: A Natural Nootropic

Lion's mane mushroom (Hericium erinaceus) is gaining popularity as a natural nootropic for its ability to support brain health and improve memory. Lion's mane stimulates the production of nerve growth factor (NGF) and brain-derived neurotrophic factor (BDNF), both of which are essential for the growth and maintenance of neurons. This unique ability makes lion's mane a powerful herb for enhancing cognitive function, supporting memory, and promoting overall brain longevity.

Emma can take lion's mane as a supplement, tea, or even incorporate it into her meals as a powder. Its versatility allows her to choose a method that best fits her lifestyle. The herb's neuroprotective properties make it an excellent choice for those like Emma who seek not only immediate cognitive benefits but also long-term brain health support. By including lion's mane in her daily regimen, Emma ensures her approach to cognitive enhancement is comprehensive and sustainable.

Ginseng: The Energy and Memory Booster

Ginseng, particularly Panax ginseng, is another herb known for its ability to enhance mental performance and support memory. Ginsenosides, the active compounds in ginseng, help improve focus, reduce mental fatigue, and enhance overall cognitive function. Ginseng also supports energy levels, providing a balanced approach to maintaining focus and mental clarity throughout the day.

For Emma, taking ginseng as a tea or supplement can be a valuable way to integrate this herb's benefits into her daily routine. Its ability to boost both energy and cognitive function makes it ideal for days when she needs to stay sharp and focused. Ginseng's reputation as a brain tonic provides Emma with confidence that she is using a well-established herb for cognitive enhancement.

These herbs offer Emma a variety of options to naturally support memory and brain performance. By integrating these into her daily wellness practices, she can enhance her cognitive function sustainably while remaining aligned with her holistic and natural approach to health. This comprehensive strategy ensures that Emma has the tools she needs to maintain mental sharpness and clarity, supporting her long-term well-being and wellness goals.

Natural Solutions for Mental Fatigue and Focus

EFFECTIVE NATURAL REMEDIES FOR COMBATING MENTAL FATIGUE AND ENHANCING FOCUS

Mental fatigue and difficulty focusing are increasingly common challenges, particularly in today's fast-paced, information-heavy world. Emma, like many individuals, may experience periods of low energy, brain fog, and difficulty maintaining concentration throughout the day. For those seeking natural and holistic approaches to manage these symptoms, several solutions offer profound benefits. Incorporating these natural remedies can help Emma restore her mental clarity, enhance focus, and maintain energy levels without relying on synthetic stimulants or pharmaceutical solutions.

Adaptogens: Nature's Stress Resilience Allies

Adaptogenic herbs, such as rhodiola and ashwagandha, play a critical role in managing stress and improving mental focus. These herbs help balance the body's response to stress, which, when unregulated, can significantly contribute to mental fatigue. Rhodiola, for instance, is known for its ability to enhance cognitive function and reduce fatigue by balancing the production of stress hormones like cortisol. By maintaining hormonal balance, rhodiola supports Emma's overall resilience, enabling her to stay focused and alert even during demanding periods.

Ashwagandha, another powerful adaptogen, not only reduces stress but also supports mental clarity and cognitive performance. Its ability to enhance energy levels naturally makes it an excellent option for those who feel mentally drained or unable to concentrate. Emma can incorporate these adaptogens into her routine through teas, capsules, or tinctures, ensuring a flexible and convenient approach to boosting her mental stamina.

Nootropic Herbs: Boosting Brain Function Naturally

Nootropics, or brain-enhancing herbs, provide Emma with a natural alternative to synthetic stimulants for improving focus and clarity. Gotu kola, for example, has been used traditionally in Ayurvedic medicine to enhance cognitive function and combat mental fatigue. It works by increasing blood circulation to the brain, improving alertness, and supporting long-term memory function. Regular use of gotu kola can help Emma feel more focused, energetic, and mentally clear, especially when she needs to manage multiple tasks efficiently.

Another effective nootropic is ginkgo biloba, which enhances blood flow to the brain and provides essential nutrients that support mental performance. For Emma, taking ginkgo biloba as a tea or supplement could be an effective strategy for boosting her cognitive function, especially when she needs to combat brain fog or maintain focus during prolonged periods of concentration. These herbs offer a balanced and sustainable way to improve mental clarity and focus without the need for caffeine or other stimulants that may lead to crashes.

Peppermint and Rosemary: Aromatherapy for Instant Clarity

Aromatherapy using essential oils like peppermint and rosemary can also be a quick and effective method for improving focus and reducing mental fatigue. Research has shown that inhaling peppermint oil can enhance alertness and reduce the feeling of mental exhaustion, making it an excellent tool for Emma when she needs an immediate boost. She can simply diffuse peppermint oil in her workspace or apply it to her wrists for quick and easy access throughout the day.

Rosemary, another aromatic herb, has been linked to improved cognitive performance and memory retention. Inhaling rosemary oil stimulates brain function and enhances mental clarity, making it ideal for Emma during periods of intense work or study. This approach offers her a practical, non-invasive way to enhance her focus using natural, accessible remedies.

Ginseng: A Natural Energy Booster

Ginseng, particularly Panax ginseng, is a powerful herb known for its ability to boost energy levels and enhance mental clarity. Ginseng works as a natural stimulant, providing a gentle increase in energy without the jitters or crashes associated with caffeine. It supports cognitive performance by improving circulation and reducing stress, making it an excellent option for Emma when she needs sustained mental energy.

Taking ginseng as a tea or supplement allows Emma to manage her energy levels and maintain focus throughout her day. This herb's adaptogenic properties also help balance her body's response to stress, ensuring that she remains calm and focused even when faced with mentally demanding tasks. The versatility of ginseng aligns with Emma's preference for natural, multi-purpose remedies that fit seamlessly into her holistic lifestyle.

Lemon Balm: A Gentle Calming Aid for Focus

Lemon balm (Melissa officinalis) is an herb traditionally used for its calming and cognitive-enhancing properties. It has the unique ability to reduce stress while simultaneously enhancing alertness, making it a perfect herb for those who struggle with maintaining focus under pressure. For Emma, who seeks a balance between calm and clarity, lemon balm offers an effective solution.

Lemon balm tea or capsules can be incorporated into her daily routine, providing her with gentle and sustained support for mental focus. By reducing anxiety levels and promoting a sense of calm, lemon balm enables Emma to concentrate better and retain information more effectively, particularly during periods of stress or fatigue.

Matcha Green Tea: Sustained Energy and Mental Focus

Matcha green tea is an excellent option for Emma when she needs a natural and sustainable energy boost. Rich in L-theanine, matcha promotes alertness without the jittery effects commonly associated with other stimulants. This compound helps to enhance focus and concentration by promoting a state of calm alertness, allowing Emma to manage her tasks efficiently.

Drinking matcha tea can provide Emma with both immediate and long-term benefits for mental clarity. The antioxidants present in matcha also protect brain cells from damage, further supporting long-term cognitive health. By replacing her typical caffeine sources with matcha, Emma can enjoy a consistent energy level and sharper focus, all while staying aligned with her holistic health practices.

Holy Basil: Balancing Mood and Enhancing Clarity

Holy basil, or tulsi, is another adaptogenic herb that supports mental clarity and reduces fatigue. It is particularly effective for those who experience mood-related cognitive issues, such as difficulty concentrating due to stress or anxiety. Holy basil works by balancing cortisol levels and enhancing the body's ability to handle stress, which in turn improves Emma's ability to focus.

Incorporating holy basil tea into her daily routine can help Emma maintain a balanced mood and clear mind throughout her day. This herb's dual effect—promoting both stress reduction and mental clarity—aligns with her holistic approach, offering a practical and natural way to support focus and manage fatigue.

By integrating these natural solutions into her lifestyle, Emma can effectively manage mental fatigue and maintain her focus throughout her daily activities. These options provide a balanced, holistic approach that empowers her to enhance her cognitive function without reliance on synthetic stimulants, aligning with her preference for sustainable and natural health practices.

Remedies for Cognitive Health

Ginkgo Biloba Memory Enhancement Capsules

INGREDIENTS

- Ginkgo biloba leaf powder
- Empty vegetable capsules

PREPARATION

1. Fill empty capsules with ginkgo biloba leaf powder.
2. Store capsules in a cool, dry place.
3. Take one capsule daily.

Benefits: Ginkgo biloba is known for improving blood flow to the brain, which enhances memory and cognitive function. It may also protect neurons from damage and improve mental clarity and focus, making it an effective supplement for boosting memory and overall brain health.

Rosemary Brain Boosting Tea

INGREDIENTS

- 1 teaspoon dried rosemary leaves
- 1 cup hot water

PREPARATION

1. Add the dried rosemary leaves to a cup of hot water.
2. Steep for 10 minutes, then strain the tea.
3. Drink once or twice daily for best results.

Benefits: Rosemary has been traditionally used to enhance memory and cognitive performance. Its antioxidants support brain health by reducing oxidative stress and inflammation, contributing to improved concentration and focus. This tea is a simple yet effective way to promote cognitive vitality.

Gotu Kola Cognitive Function Tincture

INGREDIENTS

- Fresh gotu kola leaves
- Vodka or apple cider vinegar (for tincture base)

PREPARATION

1. Place fresh gotu kola leaves in a jar and cover them with vodka or apple cider vinegar.
2. Seal the jar and let it sit for 4-6 weeks, shaking occasionally.

3. Strain the mixture and store it in a dropper bottle.
4. Take 15-20 drops daily in water.

Benefits: Gotu kola is a powerful adaptogen that supports brain function by enhancing memory and concentration. It promotes blood circulation and reduces anxiety, helping the brain operate more efficiently. Regular use can result in sharper cognitive abilities and mental clarity.

Sage and Peppermint Clarity Elixir

INGREDIENTS

- 1 teaspoon dried sage leaves
- 1 teaspoon dried peppermint leaves
- 1 cup hot water

PREPARATION

1. Combine sage and peppermint leaves in a cup of hot water.
2. Steep for 10 minutes, then strain the infusion.
3. Drink warm or cold, once daily.

Benefits: Sage is known for enhancing memory and cognitive performance, while peppermint provides an invigorating effect, boosting alertness and clarity. Together, they create a powerful blend that sharpens focus and supports overall brain health.

Bacopa Brain Function Support Capsules

INGREDIENTS

- Bacopa monnieri powder
- Empty vegetable capsules

PREPARATION

1. Fill empty capsules with bacopa powder.
2. Store in a cool, dry place.
3. Take one capsule daily for best results.

Benefits: Bacopa is an ancient herb used to support cognitive function and improve memory retention. It acts as an adaptogen, reducing stress and improving mental clarity. Regular consumption of bacopa can enhance learning capabilities and overall brain performance.

Blueberry Antioxidant Memory Smoothie

INGREDIENTS

- 1 cup fresh blueberries
- 1 cup almond milk
- 1 tablespoon flax seeds

PREPARATION

1. Combine all ingredients in a blender.
2. Blend until smooth.
3. Consume immediately for optimal freshness and benefits.

Benefits: Blueberries are rich in antioxidants, particularly anthocyanins, which protect the brain from oxidative stress and inflammation. This smoothie helps improve memory and cognitive function, providing essential nutrients that support brain health.

Ashwagandha Cognitive Support Capsules

INGREDIENTS

- Ashwagandha root powder
- Empty vegetable capsules

PREPARATION

1. Fill the capsules with ashwagandha powder.
2. Store in a cool, dry place.
3. Take one capsule daily.

Benefits: Ashwagandha is a well-known adaptogen that helps reduce stress and anxiety, both of which can impair cognitive function. It supports brain health by enhancing memory and improving focus, making it a valuable ally for cognitive enhancement.

Lemon Balm Concentration Tea

INGREDIENTS

- 1 teaspoon dried lemon balm leaves
- 1 cup hot water

PREPARATION

1. Add lemon balm leaves to hot water and steep for 5-10 minutes.
2. Strain the tea and drink it warm.

Benefits: Lemon balm is known for its calming and focus-enhancing properties. It supports concentration and reduces anxiety, making it ideal for those looking to boost cognitive performance in a relaxed and balanced way.

Holy Basil (Tulsi) Mental Clarity Drops

INGREDIENTS

- Holy basil leaves
- Vodka or apple cider vinegar (for tincture)

PREPARATION

1. Place holy basil leaves in a jar and cover with vodka or apple cider vinegar.
2. Let it steep for 4-6 weeks, shaking occasionally.
3. Strain and store in a dropper bottle.
4. Take 15-20 drops daily in water.

Benefits: Holy basil, or tulsi, is a powerful adaptogen that enhances mental clarity and focus. It helps reduce stress and improve cognitive function, supporting overall brain health. This tincture is an easy way to incorporate holy basil's benefits into your daily routine.

Schisandra Berry Focus Capsules

INGREDIENTS

- Schisandra berry powder
- Empty vegetable capsules

PREPARATION

1. Fill the capsules with schisandra berry powder.
2. Store capsules in a cool, dry place.
3. Take one capsule daily.

Benefits: Schisandra berries are known for their adaptogenic properties that support cognitive function and improve focus. They help enhance concentration, reduce mental fatigue, and boost overall cognitive performance, making them ideal for those seeking mental clarity.

Rhodiola Energy and Memory Support Capsules

INGREDIENTS

- Rhodiola rosea powder
- Empty vegetable capsules

PREPARATION

1. Fill capsules with rhodiola powder.
2. Store in a dry, cool environment.
3. Take one capsule daily, preferably in the morning.

Benefits: Rhodiola rosea is an adaptogen that boosts energy levels and supports memory retention. It helps the brain resist stress, enhancing cognitive function and overall mental performance. Regular use can result in increased clarity and focus.

Skullcap Cognitive Support Infusion

INGREDIENTS

- 1 teaspoon dried skullcap leaves
- 1 cup hot water

PREPARATION

1. Add skullcap leaves to hot water and steep for 10 minutes.
2. Strain and drink warm.

Benefits: Skullcap is traditionally used to calm the nervous system and support cognitive function. It reduces anxiety, helping improve focus and mental clarity. This infusion is perfect for those seeking a natural way to enhance cognitive performance.

Lion's Mane Mushroom Brain Health Capsules

INGREDIENTS

- Lion's mane mushroom powder
- Empty vegetable capsules

PREPARATION

1. Fill capsules with lion's mane powder.
2. Store in a cool, dry place.
3. Take one capsule daily.

Benefits: Lion's mane mushroom is known for its neuroprotective properties that enhance cognitive function and memory. It supports brain health by promoting nerve growth and reducing inflammation, making it an excellent supplement for long-term cognitive vitality.

Nettle Cognitive Function Tea

INGREDIENTS

- 1 teaspoon dried nettle leaves
- 1 cup hot water

PREPARATION

1. Steep nettle leaves in hot water for 5-7 minutes.
2. Strain and drink warm.

Benefits: Nettle leaves are rich in vitamins and minerals that support overall brain health. This tea enhances cognitive function and reduces inflammation, making it a valuable addition to a daily wellness routine focused on improving mental performance.

Brahmi Brain Power Capsules

INGREDIENTS

- Brahmi (Bacopa monnieri) powder
- Empty vegetable capsules

PREPARATION

1. Fill capsules with brahmi powder.
2. Store in a dry, cool place.
3. Take one capsule daily for optimal results.

Benefits: Brahmi is an Ayurvedic herb known for its brain-boosting properties. It improves memory retention and cognitive function, while also reducing anxiety and stress. This supplement helps enhance overall mental clarity and focus.

Oatstraw Cognitive Support Capsules

INGREDIENTS

- Oatstraw powder
- Empty vegetable capsules

PREPARATION

1. Fill capsules with oatstraw powder.
2. Store capsules in a cool, dry place.
3. Take one capsule daily.

Benefits: Oatstraw is a powerful herb for supporting cognitive health. It enhances blood flow to the brain, improves memory, and boosts concentration. Its calming properties also reduce stress, promoting a balanced and focused mental state.

Reishi Mushroom Memory Support Decoction

INGREDIENTS

- 1 tablespoon dried reishi mushroom slices
- 2 cups water

PREPARATION

1. Boil reishi mushroom slices in water for 20-30 minutes.
2. Strain and drink warm.

Benefits: Reishi mushroom supports memory and cognitive function by reducing inflammation and enhancing the immune system. It is also known to promote relaxation and reduce stress, which can have positive effects on mental clarity and focus.

Ginseng and Mint Focus Tea

INGREDIENTS

- 1 teaspoon dried ginseng root
- 1 teaspoon dried mint leaves
- 1 cup hot water

PREPARATION

1. Combine ginseng root and mint leaves in a cup of hot water.
2. Steep for 10 minutes, then strain the tea.
3. Drink once daily for best results.

Benefits: Ginseng is known for its energy-boosting and focus-enhancing properties, while mint provides a refreshing boost to cognitive function. Together, they help improve alertness, concentration, and overall mental clarity, making this tea an effective remedy for cognitive support.

Valerian Root Memory Boost Capsules

INGREDIENTS

- Valerian root powder
- Empty vegetable capsules

PREPARATION

1. Fill capsules with valerian root powder.
2. Store in a cool, dry place.
3. Take one capsule daily before bedtime.

Benefits: Valerian root not only supports relaxation and sleep, but it also aids in memory enhancement by reducing stress and promoting a calm mind. This remedy is particularly useful for those who seek to improve cognitive function through better sleep and reduced anxiety.

Eleuthero Stress and Cognitive Support Drops

INGREDIENTS

- Eleuthero root
- Vodka or apple cider vinegar (for tincture)

PREPARATION

1. Place eleuthero root in a jar and cover with vodka or apple cider vinegar.
2. Let it steep for 4-6 weeks, shaking occasionally.
3. Strain and store in a dropper bottle.
4. Take 15-20 drops daily in water.

Benefits: Eleuthero, also known as Siberian ginseng, is an adaptogen that supports cognitive function by reducing stress and enhancing mental clarity. It helps the body adapt to stress, improving focus and concentration, making it an ideal remedy for overall cognitive health.

Eyebright Vision and Clarity Infusion

INGREDIENTS

- 1 teaspoon dried eyebright leaves
- 1 cup hot water

PREPARATION

1. Add eyebright leaves to hot water and steep for 10 minutes.
2. Strain and drink warm.

Benefits: Eyebright supports eye health and vision clarity, which are essential for cognitive processing. By improving visual clarity, this infusion aids in overall cognitive function and helps maintain mental sharpness. It is especially beneficial for those who spend long hours reading or using screens.

Green Tea Cognitive Enhancement Capsules

INGREDIENTS

- Green tea extract powder
- Empty vegetable capsules

PREPARATION

1. Fill capsules with green tea extract powder.
2. Store in a cool, dry place.
3. Take one capsule daily.

Benefits: Green tea contains antioxidants and compounds like L-theanine, which enhance focus and mental alertness. This capsule provides a convenient way to enjoy the benefits of green tea, supporting cognitive function and memory while reducing oxidative stress in the brain.

Turmeric Brain Health Infusion

INGREDIENTS

- 1 teaspoon turmeric powder
- 1 cup hot water
- A pinch of black pepper

PREPARATION

1. Add turmeric powder and black pepper to hot water.
2. Stir well and let it steep for 5-7 minutes.
3. Strain and drink warm.

Benefits: Turmeric is known for its anti-inflammatory properties that protect brain cells and enhance cognitive function. The addition of black pepper increases the absorption of curcumin, the active compound in turmeric, making this infusion effective in supporting memory and brain health.

Fennel and Chamomile Mental Clarity Capsules

INGREDIENTS

- Fennel seed powder
- Dried chamomile flower powder
- Empty vegetable capsules

PREPARATION

1. Mix fennel seed powder with chamomile flower powder.
2. Fill the mixture into empty capsules.
3. Store in a cool, dry place.
4. Take one capsule daily.

Benefits: Fennel and chamomile work together to reduce stress and promote clarity of mind. Fennel supports digestion and provides mild stimulation, while chamomile calms the nervous system, enhancing overall cognitive function and reducing mental fatigue.

Burdock Root Cognitive Detox Tea

INGREDIENTS

- 1 teaspoon dried burdock root
- 1 cup hot water

PREPARATION

1. Add dried burdock root to hot water and steep for 10 minutes.
2. Strain and drink warm.

Benefits: Burdock root helps detoxify the body, supporting liver health and reducing toxins that can affect brain function. This tea promotes clarity of mind and enhances overall cognitive performance by improving metabolic processes and circulation.

Lavender and Lemon Cognitive Relaxation Oil

INGREDIENTS

- 10 drops lavender essential oil
- 10 drops lemon essential oil
- Carrier oil (e.g., jojoba or almond oil)

PREPARATION

1. Mix the lavender and lemon essential oils with the carrier oil.

2. Store the mixture in a small bottle.
3. Apply a small amount to temples and wrists for relaxation and clarity.

Benefits: Lavender and lemon oils are known for their calming and invigorating properties. When combined, they create an aromatic blend that enhances relaxation while also boosting focus and mental clarity. This oil is ideal for use during stressful times or when concentration is needed.

Elderberry Brain Function Support Syrup

INGREDIENTS

- 1 cup fresh elderberries
- 1 cup water
- 1 tablespoon honey

PREPARATION

1. Boil elderberries in water for 15 minutes.
2. Strain the mixture and add honey while warm.
3. Store in a glass bottle and refrigerate.
4. Take one tablespoon daily.

Benefits: Elderberries are rich in antioxidants that protect the brain from oxidative stress. This syrup supports immune function while also promoting cognitive health, making it an excellent remedy for overall brain vitality.

Hawthorn Berry Brain Clarity Capsules

INGREDIENTS

- Hawthorn berry powder
- Empty vegetable capsules

PREPARATION

1. Fill capsules with hawthorn berry powder.
2. Store in a cool, dry place.
3. Take one capsule daily.

Benefits: Hawthorn berries improve blood circulation, particularly to the brain, enhancing mental clarity and cognitive function. They also provide antioxidants that protect the brain from damage, supporting long-term brain health and memory enhancement.

Spearmint and Rosemary Mental Boost Tea

INGREDIENTS

- 1 teaspoon dried spearmint leaves
- 1 teaspoon dried rosemary leaves
- 1 cup hot water

PREPARATION

1. Combine spearmint and rosemary leaves in hot water.
2. Steep for 10 minutes, then strain.
3. Drink once daily for best results.

Benefits: Spearmint and rosemary work synergistically to boost mental alertness and clarity. Spearmint provides refreshing properties, while rosemary enhances memory and cognitive performance, making this tea an effective remedy for a mental boost.

St. John's Wort Mood and Memory Capsules

INGREDIENTS

- St. John's Wort powder
- Empty vegetable capsules

PREPARATION

1. Fill capsules with St. John's Wort powder.
2. Store in a cool, dry place.
3. Take one capsule daily.

Benefits: St. John's Wort supports mood regulation and improves cognitive function by enhancing neurotransmitter activity in the brain. It is particularly beneficial for those experiencing mild mood imbalances or memory issues, providing both emotional and cognitive support.

Grape Seed Extract Cognitive Support Capsules

INGREDIENTS

- Grape seed extract powder
- Empty vegetable capsules

Preparation (#p#)

4. Fill capsules with grape seed extract powder.
5. Store in a cool, dry place.
6. Take one capsule daily.

Benefits: Grape seed extract is a powerful antioxidant that supports brain health by protecting against oxidative damage. It enhances circulation and improves memory retention, making it a valuable supplement for cognitive function and clarity.

Lemon Peel Concentration Boost Capsules

INGREDIENTS

- Dried lemon peel powder
- Empty vegetable capsules

PREPARATION

1. Fill capsules with lemon peel powder.
2. Store capsules in a cool, dry place.
3. Take one capsule daily.

Benefits: Lemon peel contains compounds that support concentration and mental clarity. The natural oils and antioxidants in lemon peel enhance focus and reduce cognitive fatigue, providing a simple yet effective way to boost mental performance.

Hibiscus and Ginger Brain Tonic

INGREDIENTS

- 1 teaspoon dried hibiscus flowers
- 1 slice fresh ginger
- 1 cup hot water

PREPARATION

1. Add hibiscus flowers and ginger to hot water.
2. Steep for 10 minutes, then strain.
3. Drink warm or chilled.

Benefits: Hibiscus and ginger work together to enhance circulation and support cognitive function. Hibiscus provides antioxidants that protect brain cells, while ginger stimulates blood flow, enhancing mental clarity and alertness. This tonic is a refreshing way to boost brain health.

BOOK 25

Oral Health and Herbal Dentistry

Herbs for Healthy Gums and Teeth

NATURAL HERBS FOR GUM AND TOOTH HEALTH

Oral health is a critical component of overall wellness, and many individuals, like Emma, seek natural ways to maintain healthy gums and strong teeth without relying solely on chemical-based products. Herbs have long been used in traditional medicine for their antibacterial, anti-inflammatory, and healing properties, making them excellent natural remedies for oral care. These herbs not only support gum and tooth health but also help prevent issues such as gingivitis, tooth decay, and inflammation. Incorporating these herbs into a daily oral hygiene routine offers a holistic approach to maintaining a healthy and balanced oral environment.

Sage: The Antimicrobial Protector

Sage (Salvia officinalis) is a powerful herb known for its antibacterial and anti-inflammatory properties. Historically used in traditional medicine to treat oral infections, sage helps reduce bacteria in the mouth, making it an excellent remedy for maintaining gum health and preventing plaque buildup. The antimicrobial compounds in sage, such as rosmarinic acid, work effectively to reduce inflammation and promote healing of the gums, which is particularly beneficial for individuals experiencing gum sensitivity or early signs of gingivitis.

Emma can use sage as a mouth rinse by steeping dried sage leaves in hot water and allowing it to cool before swishing it around her mouth. This natural sage rinse can be an effective alternative to commercial mouthwashes, offering a chemical-free option to maintain oral hygiene. Additionally, brushing with a sage-infused powder can help clean teeth and support gum health, providing Emma with a versatile and effective method to incorporate this herb into her daily routine.

Myrrh: A Traditional Remedy for Gum Strength

Myrrh, derived from the resin of the Commiphora tree, has been valued for its medicinal properties for centuries, particularly in the context of oral health. Myrrh's antiseptic and anti-inflammatory effects make it ideal for strengthening gums and preventing infections. It has traditionally been used to treat gum diseases such as periodontitis, as its compounds help reduce swelling and inflammation while promoting tissue repair.

Emma can apply a myrrh tincture directly to her gums, using it as a natural remedy for strengthening her gum tissue and preventing bleeding. Alternatively, she may find it beneficial to include myrrh powder in her tooth-cleaning routine, either mixed with a natural toothpaste or used as a standalone powder. This herb's versatility and potent properties make it a valuable ally in maintaining gum health, especially for those looking for natural alternatives.

Clove: The Antibacterial Pain Reliever

Clove (Syzygium aromaticum) is another herb with a long history in dental care, particularly for its ability to relieve pain and fight bacteria. Clove oil contains eugenol, a compound that not only numbs pain but also has strong antibacterial and antifungal effects. This makes clove oil a valuable remedy for managing toothaches and reducing the risk of gum infections.

Emma can apply a small amount of diluted clove oil directly to her gums or teeth to manage discomfort and reduce bacterial presence. Chewing on whole cloves is another traditional method to maintain gum health and freshen breath naturally. For those seeking to minimize the use of synthetic pain relievers, clove offers a holistic solution, supporting oral health while providing immediate relief from pain and inflammation.

Peppermint: A Fresh Approach to Oral Health

Peppermint (Mentha piperita) is not only known for its refreshing taste but also for its antibacterial properties, making it an excellent herb for maintaining oral hygiene. The essential oil extracted from peppermint leaves contains menthol, which helps eliminate bacteria that cause bad breath and contribute to gum disease. Peppermint's cooling effect can also soothe irritated gums, making it a perfect addition to any oral care routine.

Emma can create a homemade peppermint mouthwash by diluting a few drops of peppermint essential oil in water. This simple and effective rinse provides a refreshing feeling while actively supporting gum health. Incorporating peppermint into daily oral care routines offers Emma a natural, pleasant-tasting way to enhance her oral hygiene, supporting her goals of using accessible, plant-based solutions for wellness.

Neem: The Ayurvedic Gum Protector

Neem (Azadirachta indica), often referred to as the "toothbrush tree," is a staple in Ayurvedic dental care practices. Neem has potent antibacterial, antifungal, and anti-inflammatory properties, making it particularly effective for treating gum disease and maintaining overall oral health. Its ability to inhibit the growth of harmful bacteria and reduce plaque build-up provides a comprehensive approach to dental hygiene.

Emma can use neem in various forms, such as neem oil or powder, to brush her teeth or massage her gums. Neem's bitter taste may take some getting used to, but its effectiveness in preventing cavities and reducing gum inflammation makes it a powerful addition to her natural oral care routine. By integrating neem, Emma supports her goal of using time-tested, traditional remedies that offer both preventative and therapeutic benefits.

Calendula: The Healing Gum Soother

Calendula (Calendula officinalis), commonly known as marigold, is another herb with excellent anti-inflammatory and antiseptic properties, making it beneficial for soothing sore gums and preventing infections. Calendula has been used historically to heal wounds and promote tissue regeneration, which is particularly helpful for individuals dealing with gum sensitivity or after oral surgeries.

For Emma, rinsing with a calendula tea or using a calendula-infused oil to massage her gums can help reduce inflammation and support healing. This gentle herb offers a natural way to maintain healthy gums, aligning with her preference for holistic, non-invasive remedies that integrate easily into her wellness routine.

Thyme: A Powerful Antimicrobial Ally

Thyme (Thymus vulgaris) is another potent herb for oral health, rich in thymol—a compound known for its strong antiseptic properties. Thyme can help reduce bacteria in the mouth, support healthy gums, and prevent tooth decay. It is a common ingredient in natural toothpastes and mouthwashes due to its effectiveness in maintaining oral hygiene.

Emma can prepare a thyme mouthwash by steeping thyme leaves in boiling water, then straining and cooling the infusion. This simple rinse provides a natural way to keep gums healthy and teeth clean, without relying on synthetic chemicals. Thyme's accessibility and effectiveness make it an easy addition to Emma's oral care routine, offering a practical solution that complements her holistic lifestyle.

These herbs provide a variety of natural options for maintaining healthy gums and teeth. By incorporating them into her daily oral care routine, Emma can effectively manage her oral health, preventing issues like gum disease and tooth decay while aligning with her holistic approach to wellness. Each herb offers unique benefits, allowing her to tailor her routine to her specific needs and preferences, ensuring her oral care is both effective and naturally sourced.

Remedies for Fresh Breath and Cavity Prevention

NATURAL SOLUTIONS FOR FRESH BREATH AND CAVITY PREVENTION

Maintaining fresh breath and preventing cavities are key components of oral health, and herbal remedies provide effective, natural ways to achieve both. Many individuals, including Emma, prefer these holistic approaches as they offer long-lasting benefits without the side effects associated with chemical-based products. Incorporating these remedies into a daily routine not only promotes a healthy mouth environment but also aligns with Emma's preference for sustainable, plant-based care. In this section, we explore various herbal solutions that target the causes of bad breath and cavities, ensuring comprehensive oral health.

Clove: A Potent Antimicrobial and Breath Freshener

Clove (Syzygium aromaticum) is a well-known remedy for dental issues due to its powerful antimicrobial properties. The active compound eugenol in clove is effective against the bacteria responsible for bad breath and cavities. Eugenol also provides a numbing effect, which can relieve toothaches and gum discomfort while promoting overall oral hygiene.

Emma can use clove oil as a mouth rinse by adding a few drops to water and swishing it around her mouth for a minute. This simple method helps eliminate bacteria and refreshes her breath naturally. Alternatively, she can chew on whole cloves as an instant breath freshener. The versatility of clove makes it an essential herb for anyone looking to maintain fresh breath and prevent cavities naturally.

Neem: A Traditional Ayurvedic Remedy for Cavity Prevention

Neem (Azadirachta indica), a staple in Ayurvedic medicine, has been used for centuries to promote oral health. Neem leaves and twigs are naturally antibacterial, reducing plaque buildup and preventing cavities. Its bitter properties help to neutralize acids in the mouth, protecting the enamel and maintaining a balanced pH level.

Emma can create a neem mouthwash by steeping dried neem leaves in hot water. Rinsing with neem water not only prevents bad breath but also combats the bacteria that contribute to cavities. For those comfortable with traditional methods, using a neem twig as a natural toothbrush is another effective option. This practice gently massages the gums and cleans the teeth, providing a holistic and chemical-free way to maintain a healthy mouth.

Peppermint and Tea Tree Oil: An Antiseptic Blend for Fresh Breath

Peppermint (Mentha piperita) is not only known for its refreshing taste but also for its antibacterial properties that help eliminate bad breath. Combining peppermint with tea tree oil enhances its effectiveness, as tea tree oil is a potent antiseptic that combats the bacteria causing plaque and cavities.

To prepare a natural mouthwash, Emma can mix a few drops of peppermint and tea tree oil in water. This blend, when used as a daily rinse, offers a long-lasting fresh breath effect while preventing cavity formation. The combination of these oils works synergistically, providing a powerful defense against oral bacteria and ensuring a clean, fresh mouth throughout the day.

Green Tea: A Polyphenol-Rich Solution for Cavity Defense

Green tea is a simple yet effective remedy for both fresh breath and cavity prevention. Rich in polyphenols, green tea reduces the growth of bacteria and inhibits acid production, which are major factors contributing to bad breath and tooth decay. The catechins in green tea also provide antioxidant benefits, protecting the mouth from oxidative stress and inflammation.

Drinking green tea regularly helps keep the mouth's bacteria in check, preventing cavities and promoting fresh breath. Emma can also use green tea as a mouth rinse, enhancing its protective effects. By incorporating green tea into her routine, Emma can maintain oral health effortlessly, aligning with her holistic approach to wellness.

Cinnamon: A Natural Antibacterial Agent

Cinnamon (Cinnamomum verum) is another effective herb for freshening breath and preventing cavities. The essential oil extracted from cinnamon contains cinnamaldehyde, a compound that has potent antibacterial properties. This makes cinnamon an excellent remedy for combating the bacteria responsible for bad breath and plaque buildup.

Emma can create a cinnamon-infused mouthwash by boiling cinnamon sticks in water. Using this rinse daily helps to reduce bacteria levels in the mouth and provides a warm, pleasant flavor that freshens breath. For a more portable option, chewing on cinnamon sticks can also serve as a quick solution to bad breath while providing additional antibacterial benefits.

Aloe Vera: A Soothing and Healing Solution

Aloe vera (Aloe barbadensis) is known for its soothing properties, making it a gentle and effective remedy for preventing cavities and freshening breath. Its antibacterial effects help reduce harmful bacteria in the mouth, while its anti-inflammatory properties soothe gums and support oral health.

Emma can use aloe vera juice as a mouth rinse to maintain fresh breath and protect against cavities. The gentle nature of aloe makes it suitable for those with sensitive gums or teeth. Additionally, using aloe vera gel as an ingredient in homemade toothpaste offers another way to incorporate this versatile plant into daily oral care routines.

Eucalyptus: Fighting Plaque and Freshening Breath

Eucalyptus (Eucalyptus globulus) is a powerful herb that supports oral health by reducing plaque and freshening breath. The active compounds in eucalyptus, such as eucalyptol, possess antibacterial and anti-inflammatory properties that help prevent the formation of cavities and combat the bacteria causing bad breath.

A simple eucalyptus mouthwash can be made by adding a few drops of eucalyptus oil to water. Swishing this mixture in the mouth daily can help Emma maintain a fresh and healthy oral environment. Eucalyptus oil can also be used in natural toothpaste formulations, offering a refreshing and effective solution for keeping teeth and gums in top condition.

Parsley: The Chlorophyll-Rich Breath Freshener

Parsley (Petroselinum crispum) is a natural breath freshener due to its high chlorophyll content, which neutralizes odors and helps maintain fresh breath. Parsley's antibacterial properties also contribute to cavity prevention, making it a valuable herb for oral care.

Emma can chew on fresh parsley leaves after meals to instantly refresh her breath and reduce bacteria in her mouth. For a more concentrated solution, she can prepare a parsley mouth rinse by blending the leaves with water. This easy and natural remedy aligns with her desire for accessible, plant-based solutions that are simple to integrate into daily life.

These herbal remedies offer a comprehensive approach to maintaining fresh breath and preventing cavities, ensuring Emma has a variety of natural options to choose from. By incorporating these herbs into her daily oral care routine, she can effectively manage her oral health while staying true to her holistic wellness values.

Remedies for Oral Care

Clove Oil Toothache Relief

INGREDIENTS

- Clove essential oil
- Carrier oil (e.g., coconut oil)

PREPARATION

1. Mix 2 drops of clove essential oil with 1 teaspoon of carrier oil.
2. Apply the mixture directly to the affected tooth using a cotton swab.
3. Repeat as needed for relief.

Benefits: Clove oil is well-known for its analgesic and antibacterial properties, making it effective in providing quick relief from toothache pain. It helps reduce inflammation and prevents infection, supporting overall oral health.

Peppermint Breath Freshener Drops

INGREDIENTS

- Peppermint essential oil
- Water
- Vegetable glycerin

PREPARATION

1. Mix 5 drops of peppermint essential oil with 1 tablespoon of vegetable glycerin and 1/4 cup of water.
2. Store the mixture in a small dropper bottle.
3. Use 2-3 drops directly on the tongue for fresh breath.

Benefits: Peppermint essential oil is known for its refreshing and antibacterial qualities. This breath freshener not only masks odors but also fights bacteria that cause bad breath, keeping your mouth feeling clean and fresh throughout the day.

Myrrh Gum Healing Powder

INGREDIENTS

- Myrrh resin powder
- Baking soda

PREPARATION

1. Combine 1 teaspoon of myrrh resin powder with 1 teaspoon of baking soda.
2. Apply the powder mixture directly to the gums using a finger or a soft toothbrush.
3. Rinse after a few minutes.

Benefits: Myrrh is a powerful anti-inflammatory and antibacterial agent that promotes gum healing and reduces inflammation. Combined with baking soda, it enhances oral hygiene by balancing pH levels and soothing irritated gums.

Echinacea Mouthwash for Gum Health

INGREDIENTS

- Dried echinacea root
- 1 cup water

PREPARATION

1. Boil the echinacea root in water for 10 minutes.
2. Strain and let the infusion cool.
3. Use as a mouthwash, swishing for 30 seconds before spitting out.

Benefits: Echinacea has antimicrobial and anti-inflammatory properties that help maintain gum health and prevent infections. This mouthwash supports the immune system while soothing and healing inflamed gums, contributing to overall oral health.

Sage and Thyme Antibacterial Toothpaste

INGREDIENTS

- Dried sage leaves
- Dried thyme leaves
- Baking soda
- Coconut oil

PREPARATION

1. Grind sage and thyme leaves into a fine powder.
2. Mix the powder with baking soda and coconut oil to form a paste.
3. Store in a small container and use as a toothpaste.

Benefits: Sage and thyme possess strong antibacterial properties, making them ideal for oral care. This natural toothpaste helps reduce plaque buildup, freshen breath, and promote healthy gums, all while being free from harsh chemicals.

Calendula Gum Healing Infusion

INGREDIENTS

- 1 teaspoon dried calendula flowers
- 1 cup hot water

PREPARATION

1. Steep calendula flowers in hot water for 10 minutes.
2. Strain and let the infusion cool.
3. Use as a mouth rinse twice daily.

Benefits: Calendula is known for its anti-inflammatory and healing properties. This infusion helps reduce gum inflammation, promotes healing of oral tissues, and prevents bacterial growth, making it a soothing remedy for gum health.

Neem Oil Oral Health Capsules

INGREDIENTS

- Neem leaf powder
- Empty vegetable capsules

PREPARATION

1. Fill empty capsules with neem leaf powder.
2. Store capsules in a cool, dry place.
3. Take one capsule daily.

Benefits: Neem has long been used for its antibacterial and anti-inflammatory properties in oral care. It helps reduce plaque buildup, prevents gum disease, and supports overall oral hygiene, promoting a healthy mouth from within.

Chamomile and Lemon Mouth Freshening Spray

INGREDIENTS

- Chamomile essential oil
- Lemon essential oil
- Water
- Vegetable glycerin

PREPARATION

1. Mix 5 drops of chamomile and 5 drops of lemon essential oil with 1 tablespoon of vegetable glycerin and 1/4 cup of water.
2. Store in a small spray bottle.
3. Spray directly into the mouth for freshness.

Benefits: Chamomile and lemon work together to freshen breath and reduce oral bacteria. Chamomile soothes the gums, while lemon provides a refreshing flavor and antibacterial properties, ensuring a clean and pleasant mouthfeel.

White Oak Bark Tooth Strengthening Capsules

INGREDIENTS

- White oak bark powder
- Empty vegetable capsules

PREPARATION

1. Fill capsules with white oak bark powder.
2. Store in a cool, dry place.
3. Take one capsule daily.

Benefits: White oak bark is rich in tannins that strengthen tooth enamel and support gum health. These capsules promote stronger teeth and help reduce inflammation in the gums, improving overall oral hygiene.

Turmeric and Coconut Oil Pulling Solution

INGREDIENTS

- 1 teaspoon turmeric powder
- 1 tablespoon coconut oil

PREPARATION

1. Mix turmeric powder with coconut oil until well combined.
2. Swish the mixture in the mouth for 5-10 minutes.
3. Spit out and rinse thoroughly with water.

Benefits: Turmeric has powerful anti-inflammatory and antibacterial properties, while coconut oil helps remove toxins and bacteria from the mouth. This pulling solution supports oral health by reducing inflammation, whitening teeth, and promoting gum health.

Fennel Seed Breath Freshener Capsules

INGREDIENTS

- Fennel seed powder
- Empty vegetable capsules

PREPARATION

1. Fill capsules with fennel seed powder.
2. Store capsules in a cool, dry place.
3. Take one capsule daily.

Benefits: Fennel seeds are known for their breath-freshening properties and their ability to reduce bacteria in the mouth. These capsules provide a convenient way to maintain fresh breath while promoting digestive health, which can also impact oral hygiene.

Goldenrod Gum Health Capsules

INGREDIENTS

- Goldenrod powder
- Empty vegetable capsules

PREPARATION

1. Fill empty capsules with goldenrod powder.
2. Store in a cool, dry place.
3. Take one capsule daily.

Benefits: Goldenrod has anti-inflammatory and antimicrobial properties that promote gum health and reduce inflammation. Regular use helps strengthen gums and prevent oral infections, supporting a healthy mouth.

Green Tea Antioxidant Mouthwash

INGREDIENTS

- 1 teaspoon green tea leaves
- 1 cup hot water

PREPARATION

1. Steep green tea leaves in hot water for 5-7 minutes.
2. Strain and let it cool.
3. Use as a mouthwash twice daily.

Benefits: Green tea contains antioxidants that help reduce inflammation and fight bacteria in the mouth. This mouthwash helps reduce plaque buildup and supports healthy gums, providing a natural way to enhance oral health.

Spearmint Oral Hygiene Capsules

INGREDIENTS

- Spearmint leaf powder
- Empty vegetable capsules

PREPARATION

1. Fill capsules with spearmint leaf powder.
2. Store capsules in a cool, dry place.
3. Take one capsule daily.

Benefits: Spearmint is known for its refreshing properties and ability to fight bacteria in the mouth. These capsules help maintain fresh breath and support gum health, offering a convenient way to enhance daily oral hygiene.

Thyme and Lavender Gum Healing Spray

INGREDIENTS

- Thyme essential oil
- Lavender essential oil
- Water
- Vegetable glycerin

PREPARATION

1. Mix 5 drops each of thyme and lavender essential oils with 1 tablespoon of vegetable glycerin and 1/4 cup of water.
2. Store in a small spray bottle.
3. Spray directly onto the gums for relief.

Benefits: Thyme and lavender provide powerful anti-inflammatory and antimicrobial properties that soothe gums and promote healing. This spray is perfect for reducing gum inflammation and preventing infections, making it a valuable addition to oral care routines.

Licorice Root Tooth Strengthening Drops

INGREDIENTS

- Licorice root tincture
- Water

PREPARATION

1. Mix a few drops of licorice root tincture with water.
2. Use the mixture as a rinse, swishing for 30 seconds.
3. Spit out and rinse with plain water.

Benefits: Licorice root supports oral health by reducing plaque and strengthening tooth enamel. Its antibacterial properties also help fight gum disease, making it an effective remedy for long-term dental care.

Yarrow Gum Pain Relief Capsules

INGREDIENTS

- Yarrow powder
- Empty vegetable capsules

PREPARATION

1. Fill capsules with yarrow powder.
2. Store capsules in a cool, dry place.
3. Take one capsule daily.

Benefits: Yarrow has anti-inflammatory and pain-relieving properties that are effective for managing gum pain and swelling. These capsules help reduce discomfort and promote healing, supporting overall gum health.

Hibiscus Breath Freshening Lozenges

INGREDIENTS

- Dried hibiscus powder
- Honey
- A pinch of mint powder

PREPARATION

1. Mix hibiscus powder with honey and mint powder to form a thick paste.
2. Roll the paste into small lozenges.
3. Let the lozenges air dry and store in an airtight container.
4. Use as needed for fresh breath.

Benefits: Hibiscus has natural antibacterial properties that help eliminate bad breath, while the mint provides a refreshing and cooling sensation. These lozenges support fresh breath and promote a clean oral environment, making them ideal for daily use.

Marshmallow Root Tooth Sensitivity Drops

INGREDIENTS

- Marshmallow root extract
- Water

PREPARATION

1. Mix a few drops of marshmallow root extract with water.

2. Use the mixture as a mouth rinse, swishing gently for 30 seconds.
3. Spit out and rinse with plain water.

Benefits: Marshmallow root is soothing and anti-inflammatory, making it ideal for reducing tooth sensitivity. It forms a protective barrier over the teeth and gums, providing relief from irritation and promoting overall oral health.

Holy Basil (Tulsi) Gum Health Capsules

INGREDIENTS

- Tulsi leaf powder
- Empty vegetable capsules

PREPARATION

1. Fill empty capsules with tulsi leaf powder.
2. Store in a cool, dry place.
3. Take one capsule daily.

Benefits: Holy basil (tulsi) is revered for its antimicrobial and anti-inflammatory properties. It helps maintain healthy gums by reducing inflammation and fighting harmful bacteria, supporting overall oral hygiene and gum health.

Birch Leaf Gum Strength Infusion

INGREDIENTS

- 1 teaspoon dried birch leaves
- 1 cup hot water

PREPARATION

1. Steep dried birch leaves in hot water for 10 minutes.
2. Strain and let the infusion cool.
3. Use as a mouth rinse once or twice daily.

Benefits: Birch leaves contain compounds that strengthen gum tissues and reduce inflammation. This infusion supports healthy gums and helps maintain a balanced oral environment, promoting long-term gum health.

Goldenseal Oral Healing Capsules

INGREDIENTS

- Goldenseal root powder
- Empty vegetable capsules

PREPARATION

1. Fill capsules with goldenseal root powder.
2. Store in a cool, dry place.
3. Take one capsule daily.

Benefits: Goldenseal is a powerful herb known for its antimicrobial and healing properties. These capsules help fight oral infections and promote the healing of gum tissues, supporting overall oral hygiene and health.

Lemon Verbena Toothache Relief Tincture

INGREDIENTS

- Fresh lemon verbena leaves
- Vodka or apple cider vinegar (for tincture)

PREPARATION

1. Place fresh lemon verbena leaves in a jar and cover with vodka or apple cider vinegar.
2. Seal the jar and let it steep for 4-6 weeks, shaking occasionally.

3. Strain and store in a dropper bottle.
4. Apply a few drops directly to the affected tooth for relief.

Benefits: Lemon verbena has soothing and anti-inflammatory properties that make it effective for toothache relief. This tincture helps reduce pain and inflammation, providing a natural alternative to over-the-counter pain relief options.

Rosemary Gum Health Infusion

INGREDIENTS

- 1 teaspoon dried rosemary leaves
- 1 cup hot water

PREPARATION

1. Steep dried rosemary leaves in hot water for 10 minutes.
2. Strain and allow the infusion to cool.
3. Use as a mouth rinse twice daily.

Benefits: Rosemary has antibacterial and anti-inflammatory properties that promote gum health. This infusion helps reduce inflammation, fights harmful bacteria, and strengthens gum tissues, making it an effective solution for maintaining oral hygiene.

Cinnamon and Clove Dental Powder

INGREDIENTS

- Cinnamon powder
- Clove powder
- Baking soda

PREPARATION

1. Mix equal parts of cinnamon and clove powders with baking soda.
2. Store the mixture in a small jar.
3. Use as a tooth powder for brushing.

Benefits: Cinnamon and clove are known for their antimicrobial and anti-inflammatory properties. This dental powder not only freshens breath but also helps reduce plaque and supports gum health, promoting overall oral hygiene.

Violet Leaf Mouth Freshening Spray

INGREDIENTS

- Violet leaf tincture
- Water
- Vegetable glycerin

PREPARATION

1. Mix violet leaf tincture with water and vegetable glycerin.
2. Store the mixture in a spray bottle.
3. Spray directly into the mouth as needed.

Benefits: Violet leaves provide gentle antimicrobial properties and a refreshing flavor, making them ideal for oral care. This spray freshens breath while also promoting healthy gums and reducing inflammation.

Elderflower Gum Soothing Capsules

INGREDIENTS

- Elderflower powder
- Empty vegetable capsules

PREPARATION

1. Fill capsules with elderflower powder.
2. Store in a cool, dry place.
3. Take one capsule daily.

Benefits: Elderflower has anti-inflammatory and soothing properties that help reduce gum pain and swelling. These capsules support gum health by promoting healing and reducing discomfort, contributing to overall oral wellness.

Bay Leaf Tooth Strengthening Drops

INGREDIENTS

- Bay leaf tincture
- Water

PREPARATION

1. Mix a few drops of bay leaf tincture with water.
2. Use as a rinse, swishing for 30 seconds.
3. Spit out and rinse with plain water.

Benefits: Bay leaves contain compounds that support tooth enamel strength and gum health. This tincture helps reduce inflammation and promote healthy gums, making it an effective remedy for maintaining strong teeth and oral health.

Anise Seed Oral Health Capsules

INGREDIENTS

- Anise seed powder
- Empty vegetable capsules

PREPARATION

1. Fill capsules with anise seed powder.
2. Store in a cool, dry place.
3. Take one capsule daily.

Benefits: Anise seeds have antibacterial properties that support oral hygiene by reducing bacteria in the mouth. These capsules also freshen breath and support digestive health, both of which contribute to overall oral wellness.

Aloe Vera Gum Healing Gel

INGREDIENTS

- Fresh aloe vera gel
- A drop of tea tree essential oil

PREPARATION

1. Extract fresh gel from an aloe vera leaf.
2. Mix the gel with a drop of tea tree essential oil.
3. Apply directly to the gums and leave it on for a few minutes before rinsing.

Benefits: Aloe vera is soothing and anti-inflammatory, making it ideal for treating gum irritation and swelling. Combined with tea tree oil's antibacterial properties, this gel supports gum healing and overall oral health.

Horsetail Tooth Strengthening Capsules

INGREDIENTS

- Horsetail powder
- Empty vegetable capsules

PREPARATION

1. Fill capsules with horsetail powder.
2. Store in a cool, dry place.
3. Take one capsule daily.

Benefits: Horsetail is rich in silica, which strengthens tooth enamel and supports bone health. These capsules help reinforce teeth, promoting overall oral strength and reducing the risk of decay.

Dandelion Gum Health Infusion

INGREDIENTS

- 1 teaspoon dried dandelion leaves
- 1 cup hot water (#ul#)

PREPARATION

1. Steep dandelion leaves in hot water for 10 minutes.
2. Strain and allow it to cool.
3. Use as a mouth rinse once or twice daily.

Benefits: Dandelion leaves have anti-inflammatory properties that promote gum health. This infusion helps reduce gum swelling, fights bacteria, and supports overall oral hygiene, making it a beneficial addition to daily oral care routines.

Blueberry and Mint Mouth Freshener

INGREDIENTS

- Fresh blueberries
- Fresh mint leaves
- Water

PREPARATION

1. Crush the blueberries and mint leaves in water.
2. Strain the mixture and store it in a spray bottle.
3. Spray directly into the mouth for freshness.

Benefits: Blueberries are rich in antioxidants that protect the mouth from harmful bacteria, while mint provides a refreshing flavor and cooling effect. This mouth freshener supports fresh breath and promotes a clean and healthy oral environment.

BOOK 26

Enhancing Immunity for Chronic Conditions

Immune-Boosting Herbs for Autoimmune Conditions

HERBS THAT SUPPORT AUTOIMMUNE HEALTH AND BOOST IMMUNITY

Autoimmune conditions present a unique challenge when it comes to boosting immunity. The immune system, in these cases, can become overly active and mistakenly attack healthy tissues. Therefore, the goal is not only to enhance immune function but also to regulate and balance it. Specific herbs, known as adaptogens and immunomodulators, are particularly effective for those dealing with autoimmune conditions. These herbs work by supporting the body's ability to maintain equilibrium, reducing inflammation, and promoting overall immune health. In this section, we explore various immune-boosting herbs that are both safe and effective for individuals managing autoimmune disorders.

Astragalus: Balancing and Strengthening Immunity

Astragalus (Astragalus membranaceus) is a well-known herb in traditional Chinese medicine, prized for its adaptogenic and immune-boosting properties. It helps enhance the immune system's response without overstimulating it, making it an ideal choice for individuals with autoimmune conditions. Astragalus supports the production of white blood cells, which are crucial in defending the body against infections, while also possessing anti-inflammatory effects that help modulate the immune response.

For Emma, who prefers sustainable, plant-based solutions, incorporating astragalus root into her daily routine could be an effective way to boost her immune system. She can use it as a tea, tincture, or powder mixed into soups or smoothies. This versatility allows her to adjust the dosage and form based on her needs and lifestyle, providing flexibility while maintaining immune health.

Turmeric: Reducing Inflammation While Supporting Immunity

Turmeric (Curcuma longa) is celebrated for its anti-inflammatory and immunomodulatory effects, primarily due to its active compound, curcumin. In the context of autoimmune conditions, turmeric helps reduce inflammation without suppressing the immune system entirely, striking a balance that is vital for those managing such conditions. Curcumin modulates cytokine levels, which are proteins involved in inflammation, thus helping to prevent the immune system from becoming overly aggressive.

To maximize its effectiveness, Emma can combine turmeric with black pepper, as the piperine in pepper enhances curcumin absorption. Using turmeric in her cooking, or drinking turmeric tea, can be simple yet effective ways for her to integrate this powerful herb into her daily regimen. Turmeric's accessibility and multifunctional use make it a practical option for supporting immune balance.

Reishi Mushroom: An Adaptogenic Immune Tonic

Reishi mushroom (Ganoderma lucidum) has long been revered in Eastern medicine for its immune-enhancing and balancing properties. Known as the "mushroom of immortality," reishi functions as an adaptogen, meaning it helps the body adapt to stress and maintain immune equilibrium. It is particularly effective for individuals with autoimmune conditions because it regulates immune activity, reducing overactivity while supporting overall immune health.

Emma can use reishi mushroom in powder form, adding it to her morning coffee or tea. This not only makes it easy to incorporate into her routine but also aligns with her preference for simple, natural remedies. The soothing nature of reishi, combined with its immune-balancing properties, offers a holistic approach for managing autoimmune symptoms and enhancing resilience against infections.

Ashwagandha: A Gentle, Immunomodulatory Herb

Ashwagandha (Withania somnifera) is another adaptogenic herb with immunomodulatory properties that can benefit individuals with autoimmune conditions. It supports adrenal health, helping the body manage stress, which is often a trigger for autoimmune flare-ups. Ashwagandha promotes a balanced immune response by reducing inflammation and stabilizing immune activity, making it an effective herb for those seeking long-term immune support.

Emma might appreciate the flexibility of using ashwagandha in various forms, such as capsules, powders, or teas. Its gentle nature and adaptogenic qualities make it suitable for everyday use, ensuring that she can integrate it seamlessly into her lifestyle. As Emma looks for ways to maintain her energy and reduce stress while managing her condition, ashwagandha can provide a well-rounded solution.

Licorice Root: An Anti-Inflammatory and Immune Supporter

Licorice root (Glycyrrhiza glabra) is known for its anti-inflammatory and immune-boosting effects, making it particularly useful for managing autoimmune conditions. It contains compounds that reduce inflammation and support adrenal function, which is critical for maintaining energy levels and reducing immune stress. Licorice also helps regulate cytokine production, ensuring that the immune response remains balanced rather than overly aggressive.

Emma can use licorice root as a tea or tincture, making it an easy addition to her daily routine. However, it's important to note that licorice should be used with caution, especially for those with high blood pressure or kidney issues. Consulting a healthcare professional can help Emma determine the right dosage and frequency to ensure its safe and effective use.

Holy Basil: Reducing Stress and Modulating Immunity

Holy basil (Ocimum sanctum), also known as tulsi, is an adaptogenic herb that helps manage stress and inflammation. Chronic stress can exacerbate autoimmune conditions, so using herbs like holy basil, which target both the nervous system and immune response, can be particularly beneficial. Holy basil's anti-inflammatory properties also help reduce autoimmune flare-ups, promoting a balanced immune state.

For Emma, incorporating holy basil as a tea or tincture offers a calming ritual that not only supports her immune system but also helps manage daily stress. Given her preference for plant-based, holistic care, holy basil provides a practical and effective means of supporting her overall well-being.

Echinacea: Boosting Immunity Without Overstimulation

Echinacea (Echinacea purpurea) is a popular herb for boosting immunity, but it is especially valuable for its ability to enhance immune function without overstimulating it, which is crucial for those with autoimmune conditions. Echinacea supports the body's natural defenses against infections while also exhibiting anti-inflammatory effects that can help manage symptoms associated with autoimmune flare-ups.

Emma can use echinacea as a tea or tincture during times when her immune system needs a boost, such as during flu season or when she feels run down. This approach allows her to tailor its use to her specific needs, ensuring she supports her immunity without risking overstimulation.

These herbs provide Emma with a range of options for supporting her immune system in a balanced manner, addressing the complexities of autoimmune conditions. By incorporating these herbs into her daily routine, she can maintain her health while aligning with her preference for natural, sustainable solutions.

Herbal Support for Chronic Infections and Recovery

NATURAL HERBAL REMEDIES FOR CHRONIC INFECTIONS AND RECOVERY

Chronic infections present a complex challenge, often requiring long-term management and support. They may be the result of viruses, bacteria, or fungi that the body struggles to eliminate fully, leading to persistent symptoms and a weakened immune system. Supporting recovery from such infections through herbal remedies can be highly effective when the right plants are selected. These herbs work by enhancing immunity, reducing inflammation, and directly combating pathogens while also promoting tissue repair and overall wellness. For individuals like Emma, who seek sustainable, natural solutions to manage health conditions, understanding these herbs can be transformative.

Echinacea: An Immune-Boosting Ally

Echinacea (Echinacea purpurea) is widely known for its immune-boosting properties and is particularly effective in supporting the body during chronic infections. It stimulates the production of white blood cells, enhancing the body's ability to fight off persistent pathogens. Moreover, echinacea exhibits antiviral and antibacterial properties, making it a versatile option for addressing a range of infections.

For Emma, integrating echinacea into her routine as a tea or tincture can provide a proactive approach to managing chronic infections. The herb is most effective when used at the onset of symptoms but can also be taken long-term in small doses to maintain immune resilience. This flexibility makes it a practical, easy-to-use option for her daily routine.

Garlic: Nature's Antimicrobial Powerhouse

Garlic (Allium sativum) is another potent herb renowned for its antimicrobial properties. It contains allicin, a compound with powerful antibacterial, antiviral, and antifungal effects. Studies have shown that garlic not only supports the immune system but also directly attacks pathogens, making it especially valuable for chronic infections where conventional treatments may not be as effective.

Emma could incorporate garlic into her diet by adding raw or lightly cooked cloves to her meals, or she may opt for garlic supplements if she prefers an easier method of consumption. Its versatility in use aligns with her preference for practical, everyday solutions that fit seamlessly into her lifestyle. Garlic's added benefit of promoting cardiovascular health is an extra incentive for its inclusion in a holistic wellness plan.

Goldenseal: Supporting Mucous Membranes and Immune Function

Goldenseal (Hydrastis canadensis) is a powerful herb commonly used for its antimicrobial and anti-inflammatory properties. It is particularly effective in infections affecting mucous membranes, such as respiratory or urinary tract infections. Goldenseal contains berberine, an alkaloid known for its ability to fight bacteria, fungi, and viruses.

This herb can be taken as a tincture or capsule, making it accessible for Emma's busy lifestyle. However, it is important to use goldenseal with caution, as long-term use may affect gut flora balance. Consulting a healthcare professional for dosage and duration is advisable, especially when used for chronic conditions.

Licorice Root: Anti-Inflammatory and Antiviral Benefits

Licorice root (Glycyrrhiza glabra) is an effective herb for individuals dealing with chronic viral infections. Its anti-inflammatory and antiviral properties make it useful in managing symptoms associated with long-term infections, such as fatigue and inflammation. Licorice root also supports adrenal function, helping the body cope with the stress of prolonged illness.

Emma might appreciate licorice root's versatility, as it can be consumed as a tea, tincture, or supplement. However, caution is necessary for those with high blood pressure, as licorice may exacerbate this condition. If Emma chooses this herb, consulting a healthcare provider would ensure she uses it safely and effectively.

Olive Leaf Extract: A Natural Antiviral Remedy

Olive leaf extract (Olea europaea) has been used for centuries as a natural remedy for infections due to its powerful antiviral and antibacterial properties. The active compound, oleuropein, has shown effectiveness in inhibiting the growth of various pathogens. Olive leaf extract also helps reduce inflammation, which is often present in chronic infections, and boosts overall immune function.

This extract can be taken in capsule or liquid form, providing Emma with options that suit her preference for simplicity and efficiency. Using olive leaf extract as part of a holistic approach can help her manage symptoms more effectively while avoiding synthetic medications.

Elderberry: Supporting Recovery from Viral Infections

Elderberry (Sambucus nigra) is a well-known herb for its antiviral properties, particularly in addressing respiratory infections. Rich in antioxidants and immune-boosting compounds, elderberry has been shown to reduce the duration and severity of viral infections. It is especially beneficial for those who experience recurrent colds, flu, or respiratory issues as part of a chronic condition.

Emma can take elderberry as a syrup, tea, or capsule, giving her flexibility based on her needs and preferences. Its pleasant taste also makes it an appealing option for regular use. By including elderberry in her wellness routine, Emma can enjoy both immune support and the added benefit of a tasty herbal remedy.

Pau d'Arco: A Powerful Antifungal and Antiviral Solution

Pau d'Arco (Tabebuia avellanedae) is a lesser-known herb with potent antifungal, antiviral, and anti-inflammatory properties. Traditionally used in South America, it is effective in treating fungal infections like Candida as well as chronic viral conditions. Its anti-inflammatory effects also aid in reducing the discomfort associated with prolonged infections.

Pau d'Arco can be consumed as a tea, which may appeal to Emma's preference for natural, plant-based solutions that integrate well into her lifestyle. Regular use, under the guidance of a healthcare professional, could provide her with a gentle yet effective way to combat persistent infections.

By incorporating these herbs into her daily regimen, Emma has a range of options to choose from, tailored to her specific needs and lifestyle preferences. Each herb not only supports the immune system but also provides targeted relief for chronic infections, promoting recovery and long-term wellness.

Remedies for Long-Term Immune Resilience

Elderberry Chronic Immune Support Capsules

INGREDIENTS

- Elderberry powder
- Empty vegetable capsules

PREPARATION

1. Fill empty vegetable capsules with elderberry powder.
2. Store capsules in a cool, dry place.
3. Take one capsule daily to support immune function.

Benefits: Elderberry is rich in antioxidants and has antiviral properties that support immune health. These capsules help maintain long-term immune resilience, protecting against chronic infections and boosting the body's natural defense mechanisms.

Astragalus Long-Term Immune Boost Infusion

INGREDIENTS

- 1 teaspoon dried astragalus root
- 1 cup hot water

PREPARATION

1. Add dried astragalus root to hot water and steep for 10-15 minutes.
2. Strain and drink the infusion warm.
3. Consume daily for best results.

Benefits: Astragalus is known for its immune-boosting properties, especially for long-term resilience. It enhances the body's ability to fight off infections and supports overall vitality, making it ideal for those with chronic immune challenges.

Reishi Mushroom Immune Support Capsules

INGREDIENTS

- Reishi mushroom powder
- Empty vegetable capsules

PREPARATION

1. Fill capsules with reishi mushroom powder.
2. Store capsules in a cool, dry place.
3. Take one capsule daily for immune support.

Benefits: Reishi mushrooms are adaptogens that help modulate the immune system, reducing inflammation and supporting long-term immune health. These capsules provide an easy way to incorporate reishi's benefits into your routine, promoting overall wellness and resilience.

Garlic and Ginger Immune Tonic

INGREDIENTS

- 2 cloves garlic
- 1 inch fresh ginger root
- 1 cup water

PREPARATION

1. Crush garlic and slice ginger, then add to water and boil for 10 minutes.
2. Strain and let it cool slightly before drinking.
3. Consume once daily for immune support.

Benefits: Garlic and ginger are powerful natural antibiotics with anti-inflammatory properties. This tonic boosts the immune system, helps fight off infections, and reduces inflammation, supporting long-term immune health for chronic conditions.

Echinacea Immune Modulator Capsules

INGREDIENTS

- Echinacea powder
- Empty vegetable capsules

PREPARATION

1. Fill capsules with echinacea powder.
2. Store in a cool, dry place.
3. Take one capsule daily to modulate immune response.

Benefits: Echinacea helps regulate and boost immune function, making it effective for supporting the immune system over time. These capsules aid in preventing chronic infections and maintaining a balanced immune response, promoting resilience and overall health.

Lemon Balm Long-Term Immune Support Tea

INGREDIENTS

- 1 teaspoon dried lemon balm leaves
- 1 cup hot water

PREPARATION

1. Steep lemon balm leaves in hot water for 10 minutes.
2. Strain and drink warm.
3. Consume daily for ongoing immune support.

Benefits: Lemon balm has antiviral and calming properties that support long-term immune health. This tea helps reduce stress, which can weaken immunity, while also providing antiviral support, making it an excellent choice for chronic immune conditions.

Schisandra Berry Chronic Fatigue Capsules

INGREDIENTS

- Schisandra berry powder
- Empty vegetable capsules

PREPARATION

1. Fill capsules with schisandra berry powder.
2. Store in a cool, dry place.
3. Take one capsule daily for chronic fatigue support.

Benefits: Schisandra berries are adaptogens that support the body's response to stress and fatigue. These capsules help reduce chronic fatigue symptoms and boost the immune system, promoting resilience and energy levels over the long term.

Andrographis Immune Defense Capsules

INGREDIENTS

- Andrographis powder
- Empty vegetable capsules

PREPARATION

1. Fill capsules with andrographis powder.
2. Store capsules in a cool, dry place.
3. Take one capsule daily to enhance immune defense.

Benefits: Andrographis is a potent herb known for its immune-boosting and anti-inflammatory properties. It supports the body's ability to fight chronic infections and improves immune resilience, making it effective for long-term immune support.

Ashwagandha Chronic Stress Support Tea

INGREDIENTS

- 1 teaspoon dried ashwagandha root
- 1 cup hot water

PREPARATION

1. Steep ashwagandha root in hot water for 15 minutes.
2. Strain and drink the tea warm.
3. Consume once daily for stress support.

Benefits: Ashwagandha is an adaptogen that helps the body manage chronic stress, which can impact immune function. This tea supports long-term immune health by reducing cortisol levels, enhancing resilience, and promoting overall balance in the body.

Holy Basil (Tulsi) Adaptogen Capsules

INGREDIENTS

- Tulsi leaf powder
- Empty vegetable capsules

PREPARATION

1. Fill capsules with tulsi leaf powder.
2. Store in a cool, dry place.
3. Take one capsule daily for immune modulation.

Benefits: Holy basil is a powerful adaptogen that supports the immune system and reduces inflammation. It helps the body adapt to stress and fight infections, making it a valuable ally for those managing chronic immune conditions.

Oregano Oil Chronic Immune Support Drops

INGREDIENTS

- Oregano essential oil
- Carrier oil (e.g., olive oil)

PREPARATION

1. Mix 2 drops of oregano essential oil with 1 teaspoon of carrier oil.
2. Store in a dropper bottle.
3. Take 2-3 drops daily diluted in water.

Benefits: Oregano oil is known for its powerful antimicrobial and antiviral properties. These drops help support the immune system against chronic infections, boosting overall resilience and promoting long-term health.

Thyme Long-Term Immune Strength Capsules

INGREDIENTS

- Thyme powder
- Empty vegetable capsules

PREPARATION

1. Fill capsules with thyme powder.
2. Store in a cool, dry place.
3. Take one capsule daily to strengthen immunity.

Benefits: Thyme supports immune health by providing antibacterial and anti-inflammatory properties. It helps strengthen the body's defenses against chronic infections, promoting resilience and long-term wellness.

Calendula Chronic Infection Tea

INGREDIENTS

- 1 teaspoon dried calendula flowers
- 1 cup hot water

PREPARATION

1. Steep calendula flowers in hot water for 10 minutes.
2. Strain and drink warm.
3. Consume daily for immune support.

Benefits: Calendula is a natural anti-inflammatory and antimicrobial herb that helps fight infections. This tea supports the immune system, reducing inflammation and promoting healing in cases of chronic conditions.

Milk Thistle Immune Detox Capsules

INGREDIENTS

- Milk thistle seed powder
- Empty vegetable capsules

PREPARATION

1. Fill capsules with milk thistle seed powder.
2. Store in a cool, dry place.
3. Take one capsule daily for detox support.

Benefits: Milk thistle supports liver detoxification, which is crucial for maintaining a healthy immune system. These capsules help the body eliminate toxins that can weaken immunity, promoting overall long-term immune health.

Licorice Root Immune Regulating Infusion

INGREDIENTS

- 1 teaspoon dried licorice root
- 1 cup hot water

PREPARATION

1. Steep licorice root in hot water for 10 minutes.
2. Strain and drink warm.
3. Consume daily for immune modulation.

Benefits: Licorice root has immune-regulating properties that support long-term immune balance. It helps reduce inflammation and fights off chronic infections, making it an effective remedy for those with ongoing immune challenges.

Yarrow Chronic Immune Support Capsules

INGREDIENTS

- Yarrow powder
- Empty vegetable capsules

PREPARATION

1. Fill capsules with yarrow powder.
2. Store in a cool, dry place.
3. Take one capsule daily for immune support.

Benefits: Yarrow supports immune function and reduces inflammation, helping the body fight off chronic infections. These capsules are particularly useful for maintaining a balanced and resilient immune system over time.

Turmeric and Cayenne Immune Tonic

INGREDIENTS

- 1 teaspoon turmeric powder
- A pinch of cayenne pepper
- 1 cup hot water

PREPARATION

1. Add turmeric and cayenne pepper to hot water and stir well.
2. Let the mixture steep for 5 minutes.
3. Strain and drink warm.

Benefits: Turmeric and cayenne work together to reduce inflammation and boost the immune system. This tonic supports long-term immune resilience, helping the body combat chronic conditions and maintain overall health.

Burdock Root Immune Detox Capsules

INGREDIENTS

- Burdock root powder
- Empty vegetable capsules

PREPARATION

1. Fill capsules with burdock root powder.
2. Store in a cool, dry place.
3. Take one capsule daily for detox support.

Benefits: Burdock root is a powerful detoxifier that supports liver health and helps remove toxins from the body, which can enhance immune function. These capsules aid in maintaining a balanced and strong immune system, promoting long-term resilience.

Goldenseal Chronic Inflammation Drops

INGREDIENTS

- Goldenseal root tincture
- Water

PREPARATION

1. Mix a few drops of goldenseal root tincture with water.
2. Take 15-20 drops daily diluted in water.
3. Consume daily for best results.

Benefits: Goldenseal is known for its anti-inflammatory and antimicrobial properties, making it an effective remedy for managing chronic inflammation and supporting immune health. These drops help reduce inflammation and promote long-term immune resilience.

Pine Needle Long-Term Immunity Infusion

INGREDIENTS

- 1 teaspoon dried pine needles
- 1 cup hot water

PREPARATION

1. Steep pine needles in hot water for 10-15 minutes.
2. Strain and drink the infusion warm.
3. Consume daily for ongoing immune support.

Benefits: Pine needles are rich in antioxidants and vitamin C, which support immune health and protect against chronic conditions. This infusion strengthens the immune system over time, making it a valuable ally for those seeking long-term immunity.

Olive Leaf Immune Protection Capsules

INGREDIENTS

- Olive leaf powder
- Empty vegetable capsules

PREPARATION

1. Fill capsules with olive leaf powder.
2. Store in a cool, dry place.
3. Take one capsule daily for immune protection.

Benefits: Olive leaf has antiviral and antibacterial properties that help protect the immune system. These capsules promote long-term immune resilience, supporting the body's defense mechanisms against chronic infections and improving overall health.

Skullcap Immune Calming Tea

INGREDIENTS

- 1 teaspoon dried skullcap leaves
- 1 cup hot water

PREPARATION

1. Steep skullcap leaves in hot water for 10 minutes.
2. Strain and drink warm.
3. Consume daily for immune support.

Benefits: Skullcap is a calming herb that helps reduce stress and inflammation, both of which can compromise immune function. This tea supports a balanced immune response and helps maintain long-term health, particularly for those managing chronic immune conditions.

Peppermint Immune Boost Drops

INGREDIENTS

- Peppermint essential oil
- Water

PREPARATION

1. Mix 2 drops of peppermint essential oil with water.
2. Take 5-10 drops daily diluted in water.
3. Consume as needed for immune support.

Benefits: Peppermint oil has antimicrobial properties that support immune function and promote respiratory health. These drops offer a quick boost to the immune system, helping maintain resilience and overall health.

Hibiscus and Lemon Immune Tonic

INGREDIENTS

- 1 teaspoon dried hibiscus flowers
- 1 slice fresh lemon
- 1 cup hot water

PREPARATION

1. Add hibiscus flowers and lemon to hot water.
2. Steep for 10 minutes, then strain.
3. Drink once daily for immune support.

Benefits: Hibiscus is rich in antioxidants that boost immune health, while lemon provides additional vitamin C. This tonic helps enhance immune function and protect against chronic infections, promoting overall vitality.

Ginseng Long-Term Energy Support Capsules

INGREDIENTS

- Ginseng root powder
- Empty vegetable capsules

PREPARATION

1. Fill capsules with ginseng root powder.
2. Store in a cool, dry place.
3. Take one capsule daily for energy support.

Benefits: Ginseng is an adaptogen that supports energy levels and immune function, making it effective for chronic immune conditions. These capsules help maintain stamina and resilience over time, promoting long-term immune health.

Dandelion Root Chronic Detox Capsules

INGREDIENTS

- Dandelion root powder
- Empty vegetable capsules

PREPARATION

1. Fill capsules with dandelion root powder.
2. Store in a cool, dry place.
3. Take one capsule daily for detox support.

Benefits: Dandelion root supports liver detoxification, which is crucial for maintaining immune health. These capsules help cleanse the body of toxins that can weaken immunity, promoting long-term resilience and vitality.

Nettle Immune Strengthening Tea

INGREDIENTS

- 1 teaspoon dried nettle leaves
- 1 cup hot water

PREPARATION

1. Steep nettle leaves in hot water for 10 minutes.
2. Strain and drink warm.
3. Consume daily for immune strengthening.

Benefits: Nettle is a nourishing herb that supports the immune system by providing essential vitamins and minerals. This tea helps strengthen immune function over time, promoting long-term resilience and overall health.

Red Clover Chronic Immune Support Infusion

INGREDIENTS

- 1 teaspoon dried red clover flowers
- 1 cup hot water

PREPARATION

1. Steep red clover flowers in hot water for 10 minutes.
2. Strain and drink warm.
3. Consume daily for immune support.

Benefits: Red clover is known for its anti-inflammatory properties and its ability to support immune health. This infusion helps reduce chronic inflammation and promotes long-term immune resilience, contributing to overall wellness.

Blue Vervain Immune Regulator Capsules

INGREDIENTS

- Blue vervain powder
- Empty vegetable capsules

PREPARATION

1. Fill capsules with blue vervain powder.
2. Store in a cool, dry place.
3. Take one capsule daily for immune regulation.

Benefits: Blue vervain is an immune modulator that helps balance the body's immune response, reducing inflammation and supporting resilience. These capsules are ideal for those managing chronic immune conditions and seeking long-term support.

Fenugreek Immune Support Tea

INGREDIENTS

- 1 teaspoon fenugreek seeds
- 1 cup hot water

PREPARATION

1. Steep fenugreek seeds in hot water for 10 minutes.
2. Strain and drink warm.
3. Consume once daily for best results.

Benefits: Fenugreek seeds are known for their immune-boosting properties. This tea helps enhance immune function, reduces inflammation, and supports overall health, making it a valuable remedy for chronic immune conditions.

Ginger and Lemon Immune Recovery Elixir

INGREDIENTS

- 1 inch fresh ginger root
- Juice of half a lemon
- 1 cup hot water

PREPARATION

1. Grate ginger and add to hot water.
2. Add lemon juice and let steep for 10 minutes.
3. Strain and drink warm.

Benefits: Ginger and lemon are powerful immune-boosting agents that support recovery from chronic conditions. This elixir reduces inflammation, enhances immune response, and provides antioxidants, promoting long-term immune health.

Spearmint Long-Term Immune Capsules

INGREDIENTS

- Spearmint leaf powder
- Empty vegetable capsules

PREPARATION

1. Fill capsules with spearmint leaf powder.
2. Store in a cool, dry place.
3. Take one capsule daily for immune support.

Benefits: Spearmint offers gentle immune support and anti-inflammatory properties, making it suitable for long-term use. These capsules promote a balanced immune response, supporting overall resilience and health.

Cat's Claw Immune Modulation Capsules

INGREDIENTS

- Cat's claw powder
- Empty vegetable capsules

PREPARATION

1. Fill capsules with cat's claw powder.
2. Store in a cool, dry place.
3. Take one capsule daily for immune modulation.

Benefits: Cat's claw is a powerful immune modulator that supports the body's natural defense mechanisms. These capsules help balance immune function, reduce inflammation, and support long-term health, making them ideal for those managing chronic immune conditions.

BOOK 27

Herbal Support for Liver Health

The Role of the Liver in Detoxification and Health

UNDERSTANDING THE LIVER'S VITAL ROLE IN DETOXIFICATION AND OVERALL HEALTH

The liver is one of the most essential organs in the human body, acting as the primary detoxification hub. Its intricate processes not only help filter out toxins but also play a crucial role in metabolism, digestion, and overall well-being. For individuals like Emma, who seek natural wellness strategies, understanding the liver's function is fundamental, as it directly influences her approach to health management. By comprehending how the liver supports detoxification, one can make informed decisions about incorporating herbs and natural remedies that enhance liver health.

The liver's functions are multifaceted, encompassing the breakdown of toxins, the synthesis of vital proteins, and the storage of nutrients. This organ processes everything that enters the bloodstream, including medications, food, and environmental toxins, transforming harmful substances into less toxic forms that the body can excrete through urine or bile.

The Detoxification Process: Phase 1 and Phase 2

The liver detoxifies the body through two main phases: Phase 1 and Phase 2 detoxification pathways. These phases work together to transform harmful substances into water-soluble compounds, which the body can then eliminate safely. Emma, as a wellness-conscious individual, would benefit from understanding these pathways to appreciate how herbal support aligns with her holistic lifestyle.

1. **Phase 1 Detoxification**

This is the initial step where the liver uses enzymes, primarily the cytochrome P450 enzymes, to neutralize toxins by converting them into intermediate metabolites. This phase involves oxidation, reduction, and hydrolysis reactions. However, these intermediate metabolites can sometimes be more toxic than the original substance, making it crucial for the liver to quickly move into Phase 2.

2. **Phase 2 Detoxification**

Phase 2 involves conjugation, where the liver attaches molecules like amino acids, sulfur, or glucuronic acid to the toxic intermediates produced in Phase 1. This process makes these compounds water-soluble, allowing the body to excrete them through urine or bile. This phase is particularly important for Emma as it highlights the need for balanced liver function and the importance of dietary and herbal support.

The Liver's Role in Metabolism and Digestion

Apart from detoxification, the liver is also deeply involved in the body's metabolic processes. It regulates glucose levels by storing and releasing glycogen, ensures the breakdown of fats through bile production, and plays a significant role in protein synthesis. These metabolic activities are essential for maintaining energy levels, balancing hormones, and supporting digestive health.

For someone like Emma, who prioritizes a balanced diet and wellness routine, understanding the liver's metabolic role is key. The liver's ability to regulate and maintain nutrient levels directly impacts overall vitality and energy levels, making it essential for daily functioning. A well-supported liver can optimize digestion, ensuring nutrients from her plant-based, natural diet are effectively absorbed and utilized by the body.

Environmental and Dietary Stressors on the Liver

In modern society, the liver is often overburdened by various environmental and dietary stressors. Processed foods, pollution, medications, and alcohol are just a few examples of factors that can compromise liver function. For individuals like Emma, who prefer holistic health strategies, awareness of these stressors highlights the importance of regular detoxification and liver support.

Chronic exposure to these toxins may lead to inflammation, fatty liver disease, or a reduction in the liver's ability to process and eliminate waste efficiently. As the liver becomes overwhelmed, symptoms like fatigue, digestive issues, and weakened immunity may emerge, signaling the need for proactive measures.

Supporting Liver Health with Natural Interventions

By understanding the liver's vital functions, one can better appreciate the significance of maintaining its health through natural interventions. Herbs like milk thistle, dandelion root, and turmeric are particularly beneficial for liver support, as they aid in detoxification, reduce inflammation, and promote regeneration. These herbs align with Emma's preference for sustainable, plant-based solutions and can easily be incorporated into her wellness routine.

- **Milk Thistle**: Known for its hepatoprotective properties, milk thistle helps regenerate liver cells and protects against toxin-induced damage.
- **Dandelion Root**: This herb stimulates bile production, aiding in digestion and enhancing the liver's ability to process and eliminate toxins.
- **Turmeric**: Its anti-inflammatory and antioxidant properties help reduce liver inflammation and oxidative stress, making it a powerful ally in maintaining liver health.

Incorporating these herbs, either through teas, tinctures, or supplements, can provide Emma with practical, everyday solutions that fit her holistic approach. Moreover, ensuring a balanced diet rich in antioxidants, fiber, and hydration also plays a significant role in supporting liver function.

Top Herbs for Liver Detox and Regeneration

ESSENTIAL HERBS FOR LIVER DETOXIFICATION AND REGENERATION

Liver detoxification and regeneration are fundamental aspects of maintaining overall health, particularly for individuals who are mindful of their well-being and prefer natural methods. The liver, being the primary organ for detoxifying harmful substances and regenerating itself, benefits greatly from herbal support. For individuals like Emma, who favor plant-based solutions for wellness, incorporating the right herbs into a daily routine can optimize liver function, enhance detoxification, and promote regeneration. Below are some of the top herbs known for their potent liver-supportive properties.

Milk Thistle: The Ultimate Liver Protector

Milk thistle (Silybum marianum) is often considered the gold standard when it comes to liver health. It contains a powerful compound called silymarin, which is renowned for its antioxidant, anti-inflammatory, and regenerative effects on liver cells. Silymarin not only shields liver cells from damage caused by toxins but also aids in their repair and regeneration, making it ideal for those seeking to boost their liver's resilience and recovery capacity.

- **Detoxification Support:** Milk thistle enhances the liver's Phase 1 and Phase 2 detoxification processes, ensuring harmful substances are processed efficiently and expelled from the body.
- **Regeneration:** This herb promotes protein synthesis in liver cells, accelerating the regeneration of damaged tissues and improving overall liver function. Emma would benefit from incorporating milk thistle either as a tea or supplement to maintain a robust liver.

Dandelion Root: Nature's Bile Stimulator

Dandelion root (Taraxacum officinale) is another herb that plays a significant role in liver detoxification and regeneration. Known for its ability to stimulate bile production, dandelion root supports digestion and enhances the liver's efficiency in processing fats and toxins. It is an excellent choice for individuals who want to support their liver naturally, especially those who may experience digestive issues linked to liver function.

- **Bile Production:** By increasing bile flow, dandelion root ensures that the liver can efficiently break down and excrete fats, which is crucial for detoxification.
- **Liver Cell Protection:** The antioxidants in dandelion root protect liver cells from oxidative stress and aid in the repair of damaged tissues, making it a powerful ally in liver regeneration.

Turmeric: Anti-Inflammatory Powerhouse for the Liver

Turmeric (Curcuma longa) is widely used not only for its culinary benefits but also for its profound medicinal properties. The active compound in turmeric, curcumin, has powerful anti-inflammatory and antioxidant effects that help reduce liver inflammation and prevent damage from free radicals. It's particularly beneficial for those aiming to support their liver through natural, anti-inflammatory strategies.

- **Anti-Inflammatory Action:** Curcumin reduces inflammation in the liver, which is crucial for preventing chronic liver diseases and supporting long-term liver health.
- **Regenerative Properties:** By promoting bile production and protecting liver cells from toxins, turmeric aids in both detoxification and regeneration. Emma could incorporate turmeric into her daily routine through golden milk or turmeric capsules to maximize these benefits.

Artichoke Leaf: Enhancing Liver Function and Bile Flow

Artichoke leaf (Cynara scolymus) is lesser-known but highly effective for liver support. It contains compounds like cynarin, which stimulate bile production, helping the liver process and remove toxins more efficiently. For individuals looking to maintain optimal liver function, artichoke leaf offers a natural solution that is easy to integrate into a wellness plan.

- **Bile Stimulation:** By enhancing bile flow, artichoke leaf supports digestion and ensures the liver can handle fatty substances more effectively.
- **Cell Regeneration:** Its antioxidant properties help in repairing liver cells, making it a valuable herb for liver regeneration.

Schisandra Berry: A Powerful Adaptogen for the Liver

Schisandra (Schisandra chinensis) is a potent adaptogen, meaning it helps the body adapt to stress and promotes balance. This herb is particularly beneficial for liver health, as it boosts the liver's detoxification capacity and supports its regenerative functions. Schisandra is an excellent choice for those who wish to incorporate a comprehensive approach to liver wellness.

- **Detox Enhancement:** Schisandra increases the liver's detoxification enzymes, making it more efficient at filtering and eliminating toxins.
- **Regeneration Support:** It enhances the liver's ability to regenerate by promoting cell growth and reducing oxidative damage, which is crucial for individuals like Emma who aim to sustain their liver health over the long term.

Burdock Root: Purifying the Blood and Supporting the Liver

Burdock root (Arctium lappa) is often used for its blood-purifying properties, which naturally support liver function. By cleansing the blood, burdock root lightens the liver's load, allowing it to focus on detoxification and regeneration.

- **Blood Purification:** Burdock root helps filter impurities from the bloodstream, reducing the liver's burden and enhancing its detoxification capabilities.
- **Liver Cell Protection:** With its antioxidant content, burdock root protects liver cells from damage, aiding in regeneration and improving overall liver health.

Integrating Herbs into Daily Wellness

For someone like Emma, who prioritizes holistic and sustainable approaches, integrating these herbs into her daily routine can provide consistent liver support. These herbs are available in various forms such as teas, tinctures, capsules, and even fresh preparations, making them adaptable to different preferences and lifestyles. Combining these herbs in therapeutic doses, under the guidance of a qualified herbalist, ensures she maximizes their benefits while tailoring them to her specific health needs.

Remedies for Liver Support and Detoxification

Milk Thistle Liver Detox Capsules

INGREDIENTS

- Milk thistle seed powder
- Empty vegetable capsules

PREPARATION

1. Fill the empty vegetable capsules with milk thistle seed powder.
2. Store capsules in a cool, dry place.
3. Take one capsule daily for liver support.

Benefits: Milk thistle is renowned for its liver-protective properties, primarily due to the compound silymarin. It helps detoxify the liver, promote cell regeneration, and protect against toxins and oxidative damage, making it a valuable ally for long-term liver health.

Dandelion Root Liver Cleansing Infusion

INGREDIENTS

- 1 teaspoon dried dandelion root
- 1 cup hot water

PREPARATION

1. Add the dried dandelion root to hot water and steep for 10–15 minutes.
2. Strain the infusion and drink warm.
3. Consume once daily for optimal liver cleansing benefits.

Benefits: Dandelion root is a powerful liver tonic that supports detoxification and bile production, aiding digestion and the elimination of waste. Regular consumption promotes a healthier liver and improved digestive function.

Burdock and Red Clover Liver Health Tea

INGREDIENTS

- 1 teaspoon dried burdock root
- 1 teaspoon dried red clover flowers
- 1 cup hot water

PREPARATION

1. Combine burdock root and red clover in a cup of hot water.
2. Steep for 10 minutes, then strain the tea.
3. Drink once daily for liver support.

Benefits: Burdock root and red clover work synergistically to detoxify the liver and purify the blood. This tea helps eliminate toxins and supports the liver's natural functions, promoting overall health and well-being.

Yellow Dock Liver Support Capsules

INGREDIENTS

- Yellow dock root powder
- Empty vegetable capsules

PREPARATION

1. Fill capsules with yellow dock root powder.
2. Store in a cool, dry place.
3. Take one capsule daily to support liver health.

Benefits: Yellow dock root is known for its ability to cleanse the liver and promote bile flow. It supports the elimination of toxins and enhances digestive health, contributing to improved liver function and overall detoxification.

Artichoke Leaf Liver Protection Tonic

INGREDIENTS

- 1 teaspoon dried artichoke leaves
- 1 cup hot water

PREPARATION

1. Steep the dried artichoke leaves in hot water for 10 minutes.
2. Strain and drink warm.
3. Consume once daily to protect liver health.

Benefits: Artichoke leaf has been used for centuries to support liver function and promote bile production. This tonic helps protect the liver from toxins and aids in digestion, making it a valuable addition to any liver health regimen.

Schisandra Berry Liver Health Drops

INGREDIENTS

- Schisandra berries
- Vodka or apple cider vinegar (for tincture)

PREPARATION

1. Place schisandra berries in a jar and cover with vodka or apple cider vinegar.
2. Seal and let it steep for 4-6 weeks, shaking occasionally.
3. Strain the mixture and store in a dropper bottle.
4. Take 15-20 drops daily in water for liver support.

Benefits: Schisandra berries are adaptogens that support liver health by promoting detoxification and enhancing liver enzyme production. This tincture boosts the liver's ability to process toxins and helps maintain overall vitality.

Goldenseal Liver Function Capsules

INGREDIENTS

- Goldenseal root powder
- Empty vegetable capsules

PREPARATION

1. Fill the capsules with goldenseal root powder.
2. Store capsules in a cool, dry place.
3. Take one capsule daily to support liver function.

Benefits: Goldenseal is known for its antimicrobial and anti-inflammatory properties. It supports the liver by aiding in the detoxification process, improving liver function, and promoting overall digestive health.

Nettle and Mint Liver Support Tea

INGREDIENTS

- 1 teaspoon dried nettle leaves
- 1 teaspoon dried mint leaves
- 1 cup hot water

PREPARATION

1. Combine nettle and mint leaves in hot water.
2. Steep for 10 minutes, then strain.
3. Drink once or twice daily for liver support.

Benefits: Nettle and mint provide a gentle detoxifying effect on the liver, supporting its functions and promoting bile production. This tea also soothes the digestive system, aiding in overall liver and digestive health.

Chicory Root Liver Strengthening Infusion

INGREDIENTS

- 1 teaspoon dried chicory root
- 1 cup hot water

PREPARATION

1. Steep the dried chicory root in hot water for 10 minutes.
2. Strain and drink warm.
3. Consume daily for liver strengthening benefits.

Benefits: Chicory root is a traditional remedy known for its ability to stimulate bile production and support liver function. It helps cleanse the liver, promotes digestion, and strengthens the liver's natural detoxification processes.

Licorice Root Liver Detox Capsules

INGREDIENTS

- Licorice root powder
- Empty vegetable capsules

PREPARATION

1. Fill capsules with licorice root powder.
2. Store in a cool, dry place.
3. Take one capsule daily for liver detox.

Benefits: Licorice root has anti-inflammatory and detoxifying properties that support liver health. These capsules help protect liver cells from damage, aid in detoxification, and promote overall liver function.

Blue Flag Root Liver Cleansing Capsules

INGREDIENTS

- Blue flag root powder
- Empty vegetable capsules

PREPARATION

1. Fill the capsules with blue flag root powder.
2. Store in a cool, dry place.
3. Take one capsule daily for liver cleansing.

Benefits: Blue flag root is used to cleanse the liver and promote bile flow, aiding in the elimination of toxins. Regular use supports overall liver health and improves the body's natural detoxification processes.

Calendula Liver Protection Capsules

INGREDIENTS

- Calendula flower powder
- Empty vegetable capsules

PREPARATION

1. Fill the capsules with calendula flower powder.
2. Store in a cool, dry place.
3. Take one capsule daily to protect liver health.

Benefits: Calendula has anti-inflammatory and hepatoprotective properties that support liver health. These capsules help reduce inflammation in the liver and protect against damage, promoting long-term liver function.

Fennel Seed Digestive and Liver Health Tea

INGREDIENTS

- 1 teaspoon fennel seeds
- 1 cup hot water

PREPARATION

1. Steep fennel seeds in hot water for 10 minutes.
2. Strain and drink warm.
3. Consume daily for digestive and liver support.

Benefits: Fennel seeds aid in digestion and support liver health by promoting bile production. This tea helps cleanse the liver and improve digestion, making it beneficial for maintaining overall digestive and liver wellness.

Ginger Liver Cleansing Capsules

INGREDIENTS

- Ginger powder
- Empty vegetable capsules

PREPARATION

1. Fill capsules with ginger powder.
2. Store in a cool, dry place.
3. Take one capsule daily for liver cleansing support.

Benefits: Ginger supports liver detoxification and reduces inflammation, helping the liver function more efficiently. These capsules offer a convenient way to cleanse the liver and promote overall health.

Turmeric Liver Protection Capsules

Ingredients

Turmeric powder

Empty vegetable capsules

PREPARATION

1. Fill capsules with turmeric powder.
2. Store in a cool, dry place.
3. Take one capsule daily for liver protection.

Benefits: Turmeric contains curcumin, which has powerful anti-inflammatory and antioxidant properties. These capsules help protect the liver from damage, support detoxification, and promote long-term liver health.

Holy Basil (Tulsi) Liver Support Elixir

INGREDIENTS

- Fresh holy basil leaves
- Vodka or apple cider vinegar (for tincture)

PREPARATION

1. Place fresh holy basil leaves in a jar and cover with vodka or apple cider vinegar.
2. Seal and let it steep for 4-6 weeks, shaking occasionally.
3. Strain and store in a dropper bottle.
4. Take 15-20 drops daily in water for liver support.

Benefits: Holy basil is an adaptogen that helps reduce stress and inflammation, both of which can impact liver health. This elixir supports liver detoxification and function, promoting overall liver wellness.

Reishi Mushroom Liver Health Capsules

INGREDIENTS

- Reishi mushroom powder
- Empty vegetable capsules

PREPARATION

1. Fill capsules with reishi mushroom powder.
2. Store in a cool, dry place.
3. Take one capsule daily for liver health.

Benefits: Reishi mushrooms support liver health by enhancing detoxification and reducing inflammation. These capsules help improve liver function and promote overall immune health, making them beneficial for long-term liver support.

Lemon Peel Liver Detox Drink

INGREDIENTS

- 1 teaspoon dried lemon peel
- 1 cup hot water
- A slice of fresh lemon

PREPARATION

1. Add dried lemon peel to hot water and steep for 10 minutes.
2. Strain the infusion and add a slice of fresh lemon.
3. Drink warm once daily for liver detoxification.

Benefits: Lemon peel is rich in antioxidants and vitamin C, which support liver detoxification. This drink helps cleanse the liver, promote bile production, and improve overall liver function, making it effective for long-term detox support.

Wormwood Liver Function Capsules

INGREDIENTS

- Wormwood powder
- Empty vegetable capsules

PREPARATION

1. Fill capsules with wormwood powder.
2. Store in a cool, dry place.
3. Take one capsule daily for liver function support.

Benefits: Wormwood supports liver health by enhancing bile flow and aiding in detoxification. These capsules help maintain optimal liver function and cleanse the body of toxins, promoting overall liver wellness.

Rose Hip Liver Support Capsules

INGREDIENTS

- Rose hip powder
- Empty vegetable capsules

PREPARATION

1. Fill capsules with rose hip powder.
2. Store in a cool, dry place.
3. Take one capsule daily for liver support.

Benefits: Rose hips are rich in vitamin C and antioxidants, which protect the liver and support its natural detoxification processes. These capsules help boost liver function and promote long-term liver health.

Green Tea Liver Protection Infusion

INGREDIENTS

- 1 teaspoon green tea leaves
- 1 cup hot water

PREPARATION

1. Steep green tea leaves in hot water for 5-7 minutes.
2. Strain the infusion and drink warm.
3. Consume daily for liver protection.

Benefits: Green tea contains powerful antioxidants that support liver health by reducing oxidative stress and protecting liver cells. This infusion helps cleanse the liver, supports detoxification, and promotes overall well-being.

Dandelion and Burdock Root Liver Cleanse Tea

INGREDIENTS

- 1 teaspoon dried dandelion root
- 1 teaspoon dried burdock root
- 1 cup hot water

PREPARATION

1. Combine dandelion and burdock roots in hot water.
2. Steep for 10 minutes, then strain.
3. Drink once daily for liver cleansing.

Benefits: Dandelion and burdock roots are powerful detoxifiers that work together to cleanse the liver and support its functions. This tea enhances liver health by promoting the elimination of toxins and improving digestion.

Chamomile Liver Function Capsules

INGREDIENTS

- Chamomile powder
- Empty vegetable capsules

PREPARATION

1. Fill capsules with chamomile powder.
2. Store in a cool, dry place.
3. Take one capsule daily for liver function support.

Benefits: Chamomile has anti-inflammatory and calming properties that support liver health. These capsules help reduce liver inflammation and promote overall liver function, making them suitable for long-term liver care.

Red Clover Detoxification Capsules

INGREDIENTS

- Red clover powder
- Empty vegetable capsules

PREPARATION

1. Fill capsules with red clover powder.
2. Store in a cool, dry place.
3. Take one capsule daily for detoxification support.

Benefits: Red clover supports detoxification by purifying the blood and promoting liver health. These capsules help cleanse the liver, reduce inflammation, and support the body's natural detox processes.

Peppermint Liver Support Infusion

INGREDIENTS

- 1 teaspoon dried peppermint leaves
- 1 cup hot water

PREPARATION

1. Steep peppermint leaves in hot water for 5-7 minutes.
2. Strain and drink warm.
3. Consume daily for liver support.

Benefits: Peppermint supports liver health by enhancing bile production and soothing the digestive system. This infusion aids in detoxification and promotes a healthy liver environment, making it an effective remedy for long-term liver support.

Marshmallow Root Liver Soothing Capsules

INGREDIENTS

- Marshmallow root powder
- Empty vegetable capsules

PREPARATION

1. Fill capsules with marshmallow root powder.
2. Store in a cool, dry place.
3. Take one capsule daily for liver support.

Benefits: Marshmallow root is soothing and anti-inflammatory, making it beneficial for liver health. These capsules help reduce inflammation and support the liver's natural detoxification processes, promoting overall well-being.

Sage Liver Strengthening Capsules

INGREDIENTS

- Sage leaf powder
- Empty vegetable capsules

PREPARATION

1. Fill capsules with sage leaf powder.
2. Store in a cool, dry place.
3. Take one capsule daily for liver strength.

Benefits: Sage supports liver health by reducing inflammation and enhancing bile production. These capsules help strengthen the liver, support detoxification, and promote overall digestive health, making them a valuable addition to liver care routines.

Yarrow Liver Support Tea

INGREDIENTS

- 1 teaspoon dried yarrow leaves
- 1 cup hot water

PREPARATION

1. Steep yarrow leaves in hot water for 10 minutes.
2. Strain and drink warm.
3. Consume daily for liver support.

Benefits: Yarrow is known for its anti-inflammatory properties and its ability to promote bile flow, aiding in digestion and liver health. This tea supports the liver's detoxification processes, helping maintain a balanced and healthy liver.

Lemon Verbena Liver Detox Elixir

INGREDIENTS

- Fresh lemon verbena leaves
- Vodka or apple cider vinegar (for tincture)

PREPARATION

1. Place fresh lemon verbena leaves in a jar and cover with vodka or apple cider vinegar.
2. Seal and let it steep for 4-6 weeks, shaking occasionally.
3. Strain and store in a dropper bottle.
4. Take 15-20 drops daily in water for liver detoxification.

Benefits: Lemon verbena supports liver health by promoting detoxification and reducing inflammation. This elixir helps cleanse the liver and supports its functions, making it effective for long-term detox care.

Gentian Root Liver Protection Capsules

INGREDIENTS

- Gentian root powder
- Empty vegetable capsules

PREPARATION

1. Fill capsules with gentian root powder.
2. Store in a cool, dry place.
3. Take one capsule daily for liver protection.

Benefits: Gentian root is a bitter herb that supports liver health by stimulating bile production and enhancing digestion. These capsules help protect the liver from toxins, promote detoxification, and support overall liver wellness.

Hibiscus Liver Detox Capsules

INGREDIENTS

- Hibiscus flower powder
- Empty vegetable capsules

PREPARATION

1. Fill capsules with hibiscus flower powder.
2. Store in a cool, dry place.
3. Take one capsule daily for liver detox support.

Benefits: Hibiscus is rich in antioxidants that help cleanse and protect the liver. These capsules aid in detoxification, reduce inflammation, and support overall liver health, making them ideal for long-term liver care.

Celandine Liver Health Drops

INGREDIENTS

- Fresh celandine leaves
- Vodka or apple cider vinegar (for tincture)

PREPARATION

1. Place fresh celandine leaves in a jar and cover with vodka or apple cider vinegar.
2. Seal and let it steep for 4-6 weeks, shaking occasionally.
3. Strain and store in a dropper bottle.
4. Take 15-20 drops daily in water for liver support.

Benefits: Celandine supports liver function by promoting bile flow and aiding in detoxification. This tincture helps maintain liver health, reduce inflammation, and improve overall digestive health, making it effective for liver care.

Parsley Liver Cleansing Tea

INGREDIENTS

- 1 teaspoon fresh parsley leaves
- 1 cup hot water

PREPARATION

1. Add fresh parsley leaves to hot water and steep for 10 minutes.
2. Strain and drink warm.
3. Consume daily for liver cleansing support.

Benefits: Parsley is a natural diuretic that supports liver cleansing and detoxification. This tea helps flush toxins from the liver and supports its function, promoting overall liver health and vitality.

BOOK 28

Kidney and Urinary Tract Health

Herbs for Kidney Cleansing and UTI Prevention

EFFECTIVE HERBS FOR KIDNEY CLEANSING AND UTI PREVENTION

Kidney health is crucial for the body's detoxification processes, and maintaining its function is essential for overall wellness. Similarly, urinary tract infections (UTIs) are common and can become recurrent issues if not managed properly. For individuals seeking natural, holistic ways to support their kidney and urinary health, several herbs stand out due to their cleansing, antibacterial, and anti-inflammatory properties. These herbs not only promote kidney detoxification but also help prevent and alleviate UTIs, offering a comprehensive approach to urinary health. Below are some of the most effective herbs for these purposes, tailored to fit the needs of a proactive and health-conscious individual.

Parsley: A Gentle Kidney Cleanser

Parsley (Petroselinum crispum) is more than a culinary herb; it is a powerful diuretic that can support kidney function and aid in the prevention of UTIs. Its natural diuretic effect increases urine production, which helps flush out toxins and bacteria from the urinary tract, reducing the risk of infection and promoting kidney cleansing.

- **Diuretic Properties:** By increasing urine output, parsley aids in flushing harmful substances and bacteria from the kidneys and bladder. This natural process can help prevent UTIs and support overall kidney health.
- **Antioxidant Benefits:** Rich in flavonoids and vitamin C, parsley also provides antioxidant support, which is essential for protecting kidney cells from oxidative damage.
- **Usage:** For those looking to integrate parsley into their routine, it can be consumed as a tea or added fresh to meals for both its flavor and medicinal properties.

Cranberry: Nature's UTI Preventive

Cranberries (Vaccinium macrocarpon) have long been recognized for their ability to prevent UTIs, thanks to their high concentration of proanthocyanidins. These compounds prevent bacteria, particularly *E. coli*, from adhering to the walls of the urinary tract, reducing the likelihood of infection. For individuals who are prone to recurrent UTIs, cranberry is an effective, natural preventive measure.

- **Anti-Adhesion Properties:** The unique compounds in cranberries inhibit bacteria from attaching to the bladder and urinary tract lining, making it difficult for infections to develop.
- **Kidney Health Support:** By maintaining a healthy urinary environment, cranberries indirectly support kidney function, ensuring that this vital organ continues to filter waste effectively.
- **Consumption Tips:** Cranberry juice, unsweetened and pure, or cranberry supplements are recommended to harness these benefits effectively.

Dandelion Root: Detoxification and UTI Prevention

Dandelion root (Taraxacum officinale) is a well-known herb for supporting kidney function due to its diuretic and detoxifying properties. It promotes increased urine production, which assists in flushing out bacteria and toxins, making it a great option for kidney cleansing and UTI prevention.

- **Diuretic Action:** Dandelion root stimulates the kidneys to produce more urine, aiding in the expulsion of toxins and bacteria. This natural flushing process supports both kidney health and urinary tract cleanliness.
- **Nutrient-Rich Composition:** The herb is also rich in potassium, which is crucial for balancing electrolytes when promoting diuresis. This ensures that while it increases urine flow, it does not cause potassium depletion.
- **How to Use:** Dandelion root can be consumed as a tea, tincture, or capsule, making it versatile for daily use as part of a kidney health regimen.

Corn Silk: A Traditional Remedy for UTIs

Corn silk (Stigma maydis) is a traditional herbal remedy for urinary health, known for its soothing and anti-inflammatory properties. It is particularly effective in treating and preventing UTIs, as it acts as a diuretic and reduces inflammation in the urinary tract.

- **Soothing Properties:** Corn silk calms the urinary tract lining, making it an excellent choice for individuals who experience irritation or frequent UTIs.
- **Natural Diuretic:** It helps promote urine flow, flushing out bacteria and reducing the risk of infection. This makes it an effective herb for both cleansing the kidneys and maintaining urinary health.
- **Integration:** Corn silk can be brewed into a mild tea, offering a gentle way to support kidney and urinary tract health daily.

Uva Ursi: A Powerful Antibacterial Agent

Uva ursi (Arctostaphylos uva-ursi), also known as bearberry, is a potent herb used traditionally for its antibacterial properties. It is particularly effective in treating and preventing UTIs by targeting the bacteria responsible for infections. Uva ursi contains compounds like arbutin, which is converted into an antimicrobial agent in the body, helping to cleanse the urinary tract.

- **Antimicrobial Action:** The active compounds in uva ursi are released in the urinary tract, directly attacking bacteria and reducing infection risks.
- **Anti-Inflammatory Properties:** Uva ursi also reduces inflammation in the kidneys and bladder, supporting overall urinary health and easing discomfort during infections.
- **Usage Caution:** While effective, uva ursi should be used with caution and only for short periods, as prolonged use may lead to unwanted side effects. Consulting a healthcare professional before use is advisable.

Marshmallow Root: A Mucilaginous Soother

Marshmallow root (Althaea officinalis) is another herb that supports kidney health and helps prevent UTIs through its mucilaginous properties. The mucilage content in marshmallow root coats the urinary tract, providing a protective barrier that reduces irritation and inflammation.

- **Protective Coating:** This mucilaginous effect not only soothes but also protects the urinary tract from bacteria, reducing the risk of infections.
- **Hydration Support:** Marshmallow root also promotes hydration, which is essential for kidney function and flushing out toxins. Staying hydrated is a key aspect of maintaining kidney and urinary tract health, and marshmallow root tea can be a helpful addition to a hydration routine.
- **Consumption:** Marshmallow root is best consumed as a tea to maximize its soothing and protective properties.

Integrating Herbal Kidney Support

For a comprehensive approach to kidney cleansing and UTI prevention, individuals like Emma should consider integrating these herbs into their daily routines. Herbal teas, tinctures, and supplements provide multiple ways to enjoy the benefits of these natural remedies. Regular use, along with proper hydration and a balanced diet, can significantly improve kidney function and reduce the risk of UTIs, ensuring a holistic and preventive approach to urinary health.

Natural Diuretics and Urinary Health Solutions

EFFECTIVE NATURAL DIURETICS FOR OPTIMAL URINARY HEALTH

Diuretics are substances that promote the increased production of urine, which is vital for flushing out toxins, excess fluids, and waste products from the body. They play an essential role in maintaining urinary health, supporting kidney function, and preventing urinary tract infections (UTIs). For individuals looking to maintain or improve their urinary health naturally, incorporating herbal diuretics offers a gentle, effective solution. These natural remedies are especially beneficial for those seeking alternatives to pharmaceutical diuretics, as they tend to have fewer side effects and provide additional health benefits.

Dandelion: A Potent Diuretic and Detoxifier

Dandelion (Taraxacum officinale) is one of the most well-known natural diuretics. The leaves of this plant are rich in potassium, which is essential for balancing electrolyte levels when urine production increases. Dandelion stimulates the kidneys to flush out excess water and sodium, which not only supports urinary health but also aids in detoxification.

- **How It Works:** Dandelion acts as a gentle diuretic by stimulating the kidneys, increasing urine flow without depleting essential minerals like potassium, making it a balanced solution for long-term use.
- **Additional Benefits:** Beyond its diuretic effects, dandelion also contains antioxidants and anti-inflammatory compounds, which help protect the urinary tract and support overall kidney health.
- **Usage:** Dandelion leaves can be brewed into a tea, tincture, or added fresh to salads. For maximum diuretic effects, drinking dandelion tea daily is recommended, as it provides a consistent, mild diuretic action.

Parsley: An Accessible and Effective Herbal Diuretic

Parsley (Petroselinum crispum), often seen as a simple garnish, is a powerful diuretic that supports urinary health. This herb increases urine production, helping to eliminate excess sodium and water from the body, which reduces bloating and helps prevent kidney stones.

- **Diuretic Action:** Parsley works by stimulating the kidneys to produce more urine, effectively flushing out toxins and reducing the risk of infection in the urinary tract. Its high vitamin C content also boosts immune function, further protecting the kidneys.
- **Nutrient-Rich Profile:** Loaded with antioxidants and vitamins A, C, and K, parsley supports overall kidney function while acting as a diuretic.
- **Preparation** Parsley can be consumed as a tea by boiling fresh leaves in water, or it can be added raw to meals. For those seeking a stronger effect, parsley juice is a concentrated and effective option.

Horsetail: A Traditional Remedy for Urinary Health

Horsetail (Equisetum arvense) is a traditional herb with a long history of use in supporting urinary health. Known for its silica content, which strengthens connective tissues, horsetail also has diuretic properties that help the body expel excess fluids and promote kidney function.

- **Silica and Diuretic Properties:** The high silica content in horsetail not only supports bone health but also contributes to its diuretic action, enhancing urine production and flushing the urinary system.
- **Anti-Inflammatory Effects:** Horsetail's anti-inflammatory properties help soothe the urinary tract, reducing the risk of infection and promoting overall urinary comfort.
- **Usage Guidelines:** Horsetail is commonly consumed as a tea, providing a gentle yet effective diuretic effect. It is advisable to use horsetail for short periods, as prolonged use may lead to electrolyte imbalances.

Corn Silk: A Gentle and Soothing Diuretic

Corn silk (Stigma maydis) is a lesser-known but highly effective diuretic for promoting urinary health. It acts gently, making it suitable for individuals who may have sensitive kidneys or are prone to urinary tract discomfort. Corn silk tea is often used to reduce inflammation and irritation in the urinary tract.

- **Diuretic and Soothing Properties:** Corn silk increases urine production while providing a soothing effect on the urinary tract, making it ideal for individuals who experience frequent UTIs or bladder irritation.
- **Anti-Inflammatory Action:** It contains compounds that help reduce inflammation, making it effective in supporting urinary health during infections or inflammation-related conditions.
- **Preparation** To make corn silk tea, boil fresh or dried corn silk in water and let it steep for about 10 minutes. This tea can be consumed several times a day to maintain urinary health and promote diuresis.

Nettle: A Balancing Diuretic for Long-Term Use

Nettle (Urtica dioica) is another highly effective natural diuretic. It not only increases urine production but also offers anti-inflammatory and antimicrobial properties, making it particularly beneficial for individuals prone to UTIs. Nettle is rich in vitamins and minerals, including iron and calcium, which support overall health and balance electrolyte levels during diuretic use.

- **Comprehensive Support:** Nettle's diuretic action helps eliminate excess fluids while also providing anti-inflammatory benefits, which protect the kidneys and urinary tract.
- **Mineral-Rich Composition:** The herb's mineral content ensures that electrolyte balance is maintained, reducing the risk of depletion often associated with diuretic use.
- **How to Use:** Nettle tea is a popular preparation method, offering a mild diuretic effect when consumed daily. It can also be taken as a tincture for a more concentrated dose.

Celery Seed: A Mild Diuretic with Additional Benefits

Celery seed (Apium graveolens) is a gentle diuretic that supports urinary health by encouraging the elimination of excess water and uric acid from the kidneys. It is especially useful for those dealing with conditions like gout, where reducing uric acid levels is crucial.

- **Diuretic and Detoxifying:** The compounds in celery seed promote increased urine production, helping to cleanse the kidneys and urinary tract efficiently.
- **Antioxidant Support:** Celery seed also provides antioxidants, which protect kidney cells from damage, making it a supportive herb for long-term urinary health maintenance.
- **Integration into Diet:** Celery seed can be added to meals as a spice or brewed into a tea. Consistent use in either form supports its diuretic and detoxifying properties.

Conclusion

Integrating natural diuretics like dandelion, parsley, horsetail, corn silk, nettle, and celery seed into one's wellness routine provides a comprehensive approach to maintaining urinary health. These herbs offer a balance between effective diuresis and additional health benefits, making them ideal for individuals seeking to support their kidneys and urinary tract naturally.

Remedies for Kidney and Urinary Wellness

Cranberry Urinary Tract Support Capsules

INGREDIENTS

- Cranberry powder
- Empty vegetable capsules

PREPARATION

1. Fill empty capsules with cranberry powder.
2. Store capsules in a cool, dry place.
3. Take one capsule daily for urinary tract support.

Benefits: Cranberries are well-known for their ability to prevent urinary tract infections by inhibiting bacteria from adhering to the urinary tract walls. These capsules offer a convenient way to support urinary health and prevent infections naturally.

Corn Silk Kidney Health Tea

INGREDIENTS

- 1 teaspoon dried corn silk
- 1 cup hot water

PREPARATION

1. Add dried corn silk to hot water and steep for 10 minutes.
2. Strain the infusion and drink warm.
3. Consume once or twice daily for best results.

Benefits: Corn silk is a natural diuretic that helps promote kidney health and relieve inflammation in the urinary tract. This tea supports the elimination of excess fluids, aiding in the maintenance of kidney function and overall urinary wellness.

Dandelion Leaf Kidney Detox Infusion

INGREDIENTS

- 1 teaspoon dried dandelion leaves
- 1 cup hot water

PREPARATION

1. Steep dandelion leaves in hot water for 10 minutes.
2. Strain and drink warm.
3. Consume daily for kidney detox support.

Benefits: Dandelion leaves act as a gentle diuretic, promoting urine production and assisting in the detoxification of the kidneys. This infusion helps flush out toxins and supports kidney function, enhancing overall urinary health.

Nettle Kidney Cleanse Capsules

INGREDIENTS

- Nettle leaf powder
- Empty vegetable capsules

PREPARATION

1. Fill capsules with nettle leaf powder.
2. Store in a cool, dry place.
3. Take one capsule daily for kidney cleanse support.

Benefits: Nettle leaves are known for their diuretic properties, which help cleanse the kidneys and reduce inflammation. These capsules support kidney function and promote the elimination of excess fluids, aiding in overall detoxification.

Juniper Berry Urinary Health Drops

INGREDIENTS

- Juniper berries
- Vodka or apple cider vinegar (for tincture)

PREPARATION

1. Place juniper berries in a jar and cover with vodka or apple cider vinegar.
2. Seal the jar and let it steep for 4-6 weeks, shaking occasionally.
3. Strain and store in a dropper bottle.
4. Take 15-20 drops daily in water for urinary support.

Benefits: Juniper berries possess antiseptic and diuretic properties that promote urinary health. This tincture helps cleanse the kidneys, reduce inflammation, and support overall urinary tract wellness, making it an effective remedy for long-term use.

Parsley Diuretic Support Capsules

INGREDIENTS

- Parsley leaf powder
- Empty vegetable capsules

PREPARATION

1. Fill capsules with parsley leaf powder.
2. Store in a cool, dry place.
3. Take one capsule daily for diuretic support.

Benefits: Parsley is a natural diuretic that helps increase urine production and reduce fluid retention. These capsules support kidney function, assist in detoxification, and promote overall urinary health.

Marshmallow Root Urinary Soothing Tea

INGREDIENTS

- 1 teaspoon dried marshmallow root
- 1 cup hot water

PREPARATION

1. Steep marshmallow root in hot water for 10-15 minutes.
2. Strain and drink warm.
3. Consume daily for urinary tract soothing.

Benefits: Marshmallow root has demulcent properties that soothe the mucous membranes of the urinary tract. This tea helps reduce inflammation and discomfort, supporting overall urinary health and relief from irritation.

Goldenrod Kidney Support Capsules

INGREDIENTS

- Goldenrod powder
- Empty vegetable capsules

PREPARATION

1. Fill capsules with goldenrod powder.
2. Store in a cool, dry place.
3. Take one capsule daily for kidney support.

Benefits: Goldenrod is traditionally used to support kidney health and promote urine production. These capsules help flush out toxins, reduce inflammation, and maintain overall urinary wellness, making them beneficial for long-term kidney care.

Cleavers Kidney Detox Infusion

INGREDIENTS

- 1 teaspoon dried cleavers
- 1 cup hot water

PREPARATION

1. Steep cleavers in hot water for 10 minutes.
2. Strain and drink warm.
3. Consume daily for kidney detox support.

Benefits: Cleavers is a gentle herb that supports the lymphatic and urinary systems, helping detoxify the kidneys and reduce fluid retention. This infusion aids in promoting kidney function and overall urinary health.

Uva Ursi Urinary Support Capsules

INGREDIENTS

- Uva ursi leaf powder
- Empty vegetable capsules

PREPARATION

1. Fill capsules with uva ursi leaf powder.
2. Store in a cool, dry place.
3. Take one capsule daily for urinary support.

Benefits: Uva ursi has antibacterial properties that support urinary tract health. These capsules help prevent infections, reduce inflammation, and promote a healthy urinary environment, making them effective for maintaining long-term urinary wellness.

Lemon Balm Kidney Health Drops

INGREDIENTS

- Fresh lemon balm leaves
- Vodka or apple cider vinegar (for tincture)

PREPARATION

1. Place fresh lemon balm leaves in a jar and cover with vodka or apple cider vinegar.
2. Seal and let it steep for 4-6 weeks, shaking occasionally.
3. Strain and store in a dropper bottle.
4. Take 15-20 drops daily in water for kidney support.

Benefits: Lemon balm is a calming herb that supports kidney health and promotes overall urinary function. This tincture helps reduce inflammation, supports detoxification, and aids in maintaining a healthy kidney environment.

Horsetail Diuretic Infusion

INGREDIENTS

- 1 teaspoon dried horsetail
- 1 cup hot water

PREPARATION

1. Steep horsetail in hot water for 10 minutes.
2. Strain and drink warm.
3. Consume daily for diuretic support.

Benefits: Horsetail is a natural diuretic that supports kidney function by promoting urine production. This infusion helps cleanse the kidneys, reduce inflammation, and support overall urinary health, making it effective for long-term wellness.

Ginger and Mint Kidney Cleanse Tea

INGREDIENTS

- 1 teaspoon grated fresh ginger
- 1 teaspoon dried mint leaves
- 1 cup hot water

PREPARATION

1. Add grated ginger and mint leaves to hot water and steep for 10 minutes.
2. Strain and drink warm.
3. Consume once daily for kidney cleanse support.

Benefits: Ginger and mint work together to support kidney health by promoting detoxification and reducing inflammation. This tea helps flush out toxins, enhances kidney function, and supports overall urinary wellness.

Peppermint Urinary Comfort Capsules

INGREDIENTS

- Peppermint leaf powder
- Empty vegetable capsules

PREPARATION

1. Fill capsules with peppermint leaf powder.
2. Store in a cool, dry place.
3. Take one capsule daily for urinary comfort.

Benefits: Peppermint is known for its soothing properties that can reduce discomfort in the urinary tract. These capsules support urinary health, promote relaxation, and help maintain a balanced urinary environment.

Chamomile and Lemon Kidney Support Elixir

INGREDIENTS

- 1 teaspoon dried chamomile flowers
- Juice of half a lemon
- 1 cup hot water

PREPARATION

1. Add chamomile flowers to hot water and steep for 10 minutes.
2. Strain and add lemon juice.
3. Drink warm once daily for kidney support.

Benefits: Chamomile and lemon provide anti-inflammatory and detoxifying effects that support kidney health. This elixir helps reduce inflammation, supports detoxification, and promotes overall urinary wellness.

Dandelion and Nettle Kidney Cleanse Capsules

INGREDIENTS

- Dandelion leaf powder
- Nettle leaf powder
- Empty vegetable capsules

PREPARATION

1. Mix dandelion and nettle leaf powders.
2. Fill capsules with the mixture.
3. Store in a cool, dry place.
4. Take one capsule daily for kidney cleanse support.

Benefits: Dandelion and nettle work synergistically to support kidney function and promote detoxification. These capsules help cleanse the kidneys, reduce fluid retention, and support overall urinary health.

Lemon Verbena Urinary Tract Support Drops

INGREDIENTS

- Fresh lemon verbena leaves
- Vodka or apple cider vinegar (for tincture)

PREPARATION

1. Place fresh lemon verbena leaves in a jar and cover with vodka or apple cider vinegar.
2. Seal and let it steep for 4-6 weeks, shaking occasionally.
3. Strain and store in a dropper bottle.
4. Take 15-20 drops daily in water for urinary support.

Benefits: Lemon verbena supports urinary health by reducing inflammation and promoting detoxification. This tincture helps maintain urinary tract health and supports kidney function, making it an effective remedy for long-term use.

Fennel Seed Kidney Support Tea

INGREDIENTS

- 1 teaspoon fennel seeds
- 1 cup hot water

PREPARATION

1. Steep fennel seeds in hot water for 10 minutes.
2. Strain and drink warm.
3. Consume once daily for kidney support.

Benefits: Fennel seeds help support kidney function

and promote urine production. This tea aids in detoxification, reduces inflammation, and supports overall urinary health, making it an excellent addition to kidney wellness routines.

Yarrow Urinary Relief Capsules

INGREDIENTS

- Yarrow powder
- Empty vegetable capsules

PREPARATION

1. Fill capsules with yarrow powder.
2. Store in a cool, dry place.
3. Take one capsule daily for urinary relief.

Benefits: Yarrow has anti-inflammatory and diuretic properties that support urinary health. These capsules help reduce inflammation in the urinary tract, promote urine flow, and support overall kidney function.

Cucumber and Mint Hydration Tea

INGREDIENTS

- Fresh cucumber slices
- Fresh mint leaves
- 1 cup cold water

PREPARATION

1. Add cucumber slices and mint leaves to cold water.
2. Let it sit for at least 15 minutes before drinking.
3. Drink throughout the day for hydration and kidney support.

Benefits: Cucumber and mint work together to hydrate the body and support kidney function. This refreshing tea promotes urine production and helps flush out toxins, maintaining optimal kidney health.

Blueberry and Chamomile Kidney Tonic

INGREDIENTS

- 1/2 cup fresh blueberries
- 1 teaspoon dried chamomile flowers
- 1 cup hot water

PREPARATION

1. Combine blueberries and chamomile flowers in hot water and steep for 10 minutes.
2. Strain and drink warm.
3. Consume once daily for kidney support.

Benefits: Blueberries are rich in antioxidants that protect the kidneys, while chamomile soothes inflammation. This tonic supports kidney health, reduces oxidative stress, and promotes urinary wellness.

Linden Flower Urinary Health Infusion

INGREDIENTS

- 1 teaspoon dried linden flowers
- 1 cup hot water

PREPARATION

1. Steep linden flowers in hot water for 10 minutes.
2. Strain and drink warm.
3. Consume daily for urinary health support.

Benefits: Linden flowers have diuretic properties that

promote urine flow and support kidney function. This infusion helps maintain a healthy urinary tract, supports detoxification, and reduces inflammation.

Celery Seed Diuretic Capsules

INGREDIENTS

- Celery seed powder
- Empty vegetable capsules

PREPARATION

1. Fill capsules with celery seed powder.
2. Store in a cool, dry place.
3. Take one capsule daily for diuretic support.

Benefits: Celery seeds act as a natural diuretic, supporting kidney function and promoting urine production. These capsules help flush out toxins and reduce fluid retention, aiding in overall kidney and urinary health.

Hibiscus and Lemon Kidney Support Tea

INGREDIENTS

- 1 teaspoon dried hibiscus flowers
- Juice of half a lemon
- 1 cup hot water

PREPARATION

1. Steep hibiscus flowers in hot water for 10 minutes.
2. Strain and add lemon juice.
3. Drink warm once daily for kidney support.

Benefits: Hibiscus is a natural diuretic that helps reduce fluid retention, while lemon provides vitamin C and antioxidants that support kidney health. This tea promotes detoxification and overall kidney function.

Burdock Root Kidney Detox Capsules

INGREDIENTS

- Burdock root powder
- Empty vegetable capsules

PREPARATION

1. Fill capsules with burdock root powder.
2. Store in a cool, dry place.
3. Take one capsule daily for kidney detox support.

Benefits: Burdock root supports kidney health by promoting detoxification and reducing inflammation. These capsules help cleanse the kidneys and promote urinary wellness, making them effective for long-term kidney care.

Spearmint Urinary Comfort Elixir

INGREDIENTS

- Fresh spearmint leaves
- Vodka or apple cider vinegar (for tincture)

PREPARATION

1. Place fresh spearmint leaves in a jar and cover with vodka or apple cider vinegar.
2. Seal and let it steep for 4-6 weeks, shaking occasionally.
3. Strain and store in a dropper bottle.
4. Take 15-20 drops daily in water for urinary support.

Benefits: Spearmint provides a cooling and soothing effect, helping to reduce urinary discomfort and support kidney function. This elixir helps maintain a healthy urinary tract, promoting overall comfort and wellness.

Ginger Kidney Strengthening Drops

INGREDIENTS

- Fresh ginger root
- Vodka or apple cider vinegar (for tincture)

PREPARATION

1. Place fresh ginger slices in a jar and cover with vodka or apple cider vinegar.
2. Seal and let it steep for 4-6 weeks, shaking occasionally.
3. Strain and store in a dropper bottle.
4. Take 15-20 drops daily in water for kidney support.

Benefits: Ginger supports kidney health by reducing inflammation and promoting detoxification. These drops help strengthen kidney function, support overall urinary health, and provide long-term benefits for the kidneys.

Basil and Peppermint Kidney Health Capsules

INGREDIENTS

- Basil leaf powder
- Peppermint leaf powder
- Empty vegetable capsules

PREPARATION

1. Mix basil and peppermint leaf powders.
2. Fill capsules with the mixture.
3. Store in a cool, dry place.
4. Take one capsule daily for kidney health support.

Benefits: Basil and peppermint work together to promote kidney function and reduce inflammation. These capsules help cleanse the kidneys, support detoxification, and promote overall urinary wellness.

Goldenseal Urinary Protection Capsules

INGREDIENTS

- Goldenseal root powder
- Empty vegetable capsules

PREPARATION

1. Fill capsules with goldenseal root powder.
2. Store in a cool, dry place.
3. Take one capsule daily for urinary protection.

Benefits: Goldenseal has antibacterial and anti-inflammatory properties that support urinary health. These capsules help prevent infections, reduce inflammation, and promote a healthy urinary environment, making them beneficial for long-term use.

Elderflower Urinary Tract Infusion

INGREDIENTS

- 1 teaspoon dried elderflowers
- 1 cup hot water

PREPARATION

1. Steep elderflowers in hot water for 10 minutes.
2. Strain and drink warm.
3. Consume daily for urinary tract support.

Benefits: Elderflower is known for its anti-inflammatory and diuretic properties, which support kidney function and urinary health. This infusion helps reduce inflammation, promote urine flow, and support a balanced urinary environment.

Cinnamon Kidney Support Capsules

INGREDIENTS

- Cinnamon powder
- Empty vegetable capsules

PREPARATION

1. Fill capsules with cinnamon powder.
2. Store in a cool, dry place.
3. Take one capsule daily for kidney support.

Benefits: Cinnamon supports kidney health by promoting detoxification and reducing inflammation. These capsules help maintain kidney function and promote overall urinary health, providing long-term benefits for kidney wellness.

Rosemary and Lemon Kidney Tonic

INGREDIENTS

- 1 teaspoon dried rosemary leaves (#ul#)
- Juice of half a lemon
- 1 cup hot water

PREPARATION

1. Add rosemary leaves to hot water and steep for 10 minutes.
2. Strain and add lemon juice.
3. Drink warm once daily for kidney support.

Benefits: Rosemary and lemon work together to support kidney health and promote detoxification. This tonic helps cleanse the kidneys, reduce inflammation, and support overall urinary wellness, making it beneficial for long-term use.

Oregano Kidney Health Drops

INGREDIENTS

- Fresh oregano leaves
- Vodka or apple cider vinegar (for tincture)

PREPARATION

1. Place fresh oregano leaves in a jar and cover with vodka or apple cider vinegar.
2. Seal and let it steep for 4-6 weeks, shaking occasionally.
3. Strain and store in a dropper bottle.
4. Take 15-20 drops daily in water for kidney support.

Benefits: Oregano has antimicrobial and anti-inflammatory properties that support kidney and urinary tract health. These drops help cleanse the kidneys, prevent infections, and promote a balanced urinary environment, supporting long-term kidney function.

BOOK 29

Herbal Remedies for Allergies

Understanding Allergies and Natural Prevention

EXPLORING ALLERGIES AND STRATEGIES FOR NATURAL PREVENTION

Allergies are an overreaction of the immune system to substances that are typically harmless, such as pollen, dust, pet dander, or certain foods. For individuals prone to allergic reactions, these allergens trigger a response that can range from mild symptoms like sneezing and itching to more severe reactions, including asthma or anaphylaxis. Understanding the mechanisms behind allergies is key to finding effective natural prevention strategies. By enhancing the immune system's response and reducing exposure to allergens, herbal and lifestyle approaches can provide relief and prevention without relying heavily on pharmaceutical interventions.

The Immune System and Allergic Reactions

Allergic responses occur when the immune system misidentifies a harmless substance as a threat. In response, it produces Immunoglobulin E (IgE) antibodies that trigger the release of histamines and other chemicals from cells called mast cells. This release causes inflammation and other symptoms typically associated with allergies, such as itching, sneezing, or swelling.

- **Role of Histamines:** Histamines are key players in the body's inflammatory response to allergens. They lead to symptoms such as redness, itching, and swelling, which are all common allergic reactions.
- **Immune System Imbalance:** Allergies often indicate an imbalance in the immune system, where it overreacts to non-threatening substances. This imbalance can stem from factors like genetics, environmental exposure, or a compromised immune system due to stress or poor diet.

To mitigate allergic reactions, strengthening the immune system and reducing inflammation through natural means is essential. Herbal remedies, combined with lifestyle adjustments, offer an effective path toward long-term allergy management.

The Importance of Reducing Allergen Exposure

One of the first steps in preventing allergies is minimizing exposure to common allergens. For individuals sensitive to pollen, staying indoors during peak pollen times (early morning and late afternoon) and using air purifiers can help. Similarly, for those allergic to dust mites or pet dander, frequent cleaning and using hypoallergenic bedding are practical measures.

- **Seasonal Allergies:** For pollen allergies, also known as hay fever, limiting outdoor activities during high pollen seasons and rinsing off pollen from skin and clothes after exposure can reduce symptoms. Nasal rinses and steam inhalation using anti-inflammatory herbs like eucalyptus can also clear the airways and reduce irritation.
- **Food Allergies:** Avoiding foods that commonly trigger allergic reactions (e.g., peanuts, shellfish) is crucial. Introducing anti-inflammatory herbs and foods into the diet can help strengthen the body's resilience against allergic reactions. For example, ginger and turmeric are known to reduce inflam-

mation and improve digestion, which is vital for minimizing food allergy responses.

Strengthening the Immune System with Natural Prevention

A balanced and resilient immune system is less likely to overreact to allergens. Several herbs and natural remedies support immune health, aiming to regulate the body's response rather than suppress it. These herbal solutions can help the immune system distinguish between harmful and harmless substances more effectively, reducing the frequency and severity of allergic reactions.

- **Adaptogenic Herbs**: Adaptogens like astragalus and holy basil work by regulating the body's stress response, which is often linked to immune function. By managing stress and supporting overall immunity, these herbs help the body respond appropriately to allergens.
- **Anti-Inflammatory Herbs**: Turmeric and ginger are potent anti-inflammatory herbs that reduce systemic inflammation, a common problem in allergy sufferers. Incorporating these herbs into the diet can lower the body's baseline inflammation, making it less reactive to allergens.

Antioxidant-Rich Foods for Allergy Prevention

Antioxidants play a crucial role in combating oxidative stress and inflammation, both of which can exacerbate allergic reactions. Consuming a diet rich in fruits, vegetables, and herbs high in antioxidants can bolster the immune system and reduce the frequency of allergic symptoms.

- **Quercetin**: A powerful antioxidant found in foods like apples, onions, and berries, quercetin acts as a natural antihistamine. It stabilizes mast cells, reducing the release of histamines and other inflammatory chemicals. Regular consumption of quercetin-rich foods, or supplementation during allergy seasons, can help manage and prevent allergic responses.
- **Vitamin C**: Known for its immune-boosting properties, vitamin C also acts as a natural antihistamine. Consuming citrus fruits, bell peppers, and leafy greens regularly can enhance the body's resistance to allergens.

Detoxification and Allergy Management

Detoxifying the body can also play a significant role in reducing allergy symptoms. By eliminating toxins, heavy metals, and other environmental pollutants that stress the immune system, the body is better equipped to handle allergens. Liver-supporting herbs like milk thistle and dandelion promote detoxification, ensuring that the immune system functions optimally.

- **Milk Thistle**: This herb is known for its liver-protective properties, which aid the body in detoxification. A healthy liver efficiently removes toxins, reducing the burden on the immune system and preventing overreactions to allergens.
- **Dandelion**: With its diuretic and detoxifying effects, dandelion supports the kidneys and liver, helping the body eliminate waste and maintain a balanced immune response.

Probiotics and Gut Health in Allergy Prevention

The health of the gut is directly linked to immune function. The majority of the body's immune cells reside in the gut, and an imbalance in gut bacteria (dysbiosis) can lead to an overactive immune response, increasing the likelihood of allergies. Introducing probiotics and prebiotic-rich foods into the diet can help restore gut balance, thereby supporting immune health and reducing allergic reactions.

- **Probiotic-Rich Foods**: Fermented foods like yogurt, kefir, sauerkraut, and kimchi provide beneficial bacteria that strengthen the gut lining and modulate immune responses. Consistent consumption of these foods can lower the severity of allergic reactions.
- **Prebiotics**: Foods such as garlic, onions, and bananas serve as prebiotics, feeding the beneficial bacteria in the gut. A balanced gut microbiome ensures the immune system functions correctly, making it less prone to allergies.

By understanding the immune system's role in allergies and adopting natural preventive measures, individuals can reduce their exposure to allergens and strengthen their body's defense mechanisms. Integrating herbal remedies, antioxidant-rich foods, and lifestyle adjustments provides a holistic approach to managing and preventing allergies naturally.

Herbs to Reduce Allergy Symptoms

EFFECTIVE HERBS FOR ALLEVIATING ALLERGY SYMPTOMS

Herbs have been used for centuries to manage and reduce allergy symptoms, providing a natural alternative to pharmaceutical antihistamines and decongestants. These herbs work by reducing inflammation, stabilizing immune responses, and helping the body manage histamine release. By integrating these herbs into daily routines or using them during allergy flare-ups, individuals can experience relief from common symptoms like sneezing, itching, and nasal congestion without the side effects often associated with synthetic medications.

1. Butterbur (Petasites hybridus)

Butterbur is one of the most effective herbs for managing allergic rhinitis, commonly known as hay fever. Research has shown that butterbur has antihistamine properties, comparable to over-the-counter antihistamines like cetirizine. The herb works by inhibiting leukotrienes, inflammatory molecules that play a significant role in allergic reactions.

- **Usage:** Butterbur can be taken in capsule form, especially standardized extracts that ensure it is free from pyrrolizidine alkaloids (compounds that can be harmful to the liver). Consistent use during allergy seasons helps maintain its effectiveness.
- **Benefits:** Unlike synthetic antihistamines, butterbur does not cause drowsiness, making it suitable for individuals who need symptom relief without feeling fatigued or sluggish.

2. Stinging Nettle (Urtica dioica)

Stinging nettle is another powerful herb known for its antihistamine properties. It is particularly effective for reducing symptoms such as sneezing, itching, and congestion. Nettle's effectiveness lies in its ability to inhibit histamine receptors, thereby blocking the body's allergic response.

- **Preparation** Stinging nettle can be consumed as a tea, tincture, or in capsule form. Fresh or dried leaves are brewed into a tea, which can be taken up to three times a day during allergy season.
- **Benefits:** This herb not only reduces allergic symptoms but also provides a rich source of vitamins and minerals, such as vitamin C, magnesium, and iron, which further support overall immune health.

3. Quercetin-Rich Herbs

Quercetin, a potent antioxidant and flavonoid found in several herbs and foods, is known for its ability to stabilize mast cells. Mast cells release histamines during allergic reactions, and quercetin's role in stabilizing these cells helps reduce symptoms like itching, inflammation, and nasal congestion.

- **Herbs High in Quercetin:**
- **Elderflower:** Often used in teas or tinctures, elderflower not only provides quercetin but also has anti-inflammatory properties that soothe the respiratory tract.
- **Parsley:** While primarily used as a culinary herb, parsley can be made into a tea, which delivers a dose of quercetin and helps clear up respiratory issues.
- **How It Works:** By reducing the release of his-

tamines, quercetin acts as a natural antihistamine, making it highly effective for those who suffer from seasonal allergies.

4. Eyebright (Euphrasia officinalis)

Eyebright is traditionally used to relieve eye-related allergy symptoms such as redness, itching, and swelling, commonly associated with hay fever. The herb possesses anti-inflammatory and astringent properties, making it effective for both internal and topical use.

- **Application**: Eyebright is often taken as a tea or tincture for general allergy relief. It can also be used in eye washes, but caution should be taken to ensure the solution is sterile and properly prepared.
- **Advantages**: This herb not only alleviates eye irritation but also supports the overall respiratory system, reducing nasal congestion and inflammation in the mucous membranes.

5. Turmeric (Curcuma longa)

Turmeric, a staple in Ayurvedic medicine, contains curcumin, a powerful anti-inflammatory compound. Curcumin helps reduce inflammation associated with allergic responses and can improve breathing issues related to asthma and allergic rhinitis.

- **Consumption**: Turmeric can be added to food or consumed as a tea. Mixing turmeric with black pepper enhances its absorption and effectiveness. It can also be taken in capsule form for a concentrated dose.
- **Additional Benefits**: Beyond managing allergy symptoms, turmeric supports liver health, aiding in detoxification and enhancing the body's ability to process and eliminate allergens.

6. Astragalus (Astragalus membranaceus)

Astragalus is an adaptogenic herb that strengthens the immune system, helping to prevent and reduce the severity of allergic reactions. It has been used in traditional Chinese medicine for centuries to treat respiratory ailments and boost overall immunity.

- **Usage**: Astragalus is commonly consumed as a tea or in capsule form. It is most effective when used consistently, making it a suitable option for building long-term resilience against seasonal allergies.
- **Why It Works**: As an adaptogen, astragalus modulates the immune system, preventing it from overreacting to harmless substances like pollen or pet dander. It also reduces inflammation, further easing symptoms like nasal congestion and respiratory discomfort.

7. Holy Basil (Ocimum sanctum)

Holy basil, also known as Tulsi, is another adaptogenic herb known for its ability to regulate the immune system and reduce inflammation. Its natural antihistamine properties make it effective for alleviating symptoms such as coughing, sneezing, and itchy eyes.

- **Preparation** Tulsi is often consumed as a tea or used in essential oil form. Drinking Tulsi tea daily can strengthen the immune system and provide ongoing relief from allergy symptoms.
- **Health Benefits**: Beyond its antihistamine effects, holy basil supports respiratory health, reducing asthma symptoms and improving lung function in allergy sufferers.

8. Peppermint (Mentha piperita)

Peppermint is widely used for its decongestant properties. It contains menthol, which opens up the airways, providing relief from nasal congestion and sinus pressure, common issues during allergy seasons.

- **Consumption**: Drinking peppermint tea or inhaling steam infused with peppermint oil can offer immediate relief. Peppermint essential oil is also effective when used in diffusers or applied topically (diluted) to the chest area.
- **Advantages**: In addition to its decongestant qualities, peppermint acts as an anti-inflammatory agent, soothing irritated mucous membranes and providing overall respiratory support.

Integrating Herbs into a Daily Routine

For those looking to manage allergies holistically, incorporating these herbs into daily routines can be both effective and simple. Drinking teas, using tinctures, or consuming capsules are practical methods for consistent intake. Creating a holistic plan that combines immune-boosting herbs like astragalus with anti-inflammatory and antihistamine herbs such as butterbur and stinging nettle can provide comprehensive relief throughout allergy seasons.

By understanding the specific actions of these herbs, individuals can tailor their approach to meet their unique needs, ensuring effective symptom relief and overall improved health without the need for pharmaceutical interventions.

Remedies for Allergy Relief

Nettle Leaf Allergy Relief Capsules

INGREDIENTS

- Nettle leaf powder
- Empty vegetable capsules

PREPARATION

1. Fill the empty vegetable capsules with nettle leaf powder.
2. Store capsules in a cool, dry place.
3. Take one capsule daily for allergy relief.

Benefits: Nettle leaf is a natural antihistamine that helps reduce inflammation and allergy symptoms. These capsules offer a convenient way to manage seasonal allergies and promote overall respiratory health.

Elderflower Antihistamine Tea

INGREDIENTS

- 1 teaspoon dried elderflowers
- 1 cup hot water

PREPARATION

1. Steep dried elderflowers in hot water for 10 minutes.
2. Strain the infusion and drink warm.
3. Consume once or twice daily for best results.

Benefits: Elderflower acts as a natural antihistamine, reducing the body's allergic response. This tea helps alleviate symptoms such as runny nose and watery eyes, making it an effective remedy for seasonal allergies.

Chamomile Anti-Allergy Infusion

INGREDIENTS

- 1 teaspoon dried chamomile flowers
- 1 cup hot water

PREPARATION

1. Steep chamomile flowers in hot water for 10 minutes.
2. Strain and drink warm.
3. Consume daily for anti-allergy support.

Benefits: Chamomile is known for its soothing and anti-inflammatory properties, making it effective for reducing allergy symptoms. This infusion helps calm the body's immune response, providing relief from respiratory and skin allergies.

Goldenrod Allergy Support Capsules

INGREDIENTS

- Goldenrod powder
- Empty vegetable capsules

PREPARATION

1. Fill capsules with goldenrod powder.
2. Store in a cool, dry place.

3. Take one capsule daily for allergy support.

Benefits: Goldenrod supports respiratory health and acts as a natural antihistamine. These capsules help reduce inflammation and alleviate symptoms associated with seasonal allergies, promoting overall immune balance.

Yarrow Allergy Relief Drops

INGREDIENTS

- Fresh yarrow leaves
- Vodka or apple cider vinegar (for tincture)

PREPARATION

1. Place fresh yarrow leaves in a jar and cover with vodka or apple cider vinegar.
2. Seal and let it steep for 4-6 weeks, shaking occasionally.
3. Strain and store in a dropper bottle.
4. Take 15-20 drops daily in water for allergy relief.

Benefits: Yarrow is an anti-inflammatory herb that supports the body's response to allergens. This tincture helps reduce allergy symptoms, including nasal congestion and skin irritation, providing long-term relief.

Licorice Root Immune Modulation Capsules

INGREDIENTS

- Licorice root powder
- Empty vegetable capsules

PREPARATION

1. Fill capsules with licorice root powder.
2. Store in a cool, dry place.
3. Take one capsule daily for immune modulation.

Benefits: Licorice root helps regulate the immune system, reducing the body's allergic response. These capsules support the body in managing inflammation and balancing immune function, making them effective for long-term allergy relief.

Peppermint and Thyme Allergy Elixir

INGREDIENTS

- Fresh peppermint leaves
- Fresh thyme sprigs
- Vodka or apple cider vinegar (for tincture)

PREPARATION

1. Combine peppermint leaves and thyme sprigs in a jar and cover with vodka or apple cider vinegar.
2. Seal and let it steep for 4-6 weeks, shaking occasionally.
3. Strain and store in a dropper bottle.
4. Take 15-20 drops daily in water for allergy support.

Benefits: Peppermint and thyme have anti-inflammatory and antihistamine properties that help alleviate allergy symptoms. This elixir soothes respiratory issues and supports immune balance, providing effective allergy relief.

Turmeric and Ginger Anti-Allergy Capsules

INGREDIENTS

- Turmeric powder
- Ginger powder
- Empty vegetable capsules

PREPARATION

1. Mix turmeric and ginger powders.
2. Fill capsules with the mixture.
3. Store in a cool, dry place.
4. Take one capsule daily for allergy relief.

Benefits: Turmeric and ginger are powerful anti-inflammatory agents that help reduce allergy symptoms. These capsules support the body's immune response, providing relief from respiratory and skin allergies.

Lemon Balm Allergy Comfort Tea

INGREDIENTS

- 1 teaspoon dried lemon balm leaves
- 1 cup hot water

PREPARATION

1. Steep lemon balm leaves in hot water for 10 minutes.
2. Strain and drink warm.
3. Consume once daily for allergy comfort.

Benefits: Lemon balm has calming and antihistamine properties that help reduce allergy symptoms. This tea provides relief from respiratory discomfort and skin irritation, promoting overall allergy management.

Rosehip Antihistamine Infusion

INGREDIENTS

- 1 teaspoon dried rosehips
- 1 cup hot water

PREPARATION

1. Steep dried rosehips in hot water for 10 minutes.
2. Strain and drink warm.
3. Consume daily for antihistamine support.

Benefits: Rosehips are rich in vitamin C and have natural antihistamine properties that help manage allergic reactions. This infusion supports the immune system and helps alleviate symptoms such as sneezing and itchy eyes.

Sage and Lavender Allergy Relief Balm

INGREDIENTS

- Dried sage leaves
- Dried lavender flowers
- Coconut oil

PREPARATION

1. Infuse sage and lavender in melted coconut oil over low heat for 30 minutes.
2. Strain the herbs and pour the infused oil into a container.
3. Let it cool and solidify.
4. Apply to skin as needed for allergy relief.

Benefits: Sage and lavender have anti-inflammatory and soothing properties that relieve skin irritation caused by allergies. This balm helps reduce redness and itching, providing comfort for skin allergies and rashes.

Calendula Skin Allergy Relief Lotion

INGREDIENTS

- Dried calendula flowers
- Almond oil
- Beeswax

PREPARATION

1. Infuse calendula flowers in almond oil over low heat for 30 minutes.
2. Strain the flowers and add melted beeswax to the oil.
3. Pour into a container and let it cool.
4. Apply to affected skin areas for relief.

Benefits: Calendula is known for its anti-inflammatory and healing properties. This lotion helps soothe and heal irritated skin caused by allergies, providing relief from itching and inflammation.

Blue Vervain Antihistamine Capsules

INGREDIENTS

- Blue vervain powder
- Empty vegetable capsules

PREPARATION

1. Fill capsules with blue vervain powder.
2. Store in a cool, dry place.
3. Take one capsule daily for antihistamine support.

Benefits: Blue vervain acts as a natural antihistamine, helping to reduce allergic reactions and inflammation. These capsules support respiratory health and provide relief from seasonal allergies.

Fennel Seed Digestive Allergy Relief Drops

INGREDIENTS

- Fennel seeds
- Vodka or apple cider vinegar (for tincture)

PREPARATION

1. Place fennel seeds in a jar and cover with vodka or apple cider vinegar.
2. Seal and let it steep for 4-6 weeks, shaking occasionally.
3. Strain and store in a dropper bottle.
4. Take 15-20 drops daily in water for allergy relief.

Benefits: Fennel seeds support digestive health and help manage allergic reactions related to the digestive system. These drops provide relief from symptoms such as bloating and discomfort, promoting overall allergy wellness.

Oat Straw Skin Allergy Relief Capsules

INGREDIENTS

- Oat straw powder
- Empty vegetable capsules

PREPARATION

1. Fill capsules with oat straw powder.
2. Store in a cool, dry place.
3. Take one capsule daily for skin allergy relief.

Benefits: Oat straw helps soothe skin irritations and supports the body's immune response to allergens. These capsules aid in managing skin allergies, providing relief from itching and inflammation.

Reishi Mushroom Immune Modulation Capsules

INGREDIENTS

- Reishi mushroom powder
- Empty vegetable capsules

PREPARATION

1. Fill capsules with reishi mushroom powder.
2. Store in a cool, dry place.
3. Take one capsule daily for immune modulation.

Benefits: Reishi mushrooms support the immune system by modulating its response to allergens. These capsules help reduce inflammation and support long-term allergy management, promoting overall health and resilience.

Skullcap Anti-Allergy Infusion

INGREDIENTS

- 1 teaspoon dried skullcap leaves
- 1 cup hot water

PREPARATION

1. Steep skullcap leaves in hot water for 10 minutes.
2. Strain and drink warm.
3. Consume daily for anti-allergy support.

Benefits: Skullcap has antihistamine and anti-inflammatory properties that support the body's response to allergens. This infusion helps reduce symptoms such as nasal congestion and respiratory discomfort, providing relief from allergies.

Catnip Allergy Soothing Tea

INGREDIENTS

- 1 teaspoon dried catnip leaves
- 1 cup hot water

PREPARATION

1. Steep catnip leaves in hot water for 10 minutes.
2. Strain and drink warm.
3. Consume daily for allergy relief.

Benefits: Catnip is known for its calming and anti-inflammatory properties, making it effective for soothing respiratory allergies and skin irritations. This tea provides relief from symptoms such as sneezing, itching, and inflammation.

Mullein Allergy Respiratory Support Drops

INGREDIENTS

- Fresh mullein leaves
- Vodka or apple cider vinegar (for tincture)

PREPARATION

1. Place fresh mullein leaves in a jar and cover with vodka or apple cider vinegar.
2. Seal and let it steep for 4-6 weeks, shaking occasionally.
3. Strain and store in a dropper bottle.
4. Take 15-20 drops daily in water for respiratory support.

Benefits: Mullein supports respiratory health by reducing inflammation and easing congestion. These drops help relieve symptoms associated with respiratory allergies, making them effective for long-term support.

Horehound Immune Support Capsules

INGREDIENTS

- Horehound powder
- Empty vegetable capsules

PREPARATION

1. Fill capsules with horehound powder.
2. Store in a cool, dry place.
3. Take one capsule daily for immune support.

Benefits: Horehound has expectorant and immune-supporting properties that help alleviate respiratory allergies. These capsules support the body's natural defenses and reduce inflammation, promoting overall respiratory wellness.

Basil and Lemon Antihistamine Infusion

INGREDIENTS

- 1 teaspoon dried basil leaves
- Juice of half a lemon
- 1 cup hot water

PREPARATION

1. Steep basil leaves in hot water for 10 minutes.
2. Strain and add lemon juice.
3. Drink warm once daily for antihistamine support.

Benefits: Basil and lemon both have natural antihistamine properties that help reduce the body's allergic response. This infusion provides relief from symptoms such as sneezing and nasal congestion, promoting overall comfort during allergy season.

Chamomile and Echinacea Allergy Relief Drops

INGREDIENTS

- Dried chamomile flowers
- Dried echinacea root
- Vodka or apple cider vinegar (for tincture)

PREPARATION

1. Combine chamomile flowers and echinacea root in a jar and cover with vodka or apple cider vinegar.
2. Seal and let it steep for 4-6 weeks, shaking occasionally.
3. Strain and store in a dropper bottle.
4. Take 15-20 drops daily in water for allergy relief.

Benefits: Chamomile and echinacea work together to reduce inflammation and boost the immune system. These drops help alleviate symptoms associated with allergies, such as congestion and skin irritation, providing long-term relief.

Hibiscus Allergy Comfort Capsules

INGREDIENTS

- Hibiscus powder
- Empty vegetable capsules

PREPARATION

1. Fill capsules with hibiscus powder.
2. Store in a cool, dry place.

3. Take one capsule daily for allergy comfort.

Benefits: Hibiscus has anti-inflammatory properties that help soothe allergic reactions. These capsules support the body in managing inflammation and promoting overall immune balance, making them effective for long-term allergy support.

Ginger and Lemon Respiratory Support Tea

INGREDIENTS

- 1 teaspoon grated fresh ginger
- Juice of half a lemon
- 1 cup hot water

PREPARATION

1. Add grated ginger to hot water and steep for 10 minutes.
2. Strain and add lemon juice.
3. Drink warm once daily for respiratory support.

Benefits: Ginger and lemon provide anti-inflammatory and antioxidant support, helping to reduce respiratory inflammation and improve breathing. This tea offers relief from allergy symptoms and supports overall respiratory health.

Burdock Root Allergy Support Capsules

INGREDIENTS

- Burdock root powder
- Empty vegetable capsules

PREPARATION

1. Fill capsules with burdock root powder.
2. Store in a cool, dry place.
3. Take one capsule daily for allergy support.

Benefits: Burdock root supports the immune system and helps reduce inflammation caused by allergies. These capsules aid in detoxifying the body, promoting a balanced immune response and providing relief from allergic reactions.

Elderberry Immune Modulation Capsules

INGREDIENTS

- Elderberry powder
- Empty vegetable capsules

PREPARATION

1. Fill capsules with elderberry powder.
2. Store in a cool, dry place.
3. Take one capsule daily for immune modulation.

Benefits: Elderberries are known for their immune-boosting properties, making them effective for allergy management. These capsules support immune balance and reduce inflammation, helping to alleviate symptoms associated with allergies.

Ginkgo Biloba Antihistamine Capsules

INGREDIENTS

- Ginkgo biloba powder
- Empty vegetable capsules

PREPARATION

1. Fill capsules with ginkgo biloba powder.
2. Store in a cool, dry place.
3. Take one capsule daily for antihistamine support.

Benefits: Ginkgo biloba acts as a natural antihistamine, helping to reduce allergic reactions and inflammation. These capsules support respiratory health and provide relief from seasonal allergy symptoms.

Pine Needle Allergy Defense Drops

INGREDIENTS

- Fresh pine needles
- Vodka or apple cider vinegar (for tincture)

PREPARATION

1. Place fresh pine needles in a jar and cover with vodka or apple cider vinegar.
2. Seal and let it steep for 4-6 weeks, shaking occasionally.
3. Strain and store in a dropper bottle.
4. Take 15-20 drops daily in water for allergy defense.

Benefits: Pine needles contain compounds that support respiratory health and reduce inflammation. These drops help alleviate symptoms such as nasal congestion and support the body's defense against allergens.

Gotu Kola Skin Allergy Relief Capsules

INGREDIENTS

- Gotu kola powder
- Empty vegetable capsules

PREPARATION

1. Fill capsules with gotu kola powder.
2. Store in a cool, dry place.
3. Take one capsule daily for skin allergy relief.

Benefits: Gotu kola helps soothe skin irritations and inflammation associated with allergies. These capsules promote skin healing and provide relief from itching and rashes caused by allergic reactions.

Rosemary and Mint Allergy Support Balm

INGREDIENTS

- Dried rosemary leaves
- Dried mint leaves
- Coconut oil

PREPARATION

1. Infuse rosemary and mint in melted coconut oil over low heat for 30 minutes.
2. Strain the herbs and pour the infused oil into a container.
3. Let it cool and solidify.
4. Apply to skin as needed for allergy relief.

Benefits: Rosemary and mint provide anti-inflammatory and soothing effects, making them ideal for alleviating skin allergies. This balm helps reduce redness and itching, providing comfort and relief for irritated skin.

Marigold Anti-Allergy Skin Cream

INGREDIENTS

- Dried marigold flowers
- Almond oil
- Beeswax

PREPARATION

1. Infuse marigold flowers in almond oil over low heat for 30 minutes.
2. Strain the flowers and add melted beeswax to the oil.

Pour into a container and let it cool. (#ol#)

3. Apply to affected skin areas for relief.

Benefits: Marigold is known for its anti-inflammatory and healing properties, making it effective for treating skin allergies. This cream soothes and heals irritated skin, providing relief from rashes and itching.

Holy Basil (Tulsi) Allergy Support Capsules

INGREDIENTS

- Holy basil powder
- Empty vegetable capsules

PREPARATION

1. Fill capsules with holy basil powder.
2. Store in a cool, dry place.
3. Take one capsule daily for allergy support.

Benefits: Holy basil supports immune balance and reduces inflammation, making it effective for managing allergies. These capsules help alleviate respiratory and skin symptoms associated with allergies, promoting overall wellness.

Anise Seed Digestive Allergy Relief Capsules

INGREDIENTS

- Anise seed powder
- Empty vegetable capsules

PREPARATION

1. Fill capsules with anise seed powder.
2. Store in a cool, dry place.
3. Take one capsule daily for digestive allergy relief.

Benefits: Anise seeds support digestive health and help reduce allergic reactions related to food sensitivities. These capsules provide relief from bloating and discomfort, promoting overall digestive wellness during allergy flare-ups.

BOOK 30

Integrating Herbal Wellness into Daily Life

Growing and Harvesting Your Own Medicinal Herbs

CULTIVATING AND HARVESTING MEDICINAL HERBS AT HOME

Growing and harvesting your own medicinal herbs is a rewarding and empowering journey, offering both health benefits and a deeper connection to nature. It not only provides access to fresh, potent remedies but also ensures that the herbs you use are grown organically and sustainably. Whether you have a spacious garden, a small balcony, or just a windowsill, there are ways to cultivate a variety of medicinal plants that can enhance your daily wellness routine.

1. Choosing the Right Herbs for Your Space and Climate

The first step in growing your own medicinal herbs is selecting varieties that are suitable for your environment. Herbs vary widely in their climate requirements, light preferences, and soil conditions, so it's crucial to understand what works best for your region and available space.

- **Consider Your Growing Zone**: Different herbs thrive in different climates. For instance, Mediterranean herbs like rosemary, sage, and oregano prefer warm, sunny locations, while others like mint and lemon balm thrive in cooler, shadier environments.
- **Container vs. Garden Planting**: Herbs such as basil, thyme, and lavender do well in containers, making them ideal for apartment balconies or windowsills. For those with garden space, planting directly into the soil allows for more extensive growth, which is particularly beneficial for larger plants like comfrey or echinacea.
- **Perennial vs. Annual Herbs**: Consider mixing perennial herbs (those that come back each year) such as oregano and mint with annuals like basil. This combination ensures that you have a steady supply of herbs without needing to replant everything each year.

2. Preparing the Soil and Environment

Healthy herbs begin with healthy soil. Whether you are using containers or garden beds, creating the right environment is essential for robust growth.

- **Soil Quality**: Most medicinal herbs prefer well-drained soil that is rich in organic matter. Adding compost or organic fertilizers helps provide the nutrients necessary for growth. Avoid using synthetic chemicals, as they can reduce the medicinal potency of your plants.
- **Sunlight and Watering Needs**: Most herbs require at least 6 hours of sunlight a day, but the amount varies based on the species. For instance, basil and rosemary need full sunlight, while herbs like parsley can tolerate partial shade. Proper watering is also vital; herbs generally prefer soil that is moist but not waterlogged. Using mulch can help retain moisture in the soil, especially in warmer climates.
- **Temperature Control**: For those growing herbs indoors or in containers, maintaining the right temperature is key. Herbs like basil are sensitive to cold and should be kept in a warm, sheltered environment, particularly during the colder months.

3. Propagation Techniques: Seeds, Cuttings, and Division

Knowing how to propagate herbs effectively can increase the variety and volume of your herbal garden.

- **Seeds**: Starting herbs from seeds is cost-effective and allows for a wide variety of plants. Herbs such as basil, chamomile, and dill are easy to grow from seeds. Ensure seeds are planted in a fine soil mix and kept moist until they germinate.
- **Cuttings**: Some herbs, like rosemary and mint, propagate well from cuttings. Simply snip a healthy shoot, remove the lower leaves, and place it in water or directly into the soil. Over time, roots will develop, allowing the herb to grow into a full plant.
- **Division**: Perennial herbs like oregano and lemon balm can be divided to create new plants. Dig up the plant, split the roots into sections, and replant them in different locations. This method not only increases your herb supply but also rejuvenates the original plant.

4. Harvesting Herbs: Timing and Techniques

Harvesting medicinal herbs at the right time and using proper techniques ensures that the plants retain their potency and continue to thrive.

- **Optimal Harvest Time**: The best time to harvest herbs is early in the morning after the dew has evaporated but before the sun is too intense. This preserves the essential oils, which are often the most medicinally active components. Leaves of herbs like mint and basil should be picked before the plant flowers for maximum flavor and efficacy.
- **Harvesting Methods**: When harvesting leaves, cut stems above a leaf node to encourage bushier growth. For flowers like chamomile or lavender, gently snip the blossoms when they are fully open. For root herbs such as echinacea, dig up the roots in the fall when they are the most potent.
- **Drying and Storing Herbs**: Proper drying and storage are crucial for maintaining the quality of your herbs. Herbs can be dried by hanging them in bundles in a warm, well-ventilated area or using a dehydrator. Once dried, store them in airtight containers away from light and moisture to retain their potency.

5. The Benefits of Growing Your Own Medicinal Herbs

Growing your own medicinal herbs offers multiple advantages beyond having immediate access to fresh ingredients.

- **Personal Empowerment**: Cultivating herbs allows you to take charge of your health by ensuring that the remedies you use are pure and tailored to your needs. It also provides the satisfaction of knowing exactly where your medicine comes from and how it was grown.
- **Cost-Effective**: Purchasing dried herbs or herbal supplements can be expensive over time. Growing your own significantly reduces costs, especially for herbs that are frequently used, such as basil, mint, and chamomile.
- **Sustainability and Environmental Impact**: By growing herbs organically and avoiding pesticides, you contribute to a healthier ecosystem. Plants like lavender and rosemary also attract beneficial pollinators, supporting local biodiversity.

By integrating these practices into your daily life, you can create a personalized herbal apothecary that not only enhances your well-being but also connects you to the ancient tradition of herbal medicine.

Creating Daily Rituals for Holistic Health

ESTABLISHING DAILY RITUALS FOR HOLISTIC WELLNESS

Creating daily rituals that incorporate herbal wellness practices is an effective way to promote balance and overall health. These rituals not only enhance physical well-being but also cultivate mental and emotional equilibrium. Integrating simple, consistent herbal habits into your day transforms mundane routines into moments of self-care and rejuvenation, contributing to a more centered and mindful life.

1. Morning Herbal Infusions for a Fresh Start

Beginning the day with an herbal infusion can be a powerful ritual that awakens the senses and sets a positive tone. Herbal teas made from ingredients like lemon balm, peppermint, or nettle are excellent choices.

- **Lemon Balm Tea**: Known for its calming properties, lemon balm helps reduce anxiety and uplift mood, making it an ideal herb to start the day with a sense of clarity and calm.
- **Nettle Infusion**: Rich in vitamins and minerals, nettle supports energy levels and fortifies the body, giving you a nutrient boost to begin your day.
- **Peppermint Tea**: A refreshing option that aids digestion and invigorates the senses, peppermint tea can sharpen mental focus and prepare you for a productive day.

To establish this ritual, prepare your infusion the night before by placing the herbs in a jar with hot water and letting them steep overnight. In the morning, strain and enjoy a cup of this nourishing herbal beverage as you set your intentions for the day.

2. Midday Herbal Adaptogen Break

Taking a mindful pause during the middle of the day with an adaptogen tea can provide a natural boost and help manage stress. Adaptogens like ashwagandha, holy basil (tulsi), and rhodiola are known for their ability to balance the body's response to stress, enhance energy, and stabilize mood.

- **Ashwagandha**: This adaptogen is particularly effective in reducing cortisol levels, supporting relaxation while maintaining alertness.
- **Holy Basil (Tulsi)**: Revered in Ayurvedic medicine, tulsi promotes calm and supports immune function, making it an excellent choice for midday stress management.
- **Rhodiola**: Known for its energizing properties, rhodiola helps combat fatigue, improves concentration, and balances mood swings.

Integrating this ritual into your lunch break or mid-afternoon routine can transform the day's natural energy slump into an opportunity for rejuvenation. Simply brew a cup of your chosen adaptogen tea, take a few moments to breathe deeply, and let the herbal infusion work its balancing magic.

3. Evening Winding-Down with Calming Herbs

Winding down in the evening with a ritual involving calming herbs like chamomile, lavender, or valerian root is an effective way to signal the body that it's time to relax and prepare for rest. Establishing this routine can improve sleep quality and reduce nighttime stress.

- **Chamomile Tea:** A classic choice for its mild sedative effects, chamomile promotes relaxation and can ease digestive discomfort, contributing to a more restful night.
- **Lavender Infusion:** The floral aroma of lavender not only calms the mind but also supports deep sleep. Adding a few drops of lavender tincture to warm water can amplify its soothing effects.
- **Valerian Root Tea:** This potent herb is excellent for those who struggle with insomnia or tension. A small cup of valerian root tea about an hour before bed can help the body unwind and drift into a deep sleep.

To make this ritual special, consider creating a relaxing space for yourself. Dim the lights, play soft music, or use an essential oil diffuser with calming scents like lavender or sandalwood. These small, consistent steps transform the act of preparing tea into a moment of tranquility, allowing you to disconnect from the day and connect with a sense of inner peace.

4. Incorporating Herbal Skincare Rituals

Herbal wellness isn't limited to teas; skincare rituals using natural herbs also contribute to holistic health. Herbal facial steams, masks, and oils infused with herbs like calendula, rose, and aloe vera provide nourishment for the skin and offer moments of self-care that enhance overall well-being.

- **Herbal Facial Steams:** Using herbs like chamomile, calendula, and lavender, facial steams open pores and cleanse the skin while providing an aromatic, therapeutic experience. A simple steam, using a bowl of hot water and dried herbs, can be done once a week to rejuvenate the skin and the senses.
- **Herbal Oils:** Infusing oils like jojoba or almond with herbs such as calendula or rosemary allows for an effective and natural skincare routine. Massaging these oils into the skin daily not only improves circulation but also creates a soothing ritual that nourishes both body and mind.

5. Weekend Herbal Bath Rituals for Deep Relaxation

A weekly herbal bath ritual offers an immersive way to connect with herbal wellness. Bathing with herbs like eucalyptus, rosemary, or rose petals provides a full-body experience that supports physical relaxation, respiratory health, and emotional balance.

- **Eucalyptus and Rosemary Bath:** Known for their invigorating properties, these herbs help to clear the airways and stimulate the mind while relaxing the muscles. Adding a handful of fresh or dried eucalyptus leaves and rosemary sprigs to a hot bath can create a spa-like experience at home.
- **Rose Petal and Lavender Bath:** For those seeking emotional balance, a bath infused with rose petals and lavender soothes the mind and uplifts the spirit. It's a nurturing ritual that promotes self-love and well-being.

By incorporating these simple, herbal rituals into your daily and weekly life, you create a foundation of holistic health that supports both physical and emotional well-being. These small, consistent practices enhance the connection between body, mind, and nature, promoting a life of balance, vitality, and inner peace.

Everyday Remedies for a Healthy and Balanced Life

Lemon Balm Daily Stress Relief Tea

INGREDIENTS

- 1 teaspoon dried lemon balm leaves
- 1 cup hot water

PREPARATION

1. Steep lemon balm leaves in hot water for 10 minutes.
2. Strain and drink warm.
3. Consume once or twice daily for best results.

Benefits: Lemon balm is known for its calming properties, making it ideal for relieving stress and promoting a sense of relaxation. This tea helps reduce anxiety and supports a balanced mood, making it a perfect addition to daily wellness routines.

Nettle Leaf Mineral Boost Infusion

INGREDIENTS

- 1 teaspoon dried nettle leaves
- 1 cup hot water

PREPARATION

1. Steep nettle leaves in hot water for 10–15 minutes.
2. Strain and drink warm.
3. Consume once daily for a mineral boost.

Benefits: Nettle leaf is rich in essential minerals such as iron, magnesium, and calcium. This infusion supports overall health, strengthens the body, and provides a natural boost of energy and vitality.

Calendula Skin Nourishing Oil

INGREDIENTS

- Dried calendula flowers
- Olive oil

PREPARATION

1. Infuse dried calendula flowers in olive oil over low heat for 30 minutes.
2. Strain the flowers and pour the infused oil into a container.
3. Store in a cool, dry place and use as needed on the skin.

Benefits: Calendula oil is highly nourishing and healing for the skin. It helps soothe irritation, reduce inflammation, and promote skin regeneration, making it perfect for daily skin care routines.

Chamomile and Mint Daily Digestive Tea

INGREDIENTS

- 1 teaspoon dried chamomile flowers
- 1 teaspoon dried mint leaves
- 1 cup hot water

PREPARATION

1. Combine chamomile flowers and mint leaves in hot water and steep for 10 minutes.
2. Strain and drink warm.
3. Consume once daily to support digestion.

Benefits: Chamomile and mint work together to soothe the digestive system, reducing bloating and discomfort. This tea promotes digestive health and provides relief from indigestion, making it a great addition to daily meals.

Burdock Root Detoxifying Tonic

INGREDIENTS

- 1 teaspoon dried burdock root
- 1 cup hot water

PREPARATION

1. Steep burdock root in hot water for 10 minutes.
2. Strain and drink warm.
3. Consume once daily for detox support.

Benefits: Burdock root is a powerful detoxifier that supports liver and kidney function. This tonic helps eliminate toxins from the body, promoting overall health and vitality when used as part of a daily wellness routine.

Holy Basil (Tulsi) Adaptogenic Daily Capsules

INGREDIENTS

- Holy basil leaf powder
- Empty vegetable capsules

PREPARATION

1. Fill capsules with holy basil leaf powder.
2. Store in a cool, dry place.
3. Take one capsule daily for adaptogenic support.

Benefits: Holy basil is an adaptogen that helps the body manage stress and supports overall immune health. These capsules provide a convenient way to integrate this powerful herb into daily routines, promoting balance and resilience.

Ashwagandha Energy Support Capsules

INGREDIENTS

- Ashwagandha root powder
- Empty vegetable capsules

PREPARATION

1. Fill capsules with ashwagandha root powder.
2. Store in a cool, dry place.
3. Take one capsule daily for energy support.

Benefits: Ashwagandha is an adaptogen that enhances energy levels and reduces fatigue. These capsules support overall vitality and help maintain a balanced mood, making them perfect for daily energy management.

Lavender and Rose Relaxing Bath Soak

INGREDIENTS

- Dried lavender flowers
- Dried rose petals
- Epsom salts

PREPARATION

1. Combine dried lavender, rose petals, and Epsom salts.
2. Add the mixture to warm bath water.
3. Soak for 20-30 minutes for relaxation.

Benefits: Lavender and rose provide calming and soothing effects, while Epsom salts help relax muscles. This bath soak promotes relaxation and stress relief, making it a great addition to evening wellness routines.

Ginger and Turmeric Immunity Boost Elixir

INGREDIENTS

- 1 teaspoon grated fresh ginger
- 1 teaspoon turmeric powder
- 1 cup hot water

PREPARATION

1. Add grated ginger and turmeric powder to hot water and steep for 10 minutes.
2. Strain and drink warm.
3. Consume once daily for immune support.

Benefits: Ginger and turmeric have anti-inflammatory and immune-boosting properties. This elixir supports the body's natural defenses, making it effective for maintaining health and resilience.

Oregano Oil Daily Immune Support Drops

INGREDIENTS

- Oregano essential oil
- Carrier oil (e.g., olive oil)

PREPARATION

1. Mix 2 drops of oregano essential oil with 1 teaspoon of carrier oil.
2. Store in a dropper bottle.
3. Take 2-3 drops daily diluted in water.

Benefits: Oregano oil has antimicrobial properties that support immune health. These drops help protect the body from infections, making them an effective addition to daily health routines.

Elderberry Daily Antioxidant Capsules

INGREDIENTS

- Elderberry powder
- Empty vegetable capsules

PREPARATION

1. Fill capsules with elderberry powder.
2. Store in a cool, dry place.
3. Take one capsule daily for antioxidant support.

Benefits: Elderberry is rich in antioxidants that support immune function and protect cells from damage. These capsules offer a convenient way to include elderberry in daily health routines, promoting overall vitality and wellness.

Sage Memory Support Capsules

INGREDIENTS

- Sage leaf powder
- Empty vegetable capsules

PREPARATION

1. Fill capsules with sage leaf powder.
2. Store in a cool, dry place.
3. Take one capsule daily for memory support.

Benefits: Sage has been traditionally used to enhance memory and cognitive function. These capsules help improve focus and concentration, making them a beneficial addition to daily mental wellness routines.

Hibiscus and Mint Hydration Tea

INGREDIENTS

- 1 teaspoon dried hibiscus flowers
- 1 teaspoon dried mint leaves
- 1 cup hot water

PREPARATION

1. Combine hibiscus flowers and mint leaves in hot water and steep for 10 minutes.
2. Strain and drink warm or cold.
3. Consume daily for hydration support.

Benefits: Hibiscus and mint provide a refreshing and hydrating blend that supports kidney function and overall hydration. This tea helps maintain electrolyte balance and promotes a healthy lifestyle when consumed daily.

Reishi Mushroom Longevity Capsules

INGREDIENTS

- Reishi mushroom powder
- Empty vegetable capsules

PREPARATION

1. Fill capsules with reishi mushroom powder.
2. Store in a cool, dry place.
3. Take one capsule daily for longevity support.

Benefits: Reishi mushrooms support immune function and longevity by enhancing the body's resilience to stress and inflammation. These capsules provide a convenient way to benefit from reishi's properties, promoting long-term health.

Dandelion Leaf Daily Detox Infusion

INGREDIENTS

- 1 teaspoon dried dandelion leaves
- 1 cup hot water

PREPARATION

1. Steep dandelion leaves in hot water for 10 minutes.
2. Strain and drink warm.
3. Consume once daily for detox support.

Benefits: Dandelion leaf acts as a gentle diuretic, supporting detoxification and promoting kidney function. This infusion helps cleanse the body, making it an essential part of a daily detox routine.

Fennel Seed Digestive Aid Capsules

INGREDIENTS

- Fennel seed powder
- Empty vegetable capsules

PREPARATION

1. Fill capsules with fennel seed powder.
2. Store in a cool, dry place.
3. Take one capsule daily for digestive support.

Benefits: Fennel seeds are known for their ability to aid digestion and reduce bloating. These capsules help support digestive health and provide relief from discomfort, making them perfect for daily digestive wellness.

Peppermint and Lemon Daily Refresh Tea

INGREDIENTS

- 1 teaspoon dried peppermint leaves
- Juice of half a lemon
- 1 cup hot water

PREPARATION

1. Steep peppermint leaves in hot water for 10 minutes.
2. Strain and add lemon juice.
3. Drink warm or cold as a refreshing beverage.

Benefits: Peppermint and lemon provide a refreshing and invigorating drink that supports digestion and hydration. This tea is perfect for maintaining daily vitality and refreshing the body and mind.

Chamomile Relaxing Bedtime Drops

INGREDIENTS

- Dried chamomile flowers
- Vodka or apple cider vinegar (for tincture)

PREPARATION

1. Place dried chamomile flowers in a jar and cover with vodka or apple cider vinegar.
2. Seal and let it steep for 4-6 weeks, shaking occasionally.
3. Strain and store in a dropper bottle.
4. Take 10-15 drops diluted in water before bedtime for relaxation.

Benefits: Chamomile helps to calm the mind and promote restful sleep. These drops provide an easy way to incorporate chamomile into your nighttime routine, reducing anxiety and preparing the body for sleep.

Rose Petal Skin Nourishment Lotion

INGREDIENTS

- Fresh rose petals
- Almond oil
- Beeswax

PREPARATION

1. Infuse fresh rose petals in almond oil over low heat for 30 minutes.
2. Strain the petals and add melted beeswax to the oil.
3. Pour into a container and let it cool.
4. Apply daily to nourish and hydrate the skin.

Benefits: Rose petals are known for their skin-nourishing properties, while almond oil and beeswax provide deep hydration. This lotion soothes and softens the skin, making it ideal for daily skincare routines.

Green Tea Daily Antioxidant Infusion

INGREDIENTS

- 1 teaspoon green tea leaves
- 1 cup hot water

PREPARATION

1. Steep green tea leaves in hot water for 5-7 minutes.
2. Strain and drink warm or cold.
3. Consume once daily for antioxidant support.

Benefits: Green tea is rich in antioxidants that protect cells from damage and support overall health. This infusion provides a gentle energy boost and helps maintain vitality, making it an essential part of a daily wellness regimen.

Lemon Verbena Daily Detox Elixir

INGREDIENTS

- Fresh lemon verbena leaves
- Vodka or apple cider vinegar (for tincture)

PREPARATION

1. Place fresh lemon verbena leaves in a jar and cover with vodka or apple cider vinegar.
2. Seal and let it steep for 4-6 weeks, shaking occasionally.
3. Strain and store in a dropper bottle.
4. Take 15-20 drops daily in water for detox support.

Benefits: Lemon verbena supports digestion and detoxification, helping cleanse the body and reduce inflammation. This elixir is a convenient way to integrate daily detox support into your wellness routine.

Marshmallow Root Digestive Support Capsules

INGREDIENTS

- Marshmallow root powder
- Empty vegetable capsules

PREPARATION

1. Fill capsules with marshmallow root powder.
2. Store in a cool, dry place.
3. Take one capsule daily for digestive support.

Benefits: Marshmallow root soothes the digestive tract, reducing inflammation and promoting healthy digestion. These capsules provide easy, daily support for maintaining a balanced and comfortable digestive system.

Calendula Skin Healing Balm

INGREDIENTS

- Dried calendula flowers
- Coconut oil
- Beeswax

PREPARATION

1. Infuse calendula flowers in melted coconut oil over low heat for 30 minutes.
2. Strain the flowers and add melted beeswax to the infused oil.
3. Pour into a container and let it cool.
4. Apply to skin as needed for healing.

Benefits: Calendula is a powerful skin healer that reduces inflammation and promotes regeneration. This balm helps soothe and repair irritated skin, making it essential for daily skin health.

Ginseng Daily Energy Capsules

INGREDIENTS

- Ginseng root powder
- Empty vegetable capsules

PREPARATION

1. Fill capsules with ginseng root powder.
2. Store in a cool, dry place.
3. Take one capsule daily for energy support.

Benefits: Ginseng is an adaptogen that supports energy levels and enhances stamina. These capsules provide a convenient way to maintain daily energy and vitality, helping combat fatigue and promote overall well-being.

Schisandra Berry Longevity Tincture

INGREDIENTS

- Dried schisandra berries
- Vodka or apple cider vinegar (for tincture)

PREPARATION

1. Place dried schisandra berries in a jar and cover with vodka or apple cider vinegar.
2. Seal and let it steep for 4-6 weeks, shaking occasionally.
3. Strain and store in a dropper bottle.
4. Take 15-20 drops daily in water for longevity support.

Benefits: Schisandra berries are known for their anti-aging and adaptogenic properties. This tincture supports longevity, enhances resilience to stress, and promotes overall vitality, making it a valuable addition to daily wellness practices.

Gotu Kola Daily Wellness Capsules

INGREDIENTS

- Gotu kola powder
- Empty vegetable capsules

PREPARATION

1. Fill capsules with gotu kola powder.
2. Store in a cool, dry place.
3. Take one capsule daily for overall wellness.

Benefits: Gotu kola supports cognitive function, enhances circulation, and promotes overall health. These capsules help integrate this powerful herb into daily routines, supporting wellness and longevity.

Alfalfa Mineral Boost Capsules

INGREDIENTS

- Alfalfa leaf powder
- Empty vegetable capsules

PREPARATION

1. Fill capsules with alfalfa leaf powder.
2. Store in a cool, dry place.
3. Take one capsule daily for a mineral boost.

Benefits: Alfalfa is rich in vitamins and minerals that support overall health. These capsules provide essential nutrients, enhancing energy and promoting a balanced and healthy lifestyle.

Blueberry and Hibiscus Daily Antioxidant Tea

INGREDIENTS

- 1 teaspoon dried hibiscus flowers
- 1/2 cup fresh blueberries
- 1 cup hot water

PREPARATION

1. Combine blueberries and hibiscus flowers in hot water and steep for 10 minutes.
2. Strain and drink warm or cold.
3. Consume daily for antioxidant support.

Benefits: Blueberries and hibiscus are rich in antioxidants that protect cells and support immune health. This tea helps reduce oxidative stress, promoting overall vitality when consumed daily.

Catnip Daily Calm Elixir

INGREDIENTS

- Fresh catnip leaves
- Vodka or apple cider vinegar (for tincture)

PREPARATION

1. Place fresh catnip leaves in a jar and cover with vodka or apple cider vinegar.
2. Seal and let it steep for 4-6 weeks, shaking occasionally.
3. Strain and store in a dropper bottle.
4. Take 10-15 drops daily in water for calm support.

Benefits: Catnip has calming properties that help reduce stress and promote relaxation. This elixir is perfect for integrating daily calming support into wellness routines, aiding in stress management and mental balance.

Ginger Digestive Health Capsules

INGREDIENTS

- Ginger powder
- Empty vegetable capsules

PREPARATION

1. Fill capsules with ginger powder.
2. Store in a cool, dry place.
3. Take one capsule daily for digestive health support.

Benefits: Ginger supports digestion and helps reduce inflammation in the digestive tract. These capsules provide relief from digestive discomfort and promote a balanced digestive system, making them ideal for daily use.

Horsetail Bone Support Capsules

INGREDIENTS

- Horsetail powder
- Empty vegetable capsules

PREPARATION

1. Fill capsules with horsetail powder.
2. Store in a cool, dry place.
3. Take one capsule daily for bone health support.

Benefits: Horsetail is rich in silica, which supports bone health and strengthens connective tissues. These capsules provide daily support for maintaining bone density and overall skeletal health.

Thyme Daily Respiratory Support Infusion

INGREDIENTS

- 1 teaspoon dried thyme leaves
- 1 cup hot water

PREPARATION

1. Steep thyme leaves in hot water for 10 minutes.
2. Strain and drink warm.
3. Consume daily for respiratory support.

Benefits: Thyme has antimicrobial and anti-inflammatory properties that support respiratory health. This infusion helps maintain clear airways and strengthens respiratory function, making it a beneficial addition to daily wellness.

Elderflower Daily Skin Health Capsules

INGREDIENTS

- Elderflower powder
- Empty vegetable capsules

PREPARATION

Fill capsules with elderflower powder.

1. Store in a cool, dry place.
2. Take one capsule daily for skin health support.

Benefits: Elderflower supports skin health by reducing inflammation and promoting a clear complexion. These capsules help nourish the skin from within, making them perfect for maintaining skin health and beauty as part of daily routines.

CONCLUSION

Embracing a Healthier, Balanced Future

INTEGRATING HERBAL PRACTICES FOR LIFELONG WELLNESS

Integrating herbal practices into your life for lifelong wellness is about creating a holistic lifestyle that aligns with natural rhythms and supports health at every stage. Rather than viewing herbal remedies as quick fixes, embracing them as ongoing companions in your wellness journey can transform how you live, feel, and connect with your body and nature. By incorporating simple daily, weekly, and seasonal rituals, you cultivate habits that support the body's natural healing abilities, fortify immunity, and balance physical, mental, and emotional health.

1. Creating Sustainable Daily Habits

Integrating herbs into daily routines is the foundation for long-term wellness. This begins with identifying small, consistent habits that align with your lifestyle, such as starting your day with a nutrient-rich herbal tea or ending it with a calming infusion that promotes restful sleep. Over time, these simple practices become anchors of stability and health.

- **Herbal Morning Rituals:** Consuming herbs like nettle, lemon balm, or ginger first thing in the morning can kickstart the metabolism, support digestion, and provide a steady source of energy. These herbs are easy to incorporate into daily routines through infusions or tinctures, offering a convenient way to fortify health.
- **Adaptogenic Support:** Adaptogens like ashwagandha, holy basil, or reishi mushrooms can be added to smoothies, teas, or meals, helping to manage stress levels and maintain energy balance throughout the day. These herbs enhance resilience, making it easier to handle daily challenges and adapt to stressors.

By weaving these habits into daily life, you not only gain their immediate benefits but also build a resilient foundation that supports overall health, enabling your body to respond more effectively to environmental and emotional stressors.

2. Establishing Weekly and Seasonal Rituals

Beyond daily practices, establishing weekly and seasonal rituals enriches the body's relationship with nature's cycles. Herbs are particularly effective when used in alignment with seasonal changes, as they provide targeted support that helps the body transition smoothly through different phases of the year.

- **Weekly Self-Care Rituals:** Dedicate one evening a week to a herbal bath infused with relaxing herbs like lavender, chamomile, or rose petals. This practice not only nourishes the skin but also promotes relaxation, reduces stress, and enhances emotional well-being. Similarly, incorporating a weekly herbal steam for respiratory support using eucalyptus or thyme can cleanse the airways and boost immunity.

- **Seasonal Adjustments**: Herbs can be selected based on the changing needs of each season. In winter, warming herbs like ginger and cinnamon support circulation and immunity, while cooling herbs like peppermint and lemon balm are ideal for summer heat relief. In spring, detoxifying herbs such as dandelion and burdock root help cleanse the liver, preparing the body for the renewed energy of the warmer months. Adapting your herbal routine seasonally ensures you receive the most appropriate support for the body's shifting requirements.

These practices allow for deeper engagement with herbal wellness, providing a sense of rhythm and connection to the natural world while fostering adaptability and resilience.

3. Personalized Herbal Approaches

Personalization is key to making herbal practices effective for lifelong wellness. What works for one person may not work for another, and it's essential to tailor your herbal regimen to your specific needs, preferences, and lifestyle.

- **Listening to Your Body**: The body communicates its needs through symptoms, cravings, and responses to various stimuli. Tuning into these signals can guide you in choosing the right herbs. For example, if you experience frequent stress or anxiety, herbs like passionflower or lemon balm may become a staple in your regimen. Alternatively, if digestive issues are common, herbs such as peppermint, fennel, or ginger can be integrated to enhance gut health.
- **Consultation and Education**: Working with an herbalist or engaging in ongoing education about herbal remedies can further personalize your approach. Understanding the specific properties of different herbs, their interactions, and the best forms for consumption (teas, tinctures, capsules) allows you to refine your practices over time. This adaptability ensures that herbal integration remains effective, relevant, and aligned with your evolving health goals.

4. Empowering Your Lifestyle Through Herbal Knowledge

Knowledge is power when it comes to lifelong wellness. Building a deeper understanding of herbs and their uses empowers you to make informed decisions that enhance your health. Growing your own herbs or learning basic herbal preparation techniques like infusions, tinctures, or salves can be transformative.

- **Growing Your Own Herbs**: Cultivating herbs like basil, thyme, or rosemary at home not only provides fresh ingredients for culinary use but also offers easy access to medicinal plants that can be harvested year-round. Gardening itself is a therapeutic activity that connects you with the earth, fostering mindfulness and stress relief.
- **Learning Herbal Preparations**: Knowing how to prepare your own herbal remedies, such as salves for skin healing or tinctures for immune support, expands your ability to use herbs effectively. With a few simple tools, you can create a personal apothecary that caters to your family's needs, from soothing digestive issues to addressing common colds naturally.

By investing in this knowledge, you empower yourself to integrate herbal practices confidently and effectively, transforming wellness from a passive to an active pursuit.

5. Cultivating a Holistic Perspective

Integrating herbal practices for lifelong wellness also means adopting a holistic perspective that views health as a dynamic and interconnected state of being. Herbal wellness is not just about taking remedies but understanding how herbs work synergistically with other aspects of your life, such as nutrition, exercise, and mental health practices.

- **Aligning with Nutrition**: Pairing herbs with a balanced, whole-food diet amplifies their effects. Herbs like turmeric, which is rich in anti-inflammatory compounds, work well when combined with nutrient-dense meals that support digestion and overall vitality.
- **Supporting Emotional and Mental Health**: Herbs like St. John's Wort and valerian root not only assist with physical symptoms but also support emotional balance. Integrating practices like mindfulness meditation or yoga alongside herbal routines deepens their impact, helping you build resilience and mental clarity.

Through this holistic lens, you see how herbal practices become a lifestyle rather than a series of isolated remedies. This approach fosters a balanced, adaptive, and proactive way of living that enhances longevity and quality of life.ww

Index of Recipes

C

D

E

F

G

H

J

K

L

M

N

O

S

T

U

V

W

Y

Z

Made in United States
Cleveland, OH
08 May 2025

16689818R00267